Infectious Eye Diseases - Recent Advances in Diagnosis and Treatment

Edited by Alejandro Rodriguez-Garcia and Julio C. Hernandez-Camarena

Published in London, United Kingdom

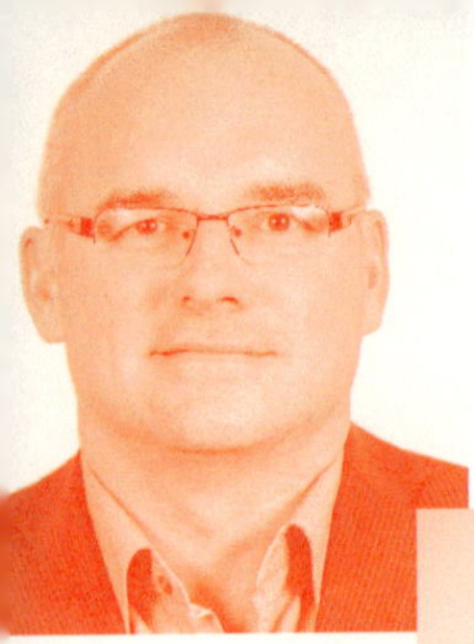
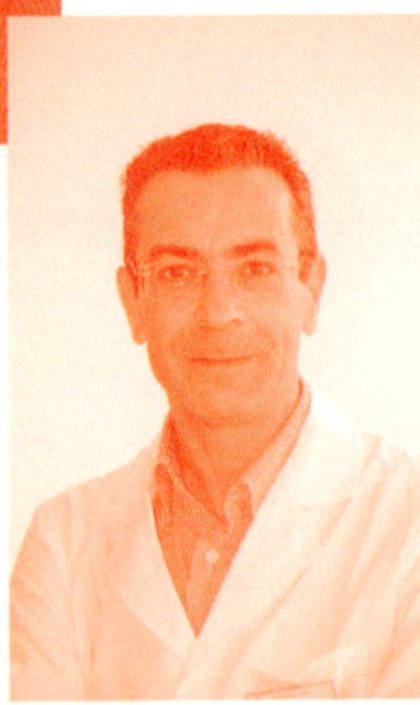
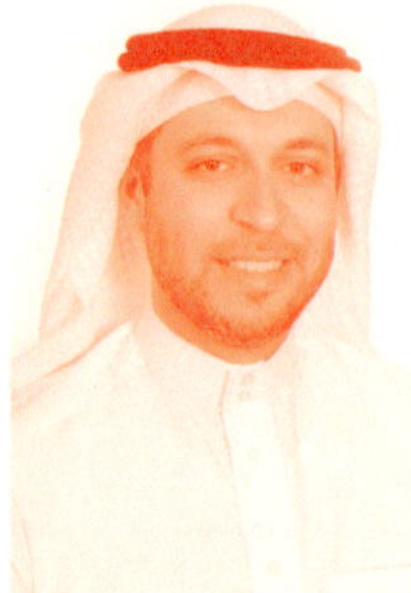
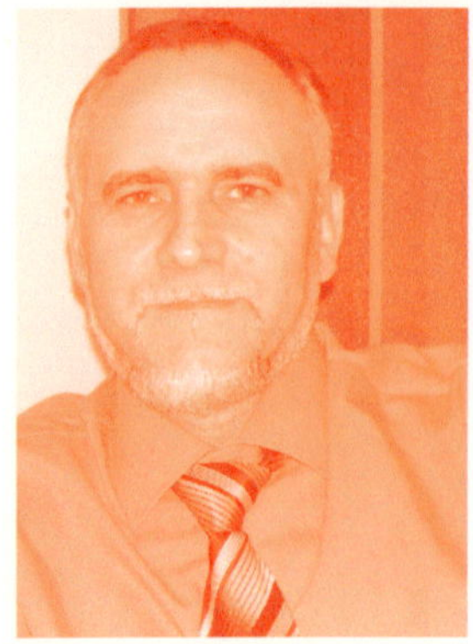
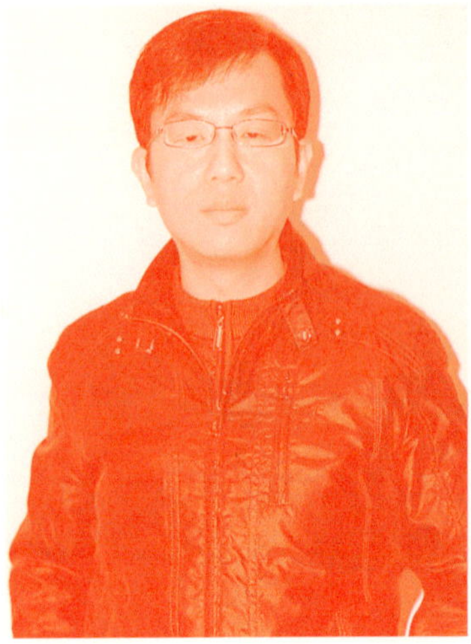
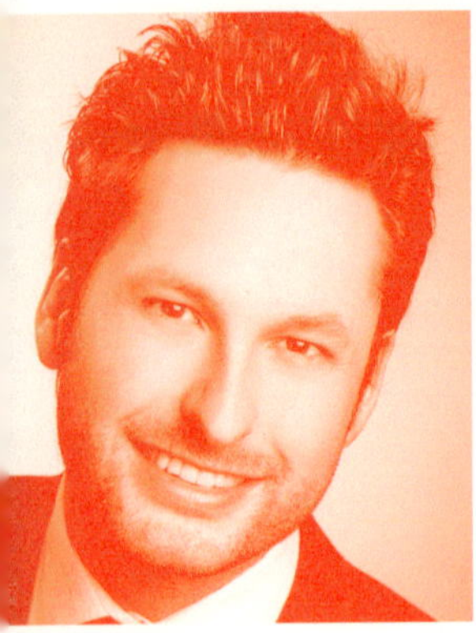
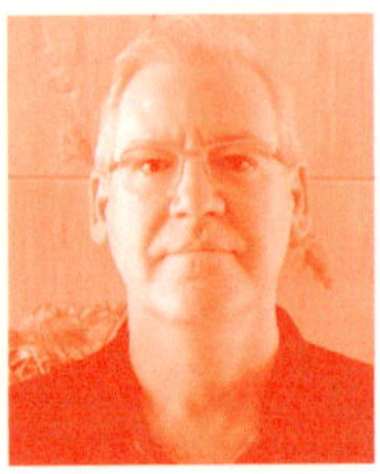

IntechOpen

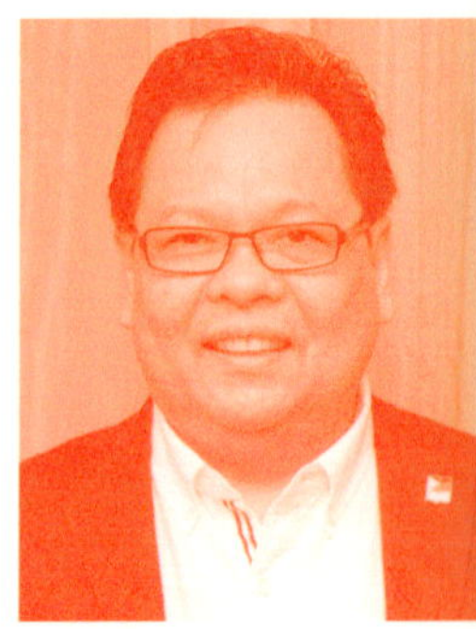
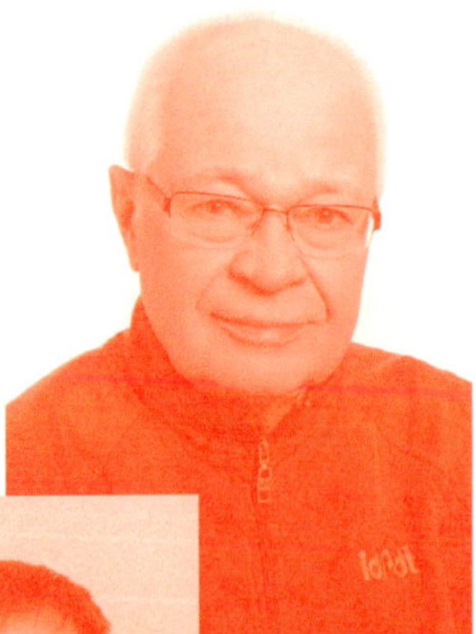
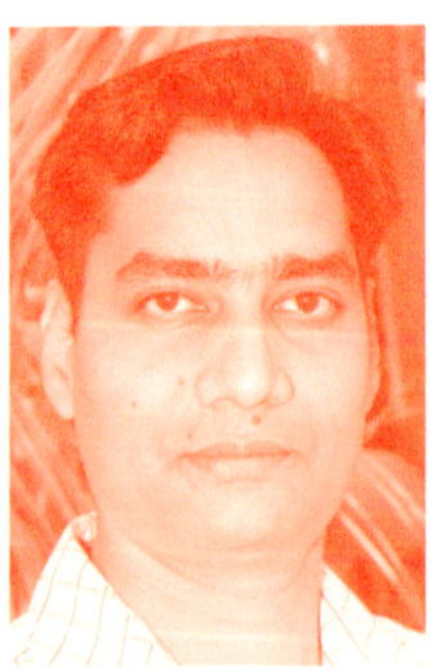
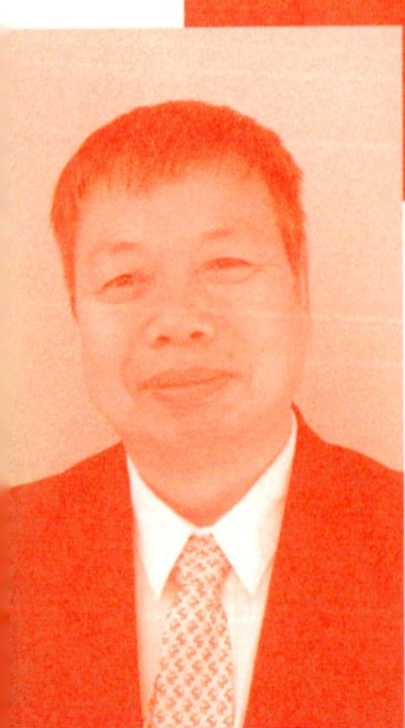
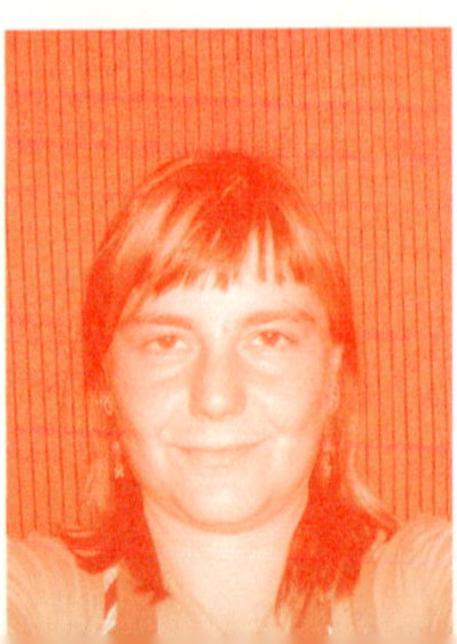
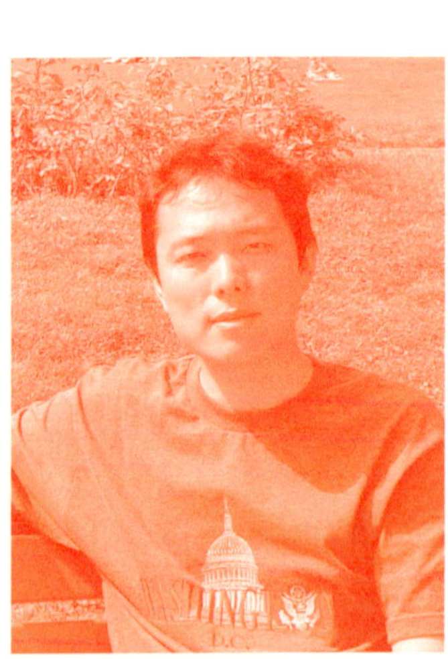

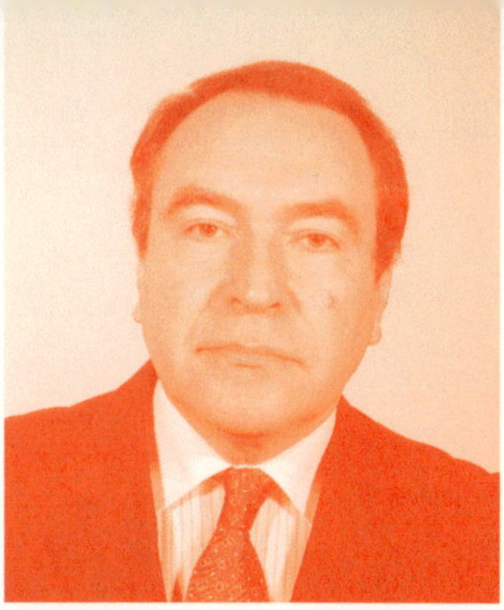
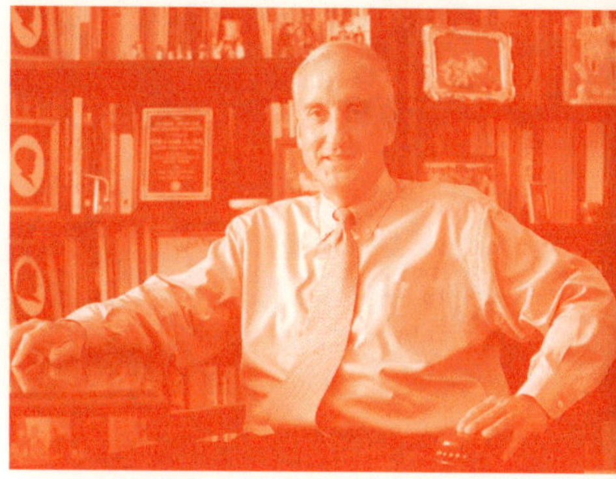
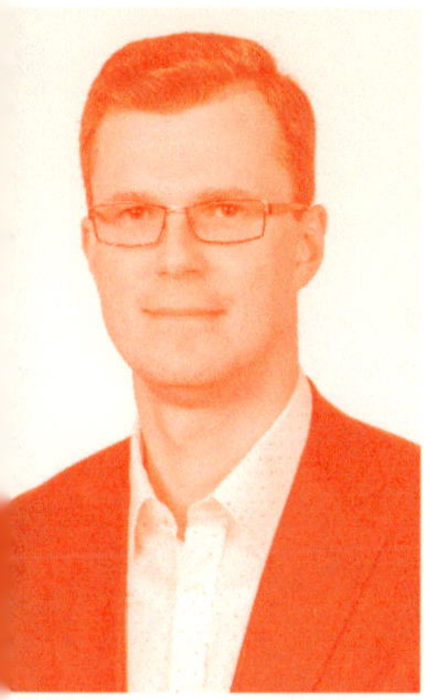
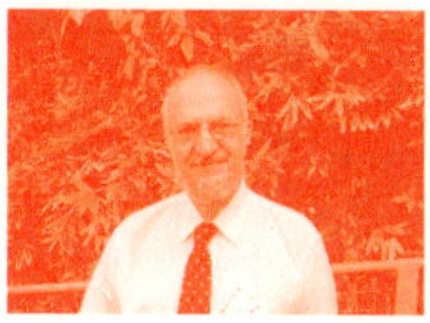
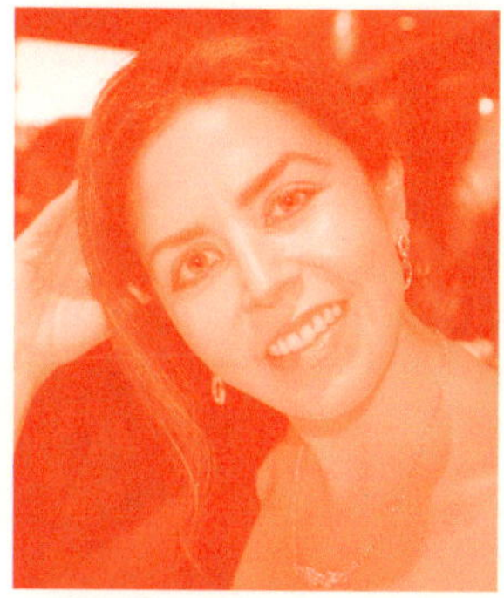

Supporting open minds since 2005

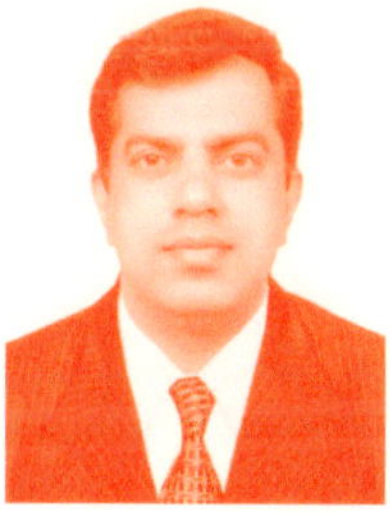
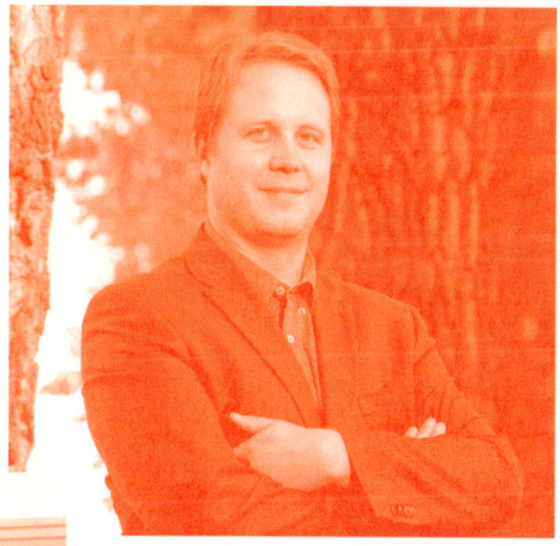
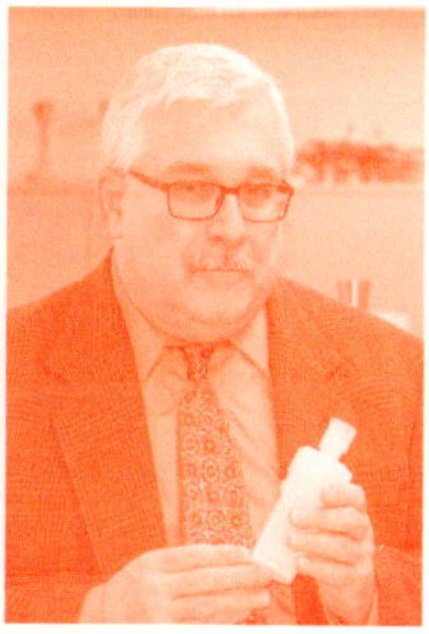
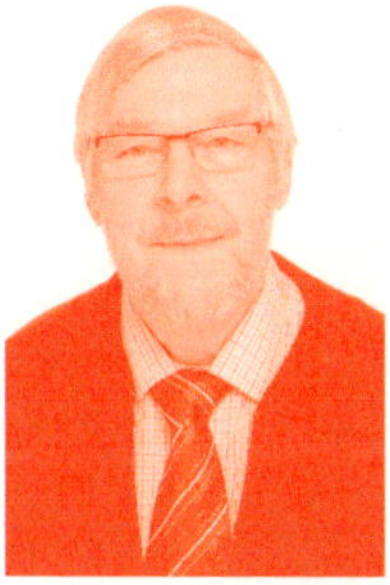
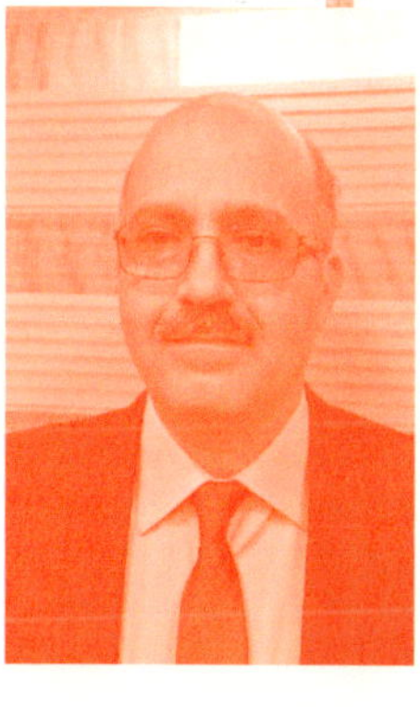
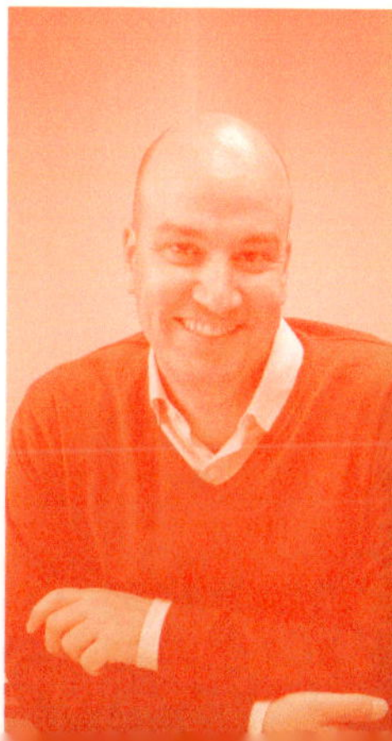
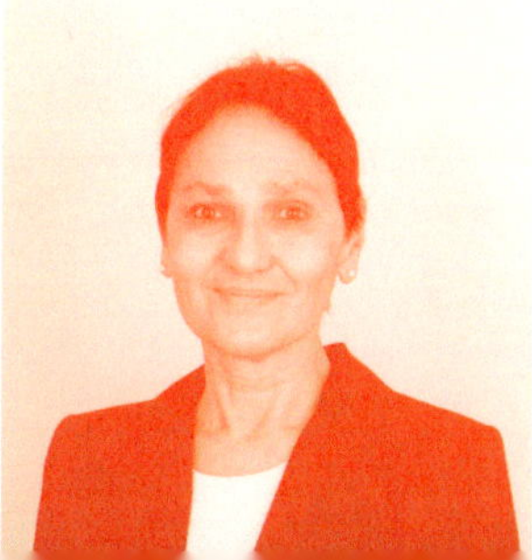

Infectious Eye Diseases - Recent Advances in Diagnosis and Treatment
http://dx.doi.org/10.5772/intechopen.91531
Edited by Alejandro Rodriguez-Garcia and Julio C. Hernandez-Camarena

Contributors
Suzana Konjevoda, Samir Čanović, Ana Didović Pavičić, Terese Kamal Gerges, Sergio E. Hernandez-Da Mota, Jesus Hernan H Gonzalez-Cortes, Jose Dalma-Weiszhausz, Jose Luis Guerrero Naranjo, Raul Velez-Montoya, Gholam A. A Peyman, Mandi D. Conway, Sami Kabbara, Neil Kelkar, Suwarna Suman, Arushi Kumar, Indu Saxena, Manoj Kumar, Sibel Çetinel Çetinel Çetinel, Ozlem Kutlu, Abuzer Alp Yetisgin, Hande Eda Sutova, Saliha Durak, Anna Karolina Nowińska, Alejandro Rodriguez-Garcia, Jimena Alamillo-Velazquez, Raul E. Ruiz-Lozano, Julio C. Hernandez-Camarena

First published in London, United Kingdom, 2021 by IntechOpen
IntechOpen is the global imprint of INTECHOPEN LIMITED, registered in England and Wales, registration number: 11086078, 5 Princes Gate Court, London, SW7 2QJ, United Kingdom
Printed in Croatia

British Library Cataloguing-in-Publication Data
A catalogue record for this book is available from the British Library

Additional hard and PDF copies can be obtained from orders@intechopen.com

Infectious Eye Diseases - Recent Advances in Diagnosis and Treatment
Edited by Alejandro Rodriguez-Garcia and Julio C. Hernandez-Camarena
p. cm.
Print ISBN 978-1-83969-319-9
Online ISBN 978-1-83969-320-5
eBook (PDF) ISBN 978-1-83969-321-2

For EU product safety concerns:
IN TECH d.o.o., Prolaz Marije Krucifikse Kozulić 3, 51000 Rijeka, Croatia, info@intechopen.com or visit our website at intechopen.com.

Meet the editors

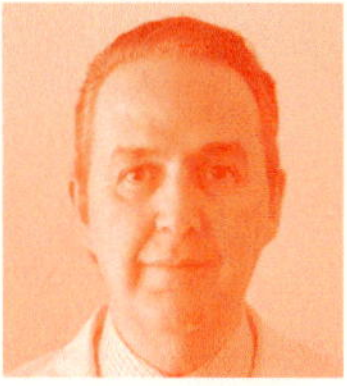

Dr. Alejandro Rodriguez-Garcia completed a Clinical and Research Fellowship in Ocular Immunology and Uveitis at the Massachusetts Eye and Ear Infirmary, Harvard Medical School. He is a Distinguished Clinical and Research Professor of Ophthalmology at Tecnologico de Monterrey School of Medicine and Health Sciences, Mexico. He is director of the Ocular Immunology and Uveitis Service at the Institute of Ophthalmology and Visual Sciences, academic director of the Ophthalmology Residency Program, and member of CONACYT National System of Researchers (Level 2). He is a former president of the Center for Ocular Inflammatory Disorders affiliated with the Mexican Society of Ophthalmology. Dr. Rodriguez is the author and co-author of more than 100 peer-reviewed scientific articles and more than thirty chapters related to inflammatory and infectious eye diseases.

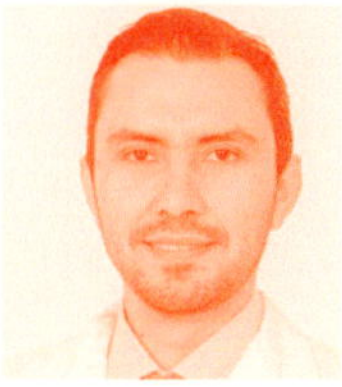

Dr. Julio C. Hernandez-Camarena completed a fellowship in Cornea and Refractive Surgery at the "Instituto de Oftalmologia Conde de Valenciana – UNAM," Mexico. He obtained a Ph.D. in Clinical Sciences at Tecnologico de Monterrey, Mexico, and is a member of the CONACYT National System of Researchers (Level 1). Dr. Hernandez is Associate Professor of Ophthalmology at Tecnologico de Monterrey School of Medicine and Health Sciences and clinical research coordinator of the Ophthalmology Residency Program. He has a special interest in clinical (keratoconus, corneal transplant, and infectious keratitis) and basic research (biopharmaceutical molecules therapy for ocular surface disease and Tissue engineering for corneal endothelium regeneration). Dr. Hernandez-Camarena is the author and co-author of more than forty peer-reviewed scientific articles related to the cornea, refractive surgery, and ocular surface disease.

Contents

Preface

Due to its evolving nature, infectious eye disease is one of the most severe sight-threatening conditions, representing a diagnostic and therapeutic challenge to ophthalmologists for centuries. Pathogens have evolved over time, producing more complex infections. Microbes such as *Treponema pallidum*, Mycobacterium *tuberculosis*, and *Toxoplasma gondii* producing syphilis, tuberculosis, and toxoplasmosis persist as important ocular pathogens. Also, the herpes viruses, the most ancestral with significant eye pathogenicity, have evolved from simple epithelial keratitis infections to devastating forms of necrotizing retinitis. During the AIDS era, characterized by a significant virally induced immune suppression, many rare opportunistic pathogens to the eye, like cytomegalovirus, atypical mycobacteria, *Coccidioides immitis*, and *Pneumocystis carinii*, among others, produced devastating infectious retinitis and panuveitis. When highly active antiretroviral therapy (HAART) was established for HIV infection, patient immune recovery drastically reduced most of these opportunistic pathogens to the eye. At present, the COVID-19 pandemic has become a new challenge for ophthalmologists, and SARS-Cov-2-related conjunctivitis has emerged.

Many pathogen microorganisms can access the eye through different routes, including invasion of the intact or damaged ocular surface, direct intraocular inoculation during surgery, penetrating trauma, or via hematogenous spread. The broad clinical spectrum produced by the different infective capabilities and tissue damage of extended genera of pathogen agents, including bacteria, fungi, viruses, and parasites, makes diagnosis a real challenge. Many ocular infectious diseases also represent a therapeutic challenge due to the microorganism's virulence, its capacity to become resistant to anti-microbial therapy, and its complex immune system interaction, characterized by an adaptive immune response to destroy the pathogen with inflammatory consequences to the infected tissue and innocent bystanders surrounding the site of infection. Another important therapeutic consideration is the potential for drug toxicity to delicate and susceptible tissues like the cornea and the retina.

This book provides the most recent advances in diagnostic methodologies and therapeutic alternatives for different infectious eye diseases. It is divided into four sections. The first section includes recent diagnostic techniques and novel treatment modalities for challenging corneal infections, from contact lens-related infectious keratitis due to a broad pathogen spectrum including bacteria, fungi, and *Acanthamoeba* spp. to herpetic and fungal corneal infections, commonly seen in general ophthalmology clinics. In the second section, an update on multimodal imaging technology for diagnosing ocular toxoplasmosis, the most common form of posterior infectious uveitis seen worldwide, is nicely illustrated with representative clinical and optical coherence tomography images at the different stages of the disease. The third section thoroughly discusses the two most important types of infectious endophthalmitis—postoperative and endogenous—from the most recent diagnostic technologic methodologies to novel therapeutic alternatives. Advanced polymerase chain reaction (PCR) techniques and another molecular sequencing, Matrix-Assisted Laser Desorption Ionization–Time of Flight Mass Spectrometry

(MALDI-TOF MS), and magneto-DNA nanoparticle systems are emerging as useful for the accurate diagnosis of infectious endophthalmitis, increasing the sensitivity and specificity of detecting pathogens. Finally, the fourth section is devoted to eye infections related to the current COVID-19 pandemic. One chapter discusses in detail the potential infectious capacity of the SARS-CoV-2 coronavirus in the ocular tissues. In another chapter, the authors bring us up to date on the most common ocular manifestation seen so far during the COVID-19 pandemic: viral conjunctivitis.

We want to congratulate all the chapter authors for their devotion in bringing us an excellent update on the most common and challenging causes of ocular infectious diseases. This book will appeal to ophthalmologists from any subspecialty since none of us are exempt from seeing and taking care of patients with such devastating sight-threatening diseases.

Alejandro Rodriguez-Garcia, M.D.
and Julio C. Hernandez-Camarena, M.D., Ph.D.
Tecnologico de Monterrey,
School of Medicine and Health Sciences,
Institute of Ophthalmology and Visual Sciences,
Monterrey, Mexico

Section 1

Infectious Keratitis

Chapter 1

Contact Lens-Associated Infectious Keratitis: Update on Diagnosis and Therapy

Jimena Alamillo-Velazquez, Raul E. Ruiz-Lozano, Julio C. Hernandez-Camarena and Alejandro Rodriguez-Garcia

Abstract

The focus of this chapter is to review the most recent advances in the diagnosis and treatment of contact-lens-related infectious keratitis, the most sight-threatening complication of contact lens wear. In the last decades, contact lenses technology has confronted several challenges, including the need for safer and more comfortable polymer materials. The development of high coefficient oxygen permeability (Dkt) and low-water content disposable contact lens translated into a significant improvement in ocular discomfort related to dry eye and allergic reactions, decreasing biofilm build-up on the external surface of the lens. Additionally, the emergence and boom-effect of corneal refractive surgery have also driven the development of better contact lens manufacturing. Despite these substantial technological advances, contact lens users continue to be at risk for developing corneal infections. We describe recent epidemiologic data, and advances in understanding the complex pathogenesis of the disease, including the clinical characteristics of the infectious process produced by bacteria, fungi, and protozoans. Finally, the recent development of diagnostic techniques and therapeutic regimens are discussed.

Keywords: contact lens, infectious keratitis, bacteria, fungi, *Acanthamoeba*

1. Introduction

Contact lenses are a useful tool for correcting refractive errors; over 125 million people wear them worldwide [1]. The widespread use of contact lenses is associated with a variable range of complications up to 39–60.99% of contact lens wearers. Complications range from mild superficial punctate keratitis to vision-threatening conditions such as contact-lens-related infectious keratitis. Infectious keratitis is a potentially blinding condition, and it rarely occurs in healthy eyes; it comprises bacterial, fungal, and *Acanthamoeba* keratitis. Contact lens wear is, in fact, the predisposing factor in up to 50.3% for infectious keratitis [2–4]. Contact lens wear is the most critical risk factor for microbial keratitis in developed countries and the second one in developing countries after trauma [5–8]. Despite different contact lens materials and wearing modalities, infectious keratitis continues to be a sight-threatening condition in contact lens wearers, with a rate of visual loss of up to

28.6% [3, 9]. The annual incidence rate for contact lens-related microbial keratitis is 2/10 000 for rigid contact lens users, 2.2–4.1/10 000 for those who use daily-wear soft contact lens, 13.3–20.9/10 000 for extended wear soft contact lens users, and 52/10 000 for patients who wear therapeutic contact lenses [10].

2. Definition

A classical definition of contact lens-associated infectious keratitis (CLAIK) includes a corneal epithelial defect or ulcer, accompanied by a stromal infiltrate, requiring corneal scraping and culturing [11]. However, corneal cultures are not readily available for all practitioners, suggesting a purely clinical definition [11]. Stapleton et al. proposed the following definition: a corneal infiltrate with an overlying epithelial defect and one or more of the following: lesions within the 4 mm of the central cornea, anterior chamber reaction, and pain [12].

3. Epidemiology

The annual incidence of CLAIK per 10 000 wearers ranges from 0.4–4.0 for rigid gas permeable (RGP) contact lenses, 2.2–4.5 for daily use of soft contact lenses, and 9.3–20.9 for overnight soft contact lenses wear [11]. Hence, daily wear of RGP contact lenses continues to have the lowest infectious keratitis rates [12]; however, the incidence of associated microbial keratitis remains unchanged despite the development of new contact lens materials [13].

Orthokeratology (ortho-K) for myopia prevention and cosmetic and decorative lenses have recently gained popularity among young wearers. On the one hand, ortho-K patients are closely monitored during treatment by their practitioners; conversely, cosmetic contact lens wear (color or party) lacks care education and professional supervision. There are reports of microbial keratitis in both wear modalities [14, 15]. In the case of cosmetic lens wear not dispensed by eye care professionals, a report shows an increased risk of infectious keratitis by a factor of 12.3 (OR 95%-CI = 4.8–31.5 Furthermore, lack of lens care education in the same study increased the risk of infectious keratitis by 26.5 times (OR 95%-CI = 10.0–70.2) [16].

4. Etiology

CLAIK is mainly attributed to bacterial pathogens with up to 90% of the cases (**Table 1**). Moreover, although fungal and protozoal infections are infrequent, they are more severe [24]. The most common bacterial agent involved in CLAIK is *Pseudomonas aeruginosa,* according to several reports (**Figure 1A** and **B**). Gram-negative bacteria are more frequently isolated in tropical climates. Gram-positive bacteria are more commonly identified in regions with temperate climates like Australia and France [2, 3, 11]. Such bacteria include coagulase-negative *Staphylococcus* (including *Staphylococcus epidermidis*), *Staphylococcus aureus,* and *Streptococcus pneumoniae*. *S. aureus* is associated with more severe disease and recurrent infections [25].

On the other hand, keratitis caused by *Acanthamoeba* and fungi has increased in the past few years [26]. In 2006, an outbreak of CLAIK caused by *Fusarium* was first reported in Singapore [27], followed by multiple reports in the United States [28–30]; these outbreaks were directly linked to a particular contact lens solution formulation reported a decreased antifungal activity [31]. In the same year,

Microorganism	Frequency (%)
Pseudomonas aeruginosa	6–55.55% [3, 17–22]
Other coagulase-negative *Staphylococcus spp.*	8–17.64% [20–22]
Serratia marcescens	2–17.1% [3, 17–22]
Staphylococcus aureus	2–12.5% [3, 19–22]
Acanthamoeba spp.	1.96–12.5% [3, 19, 21]
Fusarium spp.	2–12.5% [19, 21, 22]
Propionibacterium acnes	11.76% [21]
Mycobacterium chelonae	6.4% [23]
Streptococcus spp.	3.92–5.9% [20, 21]
Nocardia spp.	1–1.96% [21, 22]
Klebsiella spp.	0–1% [22]

Table 1.
Prevalence of causal microorganisms of contact lens-associated infectious keratitis.

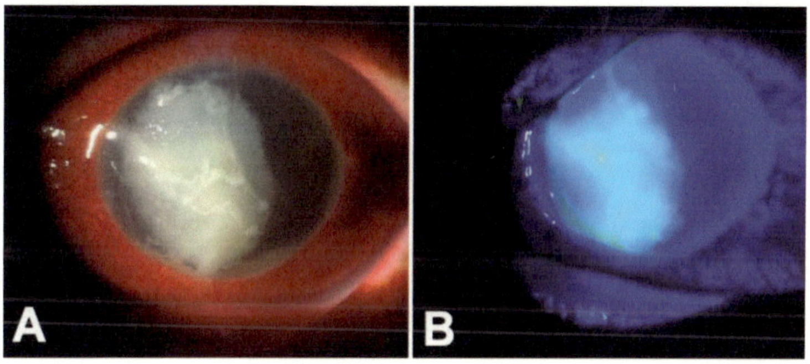

Figure 1.
A. The left cornea of a patient with a five day-history of red eye, discharge, and pain after wearing disposable contact lenses overnight. Conjunctival chemosis and ciliary injection are present; a dense stromal infiltrate, 2 mm hypopyon, and a shallow anterior chamber are observed. B. Fluorescein staining shows an extensive overlying epithelial defect. The smear staining revealed a Gram-negative rod, and the culture confirmed the diagnosis of Pseudomonas aeruginosa.

outbreaks of *Acanthamoeba* keratitis were also reported and partly associated with another contact lens solution [32].

It is noteworthy to mention the occurrence of CLAIK associated with multiple microorganisms. A retrospective analysis of CLAIK, performed by Karaca et al., demonstrated that 20% (12 cases) were mixed infections. All of them were mixed bacterium-bacterium infections. *P. aeruginosa* was involved in eight cases [33]. Regarding mixed fungi-bacterial infections, Ahn et al. reported a prevalence of 4.4% (33/757). Ocular trauma (45.5%) and diabetes mellitus (18.2%) were the most frequent associated risk factors for mixed bacterial and fungal keratitis, and *Fusarium spp.* and *Staphylococcus spp.* were the most frequent fungi and bacteria isolated, respectively [34].

5. Risk factors

Among the many different risk factors predisposing to CLAIK, overnight wear and poor hygiene are the two most frequent ones, accounting for 43% and 33%

Risk factors	Highest risk	Lowest risk
Modifiable		
Wear schedule	Overnight use	Daily wear only
Days of weekly use	6–7 days	≤ 2 days
Hand washing before cleaning	Not always	Always
Contact lens type	Daily disposable	Rigid lenses [36]
Current smoker	Yes	No
Case hygiene/replace time	Poor	Excellent
Purchase of contact lens	Internet/mail order	Optometrist [12]
Showering with lenses	Yes	No [40]
Water exposure[1]	Yes[2]	No [41]
Ocular surface and systemic diseases	Presence	absence [42]
Non-modifiable		
Gender	Male	Female
Age	≤ 49 years	≥ 50 years [36]
Socioeconomic status[3]	High [12]	Low [3]
Caucasian race[1]	Yes	No [41]
Previous ocular trauma	Presence	Absence [42]

[1]*Especially related to Acanthamoeba keratitis.*
[2]*High risk when exposure to ocean/sea/river/lake water and highest risk when swimming in public or private pool and hot tub.*
[3]*Low socioeconomic status is associated with higher risk of Acanthamoeba keratitis.*

Table 2.
Modifiable and non-modifiable risk factors associated with contact lens-associated infectious keratitis.

of the cases, respectively [35]. Regarding corneal infection in overnight wear, the risk is higher with increased extended wear and inexperienced patients [36, 37]. Interestingly, in severe keratitis, mishandling of the contact lens case (poor hygiene and lack of replacement) accounts for 63% of the population-attributed risk for bacterial and fungal infection. Moreover, swimming with contact lenses on and traveling are also risk factors for infection. The former for *Acanthamoeba* keratitis, and the latter related to routine wearing changes [3, 38].

Other risk factors of infectious keratitis in contact lens wearers include being a male, probably related to poor compliance and reluctance to seek regular care attention [39]. Genetic susceptibility related to small mutations of defensins, interleukins, and other inflammatory mediators seems to play a role in CLAIK (**Table 2**) [43].

6. Pathogenesis

The primary vector for bacterial transmission in CLAIK is the contact lens through various contaminants, including the eyelids, hands, storage case, cosmetics, and contaminated water or lens solutions [44, 45]. Contact lenses wear alone alters the normal physiology of the cornea. To a greater or lesser extent, the local hypoxia induced by contact lenses causes a decreased epithelial metabolic rate, resulting in epithelial thinning, loss of tight cell junctions, and hemidesmosomes, which lead to epithelial abrasions predisposing to opportunistic infections. Other corneal hypoxic effects include vascularization and hypoesthesia.

The understanding of CLAIK pathogenesis has changed over time as contact lens materials evolved. Contact lens wear increased in popularity when soft hydrogel contact lenses were introduced, given a higher comfort for the wearer [46]. However, their intrinsic low-oxygen transmissibility was demonstrated to be problematic. It is well-known that lower oxygen transmissibility is related to a higher rate of bacterial binding to the corneal surface; hypoxic conditions in human corneas increase wild-type cystic fibrosis transmembrane conductance regulator (CFTR) expression, which is the cellular receptor for *Pseudomonas aeruginosa*. Hence a lower bacterial load can induce infectious keratitis and inflammatory responses in this type of contact lenses [47]. Previous reports show that decreasing oxygen permeability of contact lenses is associated with increased desquamation of superficial epithelial cells of the cornea [48–50]. These observations led to development and innovation in contact lens materials to address the problem of hypoxia, which led to the advent of highly oxygen-transmissible, soft silicone hydrogel contact lenses. With the introduction of silicone hydrogel soft contact lenses, a decrease in infectious keratitis cases was anticipated; this was hypothesized because of their increased oxygen permeability and decreased bacterial binding [50]. However, no difference in the incidence of infectious keratitis was observed; clinical characteristics, pathogens, and rate of vision loss also remained unchanged despite the new contact lens material [1].

Because solving the hypoxia mechanism did not result in a reduced incidence rate of microbial keratitis, other alternative pathogenic mechanisms are suggested for corneal infection, including inadequate tear exchange. Deficient tear exchange leads to the entrapment of debris and microbes on the posterior surface of contact lenses and hinders the natural antimicrobial functions of the tear film. In fact, there is a reduction in the antimicrobial activity of the tear film on the posterior surface of silicone hydrogel soft contact lenses after 8 hours of wearing them [51]. This mechanism could explain why soft contact lenses are associated with a higher risk of infectious keratitis than rigid gas permeable lenses, given the inadequate tear exchange in the former [52, 53].

Microbes responsible for infectious keratitis may come from the lid margins, the wearers' fingers upon contact lens insertion, or removal, directly from the contact lens or indirectly from the storage case or the lens care solution [54]. Contact lens case contamination has been reported in up to 80% of contact lens wearers, despite adequate compliance with care regimens [55, 56]. The formation of bacterial biofilm on the contact lens surface and storage cases has been previously reported, and it may also play a role in the pathogenesis of microbial keratitis [56]. Bacterial cells within a biofilm show increased resistance to antimicrobial agents [57]. Moreover, multiple biguanide-based contact lens solutions have no effect against biofilms of *Serratia marcescens, Staphylococcus aureus,* and *Pseudomonas aeruginosa* formed in silicone hydrogel contact lenses [58]. Also, outbreaks of keratitis caused by *Acanthamoeba* and *Fusarium spp* have been linked to specific contact lens solutions [26, 27, 32].

Animal models have also been used to improve understanding CLAIK. In mouse and guinea pig models, a corneal erosion must occur to produce infectious keratitis; animals with non-scratched corneas only show non-infectious inflammatory responses [59]. This has led to the hypothesis that a corneal defect or erosion is a prerequisite for CLAIK to occur and not microbial contamination alone [60]. Corneal erosions are known complications in contact lens wearers, especially on extended wear schedules [61, 62].

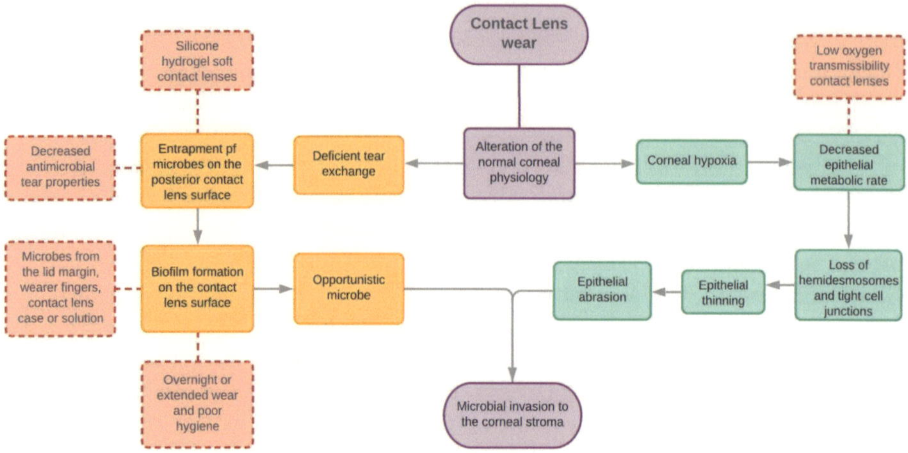

Figure 2.
Flow chart showing the relationship between the risk factors and the main events involved in the pathogenesis and development of contact lens-associated infectious keratitis.

Several risk factors have been associated with microbial keratitis. The most consistent factor is overnight wear, which increases the risk for microbial keratitis by 10 to 15 times compared to daily wear, irrespective of lens type [9, 12, 50, 63–65]. The extended wear risk of infectious keratitis also increases by 9 times with aphakia correction in elderly patients; 12 times greater in patients misusing daily-wear lenses for overnight wear. Other risk factors include contact lens case hygiene, inadequate or lack of handwashing, infrequent case replacement, and smoking; wearing contact lenses while swimming or showering also increases the risk [27, 17, 66–71]. Contact lens wearers who live or travel to tropical locations also have a higher risk for microbial keratitis [18]. According to the lens type, the risk for microbial keratitis is as follows: daily disposable < rigid gas permeable < daily wear of soft contact lens < extended wear of soft contact lens [3, 35, 72].

Furthermore, contact lens wear results in a decrease in basal cell proliferation on the cornea and vertical migration of differentiated cells to the surface of the epithelium, and an abnormal accumulation of older epithelial cells [73, 74].

The pathogenesis of CLAIK is complex and involves intrinsic lens properties, including lens material and oxygen transmissibility and environmental variables such as bacterial contamination; user behavior, such as schedule wear and poor hygiene coupled with the alteration of normal corneal physiology, loss of epithelial adherence mechanisms and corneal erosions, lead to the development of microbial keratitis [12]. In summary, microbial contamination of the lens is followed by microbial adhesion to the corneal epithelium; then microtrauma or erosion to the epithelium occurs, resulting in the microbial invasion of the corneal stroma (**Figure 2**) [75].

7. Diagnosis

Proper diagnosis of CLAIK is based on a complete ocular history of contact lens wear, patient's symptoms, a complete ophthalmological examination, corneal scrape, and culture, including the removed contact lens, the case, and solution [66].

7.1 Symptoms and signs

Symptoms common to microbial keratitis include a rapid onset of ocular pain, red eye, tearing, foreign body sensation, conjunctival mucopurulent discharge, and

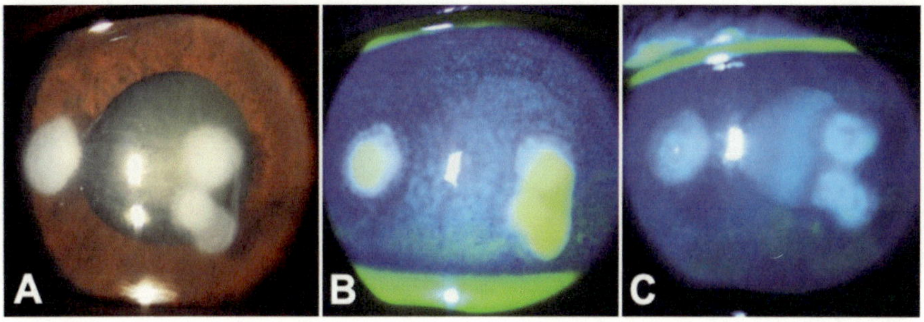

Figure 3.
53 years-old diabetic female using a one-month schedule silicone hydrogel disposable soft contact lenses in an overnight extended wear mode. The patient had been treated with 0.3% ciprofloxacin and prednisolone acetate 1% for one week. One day after stopping medications, a scrape and culture confirmed Staphylococcus spp. infection A. Left cornea showing three round dense stromal infiltrates with moderate stromal edema and Descemet folds. B. Positive fluorescein staining (>80% lesion surface) demarcating extensive corneal ulceration in all lesions. C. Three weeks on intense topical regime of 0.5% moxifloxacin and fortified vancomycin (50 mg/ml), the ulcers resolved.

photophobia with a variable degree of vision loss. These symptoms are be accompanied by prominent signs including, eyelid swelling, ciliary injection, conjunctival chemosis, a corneal epithelial defect or ulceration, stromal inflammatory/microbial infiltrate, edema, endothelial keratic precipitates (KPs), and anterior chamber reaction (inflammatory cells, flare, fibrin, plasmoid bodies, hypopyon) [11, 76–78].

There are clinical features that may guide the clinician to a possible etiological agent. Bacterial keratitis is characterized by a round, or oval epithelial defect with an underlying stromal infiltrate and anterior chamber reaction or hypopyon (**Figure 3A–C**) [66].

The classical findings in *Acanthamoeba* keratitis are severe pain that is disproportionate to the clinical signs, ring-shaped corneal infiltrates, and radial perineuritis [69, 75]. Fungal keratitis may present with a grayish, deep infiltrate with feathery borders and satellite lesions or an endothelial plaque and usually has a more insidious course [27, 66, 69]. However, these clinical findings are often misleading; in fact, cornea specialists distinguish correctly bacterial from fungal keratitis only 66% of the time in a photographic survey [79]. Thus, corneal scrapings and cultures remain the gold standard for microbial identification and the only method for determining antibiotic sensitivity [80].

7.2 Smear staining and culture

Corneal scrapings are obtained in the office under the slit lamp. A topical anesthetic agent is instilled, ideally proparacaine hydrochloride 0.5% or a preservative-free anesthetic [81]. The corneal material is obtained with a sterile platinum spatula, blade, forceps, or a calcium alginate swab moistened in thioglycolate broth. The smear stains helpful in identifying the causative organism are Gram stain, Giemsa stain, and Acridine orange are the most frequently used for detecting bacteria. The Gram stain permits identification of gram-positive and -negative coccus and rods, which is essential to choose the initial antibiotic type before the antibiogram and sensitivity profile of the microorganism in question is available. For example, cephalosporins are more appropriate for gram-positive and aminoglycosides for gram-negative bacteria [82].

In case of presumptive fungal infection, special stains like potassium hydroxide (KOH) and calcofluor white (CFW) are more reliable to initiate antifungal therapy than Gram staining is for bacterial infection (**Figure 4A** and **B**) [82, 83].

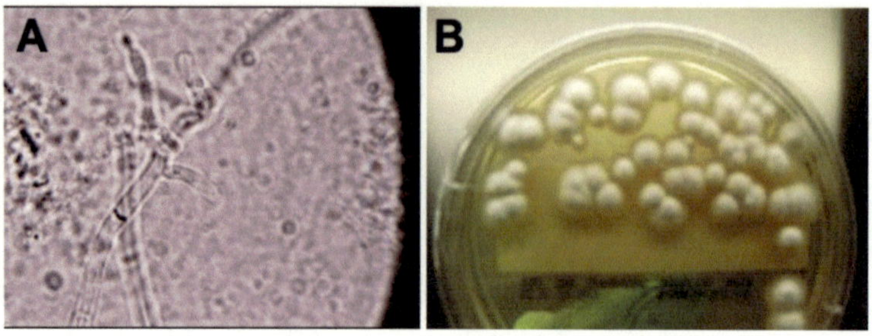

Figure 4.
A. Potassium hydroxide (KOH) preparation of a corneal smear from a fungal CLAIK patient, showing septate, branched, hyaline hyphae characteristic of filamentous fungus. B. Sabouraud dextrose agar (SDA) plate showing white, cottony colonies consistent with Fusarium solani.

Staining technique	Visualized microorganisms
Gram	Bacteria, fungi and *Acanthamoeba*
Giemsa	Bacteria, fungi and *Acanthamoeba*
Potassium hydroxide (KOH)	Fungi
Acridine orange	Bacteria, fungi and *Acanthamoeba*
Calcofluor white (CFW)	Fungi and *Acanthamoeba*
Acid fast (modified Ziehl-Neelsen)	Mycobacteria and *Nocardia* [82, 84]

Table 3.
Most used microorganism identification staining techniques for the diagnostic confirmation of contact lens-associated infectious keratitis.

Mycobacterial or *Nocardia* infection will require the acid-fast or modified Ziehl-Neelsen (1% H2SO4, cold) staining (**Table 3**).

According to the American Academy of Ophthalmology Bacterial Keratitis Preferred Practice Pattern, cultures and smears should be obtained in cases of suspected microbial keratitis in the following conditions:

- the presence of a large, central infiltrate and/or accompanied with stromal melting
- chronic or unresponsive infection despite broad-spectrum antibiotic therapy
- atypical clinical findings suggestive of fungal, protozoal, or mycobacterial agents
- multifocal infiltrates or a history of corneal surgery [82].

Corneal scrapings should be directly inoculated into the culture media at room temperature and immediately taken to the laboratory for further processing. If culture media are not readily available, scrapings should be inoculated into transport media, including brain-heart infusion media and amies medium with charcoal. Both transport media may be used for aerobic and facultative anaerobic bacteria and, the latter, also for fungi [82]. Standard culture media include blood agar, chocolate agar, Sabouraud dextrose agar, thioglycolate broth, and mannitol salt agar. If *Acanthamoeba* is the suspected pathogen, a non-nutrient agar with *Escherichia coli* overlay must be used (**Table 4**) [82, 85]. In addition to culturing corneal scrapings, cultures of the contact lens and case can also yield positive results. Corneal scrapings

Standard media	Isolates
Blood agar	Aerobic, anaerobic, and facultative anaerobic bacteria. *Pseudomonas aeruginosa, Staphylococcus aureus, Staphylococcus epidermidis, Streptococcus pneumoniae* Saprophytic fungi and *Nocardia*.
Chocolate agar	Aerobic, anaerobic, and facultative anaerobic bacteria. Ideal for isolation *Haemophilus influenzae, Neisseria gonorrhoeae,* and *Moraxella.*
Sabouraud dextrose agar	Fungi and *Nocardia*
Mannitol-salt agar	*Staphylococcus spp.*
Thioglycolate broth	Aerobic and anaerobic bacteria
Supplemental media	**Isolates**
CDC anaerobe blood agar	*Propionibacterium acnes, Peptostreptococcus spp.*
Non-nutrient agar with *E. coli*	*Acanthamoeba spp.*
Transport media	**Isolates**
Brain-heart infusion broth	Filamentous fungi and yeasts. Aerobic and facultative anaerobic bacteria.
Amies medium without charcoal	Aerobic and facultative anaerobic bacteria. Fungi [66, 82, 84, 85]

Table 4.
Respective culture media type used for microorganism isolation in contact lens-associated infectious keratitis.

culture provides positive results in 34–44% cases [67, 86–88], while cultures of contact lenses are positive in 67–92%, and 80–85% for contact lens cases [66]. Studies have found an association between cultures of corneal scrapings and of contact lenses, with a concordance of up to 84% [67, 89]. Therefore, contact lens culture may guide in the identification of the causative organism in cases in which the corneal scraping culture is negative; however, contact lens cultures do not replace corneal cultures as the gold standard for the etiologic diagnosis of microbial keratitis [67].

7.3 Tissue biopsy

A corneal biopsy may be performed if there is an inadequate response to treatment or if cultures are repeatedly negative, particularly for suspicious *Acanthamoeba* keratitis (**Figure 5A–C**). It can be performed at the slit-lamp or in the operating room using topical anesthesia and a small 2 or 3-mm dermatologic trephine punch; the tissue obtained is then bisected and sent for culture and histopathologic analysis. A section of the corneal specimen is homogenized with trypticase soy broth and cultured on conventional blood and chocolate agar, anaerobic media, Sabouraud agar, and thioglycolate broth; in specific cases, the corneal specimen may also be plated on a non-nutrient agar with *E. coli* or Lowenstein Jensen media. The specimen section that is sent for histopathologic analysis may be processed with standard stains for bacteria, fungi, acid-fast-bacilli, and *Acanthamoeba* such as Gram and Giemsa stain, potassium hydroxide, calcofluor white and, Ziehl-Neelsen [90]. Several considerations should be taken into account to maximize the diagnostic yield of a corneal biopsy [90–92]:

- To obtain the tissue specimen, topical antibiotics must be suspended at least 24–48 hours before the procedure [90]. Also, appropriate planning and consultation with the microbiologist and pathologist is recommended (i.e., need for special stains for fastidious organisms, appropriate fixatives if electron microscopy is required) [91].

- The biopsy must be performed under appropriate magnification at either the operating room or under the slit lamp, with free lamellar dissection using a diamond-sharp blade, set at 0.2 to 0.3 mm depth, or a 3 to 5 mm diameter trephine (skin biopsy punches), cutting to approximately 0.2 to 0.3 mm depth to avoid corneal perforation [92]. After trephination, the base of the tissue block must be gently pulled upward and sideways with a Colibri 0.12 mm tooth forceps to cut it off with a sharp knife (i.e., Grieshaber knife, Beaver blade No.66) or a Vannas scissors, completing the lamellar keratectomy [92].

- The tissue biopsy must include a leading edge of the infiltrate or ulcer, including an uninvolved tissue margin [91].

- The tissue sample's processing technique (i.e., electron and light microscopy histopathologic analysis, immunofluorescence, or histochemistry) depends on the clinical features and the amount of tissue available. For small specimens (<3 mm), it is suggested to use only the technique potentially yielding the best result, which must be selected based on a clinical suspicion [91].

- If a large sample is obtained, the specimen is divided under sterile technique with a sharp #11 or a 15° knife. Each portion is placed in the appropriate fixative [92].

- With a cotton-tipped applicator or a moistened cellulose (Weck-cel) sponge, swab the base of the keratectomy and streak the culture material on plates containing transport media [92].

7.4 Molecular biology techniques

The most common approach to diagnose CLAIK is to culture microorganisms from corneal scrapings. However, more than 99% of the biosphere's microbes are

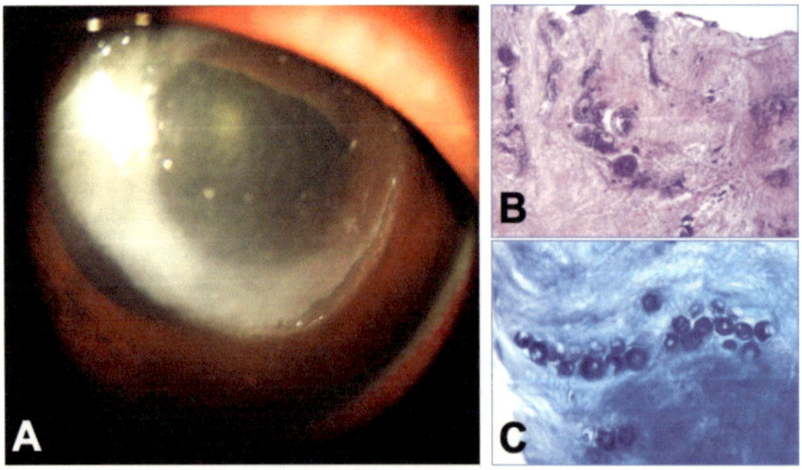

Figure 5.
Left cornea from a hardware store worker with keratoconus fitted with RGP contact lenses used to wash his face with stagnant water in an open tank deposit. A. Dense ring infiltrate with multiple stromal satellite nummular lesions and anterior chamber reaction. B. A 3 mm diameter corneal biopsy stained with H&E (mag. 40x), showing multiple Acanthamoeba cysts in the corneal stroma. C. Modified Giemsa stain from the same biopsy piece enhancing the presence of multiple Acanthamoeba cysts.

not cultivable using standard laboratory culture techniques [93]. Furthermore, identifying slow-growing bacteria (e.g., atypical mycobacteria) or fungi with atypical phenotypes is tedious and time-consuming [94]. The advent of molecular culture-independent high-throughput sequencing approaches has allowed further identification and characterization of microorganisms that cause CLAIK [95].

7.4.1 Polymerase chain reaction (PCR)

PCR is a highly sensitive technique that allows rapid amplification of tiny samples of DNA. In the context of infection, it may be used to detect the presence of pathogenic DNA of specific microorganisms [96]. The 16S and 18S rRNA are the most frequently used marker genes for assessing bacterial and fungal profiles, respectively. They are found in all respective microorganisms and have enough variation for phylogenetic analysis and sequence conservation for accurate alignment [97]. The 16S rRNA gene sequence is 1,550 bp long, and it is composed of nine variable regions (V1-V9) interspaced in more conserved regions. By amplifying the 16S rRNA region with PCR, the background host contamination encountered in routing culturing techniques is reduced significantly [98].

Kim et al. compared the detection rate of PCR compared with traditional cultures in patients with infectious corneal ulcers [99]. Of 108 samples taken from ulcers, 52% were culture-positive and 89% PCR-positive for fungal primers (18S rRNA), bacterial primers (16s rRNA), or both. Of note, other nonpathogenic organisms (i.e., *Ralstonia, Oerksovia,* and *Leclercia* species) were also identified in 60% and 52% of the PCR samples and control swabs, respectively. Airborne contamination and false-positive results for pan-fungal and pan-bacterial PCR constitute a significant limitation of the technique [100]. Moreover, when analyzing culture-positive samples, 24% and 6.5% were PCR negative for bacteria and fungi, respectively, suggesting that PCR does not replace traditional culturing. PCR, however, accurately distinguishes fungal from bacterial pathogens [99]. In patients with suspected *Acanthamoeba* keratitis, PCR and *in-vivo* confocal microscopy (IVCM, see Section 7.5) are preferred over conventional cultures since the latter has a low sensitivity and requires special media and extended incubation periods [101]. Goh et al. compared traditional cultures, PCR, and IVCM in the early diagnosis of *Acanthamoeba* keratitis. All methods exhibited a specificity and positive predictive value of 100%. However, the diagnostic sensitivities were 100% for IVCM, 71.4% for PCR, and 33.3% for traditional cultures. Since IVCM is an expensive device and requires an experienced operator, PCR is considered as a valuable adjunct to cultures when *Acanthamoeba* is suspected [101].

7.4.2 Next-generation sequencing (NGS)

NGS encompasses an evolving group of high-throughput sequencing technologies which allow massive sequencing of nucleic acid. The Sanger (1970s), a precursor to NGS, is a first-generation sequencing platform with high accuracy when dealing with one bacterium. In fact, the Human Genome Project (2003) was completed with the automatization of this technique. Isolated bacterial sequencing required multiple reactions with the Sanger platform, and thus, it was complex and time consuming [102]. Second-generation platforms (Illumina HiSeq 2500), although able to generate high sequence throughput data in a single reaction, they only sequenced part of the 16S gene [94, 103, 104]. Current third-generation platforms use nanopore sequencing technology directly from clinical samples to diagnose bacterial keratitis in real time and with higher accuracy [98].

Metagenomic NGS (mNGS) is an emerging approach that analyzes microbial, and host's genetic material (DNA and RNA) in samples from patients [105]. mNGS may detect all potential pathogens (bacteria, fungi, parasites, and viruses) in a clinical or environmental sample and simultaneously interrogate host responses by performing billions of reads in a single run [105, 106]. Unfortunately, the untargeted nature of this approach most likely results in host-derived reads [102].

Obtaining a rapid, real-time diagnosis of the causative microbe in bacterial keratitis will allow the ophthalmologist to initiate prompt and adequate antibiotic therapy; thus, improving the visual outcome and reducing antibiotic resistance [107]. However, test validation, reproducibility, high costs, among others, are significant drawbacks for the routine use of NGS and mNGS in clinical settings. Nevertheless, they must be considered in refractory difficult-to-identify cases of infection.

7.5 In vivo confocal microscopy (IVCM)

IVCM is a non-invasive imaging technique that allows dissection of the corneal architecture at a cellular level, providing real-time images equivalent to those obtained from ex-vivo histopathological techniques (tissue biopsy) [108]. It is currently used to evaluate corneal nerves in healthy eyes and those affected by ectatic corneal diseases, neurotrophic keratopathy, corneal dystrophies, ocular surface inflammation, contact lens wear, and infectious keratitis [108–110].

The role of IVCM in CLAIK relies on the identification of fungal hyphae and *Acanthamoeba* cysts; bacteria are too small to be visualized by IVCM [111]. Chidambaram et al. evaluated the IVCM cellular features in patients with bacterial, fungal, and *Acanthamoeba* keratitis [112]. A honeycomb-like distribution of anterior inflammatory cells in the corneal stroma was distinctive of fungal keratitis. *Aspergillus* and *Fusarium* ulcers were also associated with stromal dendritiform cells and interconnected cell processes with a stellate appearance, respectively. Bacterial keratitis was significantly associated with anterior stromal bullae and basal dendritiform cells. Normal keratocyte-like morphology was found in most eyes with both bacterial and fungal keratitis. Distinguishing features of *Acanthamoeba* included double-walled cysts, bright spots, and clusters after topical steroid use. While the keratocyte morphology was altered in 82% of bacterial (82%) and 77% of fungal keratitis, it was only abnormal in 39% of *Acanthamoeba* cases [112].

Although IVCM may be used in culture-negative cases or when the clinical diagnosis is unclear, this technique requires an experienced examiner. The rearmost since cellular features exhibited in microbial keratitis may be easily confused with nerve fibers, activated stromal keratocytes, and Langerhans cells [111]. Moreover, its small field of view precludes fair dismissal of *Acanthamoeba* cysts [113].

8. Differential diagnosis

8.1 Microorganism profile

According to the clinical features of the infectious/inflammatory process seen in CLAIK, specific differences, although not compelling, help identify the infectious agent involved in the process. For example, Gram-negative bacteria are usually associated with a significant anterior chamber reaction and larger ulcers compared to Gram-positive ones. Also, *Pseudomonas aeruginosa* tends to produce larger stromal inflammatory infiltrates [2, 40]. A study analyzing the causative microorganism involved in CLAIK found moderate positive prediction for *Acanthamoeba* annular

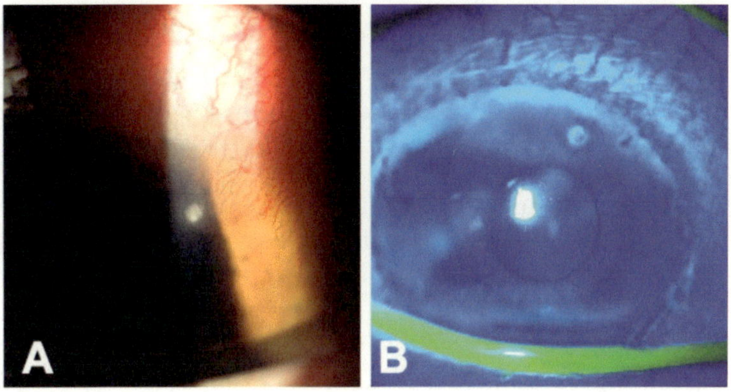

Figure 6.
A. Sterile peripheral inflammatory infiltrate in the right eye due to corneal hypoxia and a tight lens fitting of a 26-year-old female wearing hydrogel-silicone, one-month schedule disposable contact lenses complaining of red-eye, foreign body sensation, and tearing from the past three days. B. Fluorescein staining shows a slight epithelial defect at the infiltrated site and superficial punctate keratitis.

stromal infiltrate at 89% (95% CI = 52–100) and *Pseudomonas* larger ulcer at 65% (95% CI = 43–84) [114]. On the other hand, pseudo-dendrites, epitheliopathy, and stromal infiltrate found in *Acanthamoeba* keratitis may confuse herpetic keratitis [115]. Serrated (feathery) ulcer margins with raised and dry texture infiltrate and satellite lesions are common features of fungal keratitis [116].

8.2 Infectious versus inflammatory keratitis

One of the first dilemmas confronted by professionals taking care of patients wearing contact lenses is to know if the corneal lesion is infectious or inflammatory (**Figure 6A** and **B**). The difficulty arises because the ocular immune response to foreign stimuli, including microbes and their products, foreign bodies, trauma, allergic and toxic reactions, is non-specific inflammation, which may be indistinguishable from infection in that respect [78, 117, 118]. A study asking ophthalmologists to identify sterile from culture-proven CLAIK found good predictability (76%, 95% CI = 67–84) with 79 cases classified correctly [114].

Some key clinical features help to differentiate between sterile from infectious keratitis. In sterile inflammation, the absence of eyelid edema, no conjunctival discharge, peripheral location of the lesion, and minimal or no anterior chamber reaction contrast with significant eyelid edema, abundant mucopurulent discharge, central/paracentral lesions, and severe reaction and hypopyon formation in infectious keratitis [78].

9. Management

First and foremost, efforts should be focused on the prevention of CLAIK. Wearers should be educated on the proper use of contact lenses. They should be counseled to avoid overnight wear and exposure to water and be educated on appropriate hygiene practices when handling contact lenses and timely contact lens replacement [35].

To make the right management decisions, recognizing the risk factors for CLAIK, its different clinical infectious patterns, and getting the causal microorganism identification/isolation are critical to obtaining an optimal therapeutic response, avoiding sight-threatening severe complications.

9.1 Bacterial keratitis

An early diagnosis and appropriate treatment of infectious keratitis are essential. Broad-spectrum topical antibiotics are the first-line therapy for bacterial keratitis and should be initiated immediately after cultures are obtained, while waiting for the results. Antibiotics should be indicated, taking into consideration the local epidemiological data, frequency of specific pathogens, and antibiotic sensitivities (**Table 5**) [82, 119]. Severe keratitis should be treated with an initial loading dose every 5 to 15 minutes for the first hour, followed by hourly instillation for 24 to 48 hours; a topical fortified antibiotic or fluoroquinolone may be used [119].

In a recent meta-analysis, no difference in effectiveness, defined as complete corneal re-epithelialization, was observed between the use of commercially available fourth-generation topical fluoroquinolones and aminoglycoside-cephalosporin fortified combinations; there was no difference in time to resolution either. However, symptoms of ocular discomfort and toxic conjunctivitis were more frequent when using fortified aminoglycoside-cephalosporin combinations (see Appendix 1) [119].

Treatment should be tapered according to response to a minimum of four times a day, avoiding toxicity from prolonged and unnecessary use of antibiotics [112]. If no clinical stabilization or improvement is observed after the first 48 hours of treatment, the therapeutic regimen should be modified; culture results and antibiotic sensitivity should guide the clinician under these conditions. Good therapeutic response features include decreased pain, conjunctival discharge, eyelid edema, reduced corneal stromal edema, a decreased anterior chamber response, and signs of re-epithelialization. Patients with severe keratitis should be followed daily until clinical improvement is observed. Cycloplegic agents may be indicated in cases of severe keratitis with significant anterior chamber reaction to prevent the formation of irissynechiae and reduce the pain [63].

The use of topical corticosteroids is controversial but may have a role in treating certain bacterial keratitis to reduce corneal scarring. According to a subgroup analysis of the Steroids for Corneal Ulcers Trial (SCUT) in non-*Nocardia* bacterial keratitis, topical corticosteroids within two to three days of topical antibiotic therapy resulted in a one-line improvement in visual acuity compared to placebo [120]. However, topical corticosteroid use in *Nocardia* ulcers was associated with larger scars at 12 months, and therefore, it is not recommended for these cases [121]. Other well-designed randomized clinical trials are necessary to confirm these findings [122] .

9.2 Fungal keratitis

Fungal keratitis is often more aggressive than bacterial keratitis. However, there is no consensus on standard treatment, and randomized clinical trials on this subject are scarce [122]. Most antifungal medications available for ocular infections have significant limitations, including low bioavailability and limited ocular penetration in deep-seated lesions (**Table 6**) [123–125]. Furthermore, antifungal susceptibility testing has limited availability and is rarely used in ordinary contact lens and cornea clinics [126]. The Mycotic Ulcer Treatment Trial I (MUTT I) showed that topical natamycin is superior to topical voriconazole treating fungal keratitis in general, particularly in those caused by *Fusarium* [127]. According to the MUTT II results, there is no difference in perforation rate or need for therapeutic penetrating keratoplasty in fungal ulcers treated with oral voriconazole combined with topical antifungal agents compared to oral placebo and equal antifungal topical therapy. However, systemic adverse events were more frequent in the oral voriconazole group

Drug	Topical concentration	Subconjunctival dose	Activity
Cephalosporins: Inhibit bacterial cell wall formation by disrupting the synthesis of peptidoglycans. Less susceptibility to β-lactamases compared with penicillins.			
Cefazolin[1]	50 mg/mL	100 mg in 0.5 mL	Gram-positive cocci
Ceftriaxone	50 mg/mL	100 mg in 0.5 mL	Gram-negative cocci[2]
Ceftazidime	50 mg/mL	100 mg in 0.5 mL	Gram-negative cocci / rods
Fluoroquinolones[1]: Inhibit bacterial DNA gyrase and topoisomerase IV, enzymes required for bacterial DNA synthesis.			
Ciprofloxacin	3–6 mg/mL	Not available	Gram-negative cocci / rods
Ofloxacin	3–6 mg/mL	Not available	Gram-negative cocci / rods
Levofloxacin	5–15 mg/mL	Not available	+ gram-positive cocci
Moxifloxacin	5–6 mg/mL	Not available	+ gram-positive cocci and NTM
Gatifloxacin	5–6 mg/mL	Not available	
Besifloxacin	5–6 mg/mL	Not available	
Aminoglycosides: Bind to ribosomal subunits, resulting in defective mRNA translation and inhibition of protein biosynthesis.			
Gentamicin[1]	9–14 mg/mL	20 mg in 0.5 mL	Gram-negative rods
Tobramycin[1]	9–14 mg/mL	20 mg in 0.5 mL	Gram-negative rods
Amikacin	20–40 mg/mL	20 mg in 0.5 mL	NTM / *Nocardia*
Penicillins: Inhibit bacterial cell wall formation by disrupting the peptidoglycan synthesis.			
Penicillin G	100,000 U/mL	1,000,000 U/mL	Nonpenicillinase producing gram-positive organisms
Methicillin	50 mg/mL	200 mg/mL	Penicillinase-producing gram-positive organisms
Piperacillin	7 mg/mL	200 mg/mL	Gram-positives and some gram-negatives, including *Pseudomonas*
Glycopeptides: Inhibit cell wall formation of gram-positive bacteria			
Vancomycin[3]	15–50 mg/mL	25 mg in 0.5 mL	Gram-positive cocci
Macrolides: Inhibit bacterial protein synthesis by binding to the 50S ribosomal subunit.			
Erythromycin[4]	5 mg/gram	Not available	Gram-positive bacteria
Clarithromycin	10 mg/mL	20 mg in 0.5 mL	NTM
Bacterial folic acid inhibitors: Folic acid, used in DNA synthesis is required by bacteria for growth and replication.			
Sulfacetamide[5]	100 mg/mL	20 mg in 0.5 mL	*Nocardia*
TMP-SMX[6]	16 mg/mL 80 mg/mL	20 mg in 0.5 mL	*Nocardia*

Adapted and modified from Mannis MJ and Holland EJ (Eds.). (2017). Cornea. Elsevier.
NTM, non-tuberculous mycobacteria; TMP-SMX, trimethoprim-sulfamethoxazole.[1]*Also used when no organism or multiple types or organisms are identified.*
[2]*Systemic therapy is required for suspected gonococcal infection.*
[3]*Potent activity against methicillin-resistant Staphylococcus aureus; used for resistant Enterococcus species and penicillin allergy. Must not be used as single therapy against bacterial keratitis due to poor gram-negative activity.*
[4]*Mostly used in ointment presentation for the management of blepharitis, rarely used in keratitis due to poor corneal penetration.*
[5]*Active against gram-negative and -positive bacteria; however, used because bacteria become highly resistant during therapy.*
[6]*Rarely used in bacterial keratitis due to poor corneal penetration when intact epithelium.*

Table 5.
Topical and subconjunctival antibiotics and their indication for microbial keratitis.

Drug	Topical concentration	Coverage
Polyenes: bind to ergosterol in the fungal cell wall; disruption of cell wall Dose: initial dose of one drop every 30 minutes with tapering to every 3 to 6 hours		
Amphotericin B	0.05%–0.50%	First-line therapy for *Candida;* good activity against *Aspergillus* and *Fusarium.*
Natamycin	2.5%–5%	*Aspergillus, Fusarium*; moderate for *Candida*
Azoles: inhibit the synthesis of ergosterol through the cytochrome P-450-dependent enzyme Dose: undetermined		
Clotrimazole	1%	*Candida, Aspergillus*
Econazole	0.02%–2%	*Fusarium, Aspergillus, Candida*
Voriconazole	1%–2%	*Candida, Aspergillus*
Itraconazole	1%	*Candida, Aspergillus*
Fluconazole	0.5%–1%	*Candida* and other yeasts
Ketoconazole	1%–2%	*Candida* and *Aspergillus*
Echinocandins: block beta-glucan synthesis Dose: undetermined		
Caspofungin	0.5%	*Candida, Aspergillus*
Micafungin	0.1%	*Candida, Aspergillus*
Allylamines: block ergosterol biosynthesis by inhibition of squalene epoxidase Dose: undetermined		
Terbinafine	0.25%	*Aspergillus, Fusarium and Candida*
Adapted and modified from Mannis MJ and Holland EJ (Eds.). (2017). Cornea. Elsevier.		

Table 6.
Topical antifungals formulations for the treatment of mycotic keratitis.

[128]. According to a metanalysis of the available randomized clinical trials, there is still limited evidence to support using any particular drug or combination of drugs to treat fungal keratitis [129]. In general, topical treatment may include natamycin 5%, amphotericin-B 0.15% to 0.5 %, or voriconazole 1% or 2% [122].

9.3 Acanthamoeba keratitis

There is no consensus on the standard treatment for *Acanthamoeba* keratitis. Trophozoites are sensitive to a variety of antibiotics, antifungals, antiseptics, and antineoplastic agents. In contrast, cysts are highly resistant to a number of these drugs [113]. Effective topical treatment for *Acanthamoeba cysts* may include diamidines and biguanides such as propamidine-isethionate 0.1%, hexamidine-diisethionate 0.1%, dibromopropamidine 0.1%, polyhexamethylene-biguanide 0.02%, or chlorhexidine 0.02% [130]. A combination therapy of a biguanide and a diamidine is often used initially on an hourly schedule for the first 48 hours; treatment is then tapered according to the clinical response and potential epithelial toxicity and may be continued for several months. The objective is to eradicate *Acanthamoeba* trophozoites and cysts, with the resolution of the corneal inflammatory response [113].

9.4 Topical corticosteroids in infectious keratitis

The use of topical corticosteroids in infectious keratitis remains controversial [131]. Some authors advocate their use suggesting corticosteroids minimize corneal inflammation, opacification, and neovascularization. Others oppose their use, claiming that they might exacerbate microbial replication, delay epithelial healing, accelerate stromal melting, and increase the risk of perforation [132]. Several authors have demonstrated in non-controlled studies that prior corticosteroid use in bacterial keratitis significantly increases the risk of antibiotic failure and corneal ulceration [132, 133]. A Cochrane review of three small randomized trials found no benefit in healing times or visual acuity outcomes with adjuvant corticosteroid treatment [134]. The Steroids for Corneal Ulcers Trial (SCUT), the largest randomized controlled trial to date, showed no overall benefit of steroid use in visual acuity, scar size, or perforation rate at 3-months follow-up [121]. Of note, steroids (prednisolone sodium phosphate 1%) or placebo were started after 48 hours of topical 0.5% moxifloxacin. The SCUT also demonstrated that adjuvant corticosteroids, compared to placebo, resulted in one-line improvement in visual acuity in non-*Nocardia* ulcers and more extensive scars in *Nocardia* ulcers at one year [121]. In a recent report by the American Academy of Ophthalmology, authors suggest using topical corticosteroids after 48 hours of antibiotic therapy in culture-positive non-*Nocardia* bacterial keratitis [122].

Similar results were described by Wouters et al. in eyes with *Acanthamoeba* keratitis [135]. Topical corticosteroid use was associated with a delay in diagnosis (23 *vs.* 62 days, $p < 0.001$), increased disease severity, worst visual outcomes ($\leq$20/80, $p = 0.03$), and the need for an urgent corneal transplant [135].

In a recent murine model of *Candida albicans*, topical 0.1% dexamethasone exacerbated fungal keratitis by increasing the aggressivity of the pathogen, reducing the neutrophil infiltration, and inhibiting the formation of neutrophil extracellular traps [136].

9.5 Corneal collagen crosslinking (CXL)

Corneal CXL is a therapeutic modality consisting of photoactivation of a chromophore, riboflavin (vitamin-B_2), by ultraviolet (UVA) light at a wavelength of 370 nm. This technique is mainly used for stabilizing the corneal curvature and vision in patients with keratoconus and ectatic disorders [137, 138]. Studies suggest that guanine oxidation of nucleic acids and reactive oxygen species generation by activated riboflavin results in nucleic acid destruction with subsequent microbial proliferation. In 2013, the term photoactivated chromophore for infectious keratitis-corneal collagen crosslinking (PACK-CXL) emerged [137].

Price et al. performed the first prospective study assessing the efficacy of CXL in infectious keratitis [139]. PACK-CXL was deemed more effective for bacterial keratitis involving the superficial layers of the corneal stroma [139]. Another prospective clinical trial randomized 40 eyes to receive either PACK-CXL in addition to antimicrobial therapy or antimicrobial therapy alone [140]. Although PACK-CXL did not shorten the corneal healing time compared to the control group, it did result in an absent incidence of corneal perforation or recurrence of infection (0% *vs.* 21%) [140]. A recent meta-analysis performed by Ting et al., including four randomized-control trials, demonstrates that adjuvant PACK-CXL results in shorter mean healing times and quicker resolution of infiltrates when comparing with antimicrobial treatment alone. Despite the latter, high-quality randomized controlled trials are required to establish PACK-CXL's efficacy in infectious keratitis fully [141].

9.6 Rose bengal photodynamic antimicrobial therapy (RB-PDAT)

RB-PDAT is an emerging therapeutic modality for the management of infectious keratitis [142]. It was first introduced by Amescua et al. in 2017 for the management of a patient with multidrug-resistant *Fusarium keratoplasticum* keratitis [143]. In this therapeutic modality, rose bengal, a routinely used dye in ophthalmology, is excited with a green light at a wavelength of 500–550 nm to generate reactive oxygen species [144]. Rose bengal is a type II photosensitizer that, when activated, induces cellular apoptosis by converting triplet oxygen to singlet oxygen [142]. A pilot study performed by Naranjo et al. including *Acanthamoeba* keratitis (10 cases), *Fusarium spp.* (4 cases), *Pseudomonas aeruginosa* (2 cases), and *Curvularia spp.* (1 case), evaluated the clinical outcomes of RB-PDAT. One patient had no microbiological diagnosis [144]. Most individuals (14/18, 79%) were contact-lens wearers. Successful therapy, defined as avoiding therapeutic keratoplasty, was achieved in 72% of the cases. Although adequately powered randomized controlled trials are required to ascertain the efficacy of RB-PDAT, preliminary results are promising.

9.7 Future drug-delivery systems

Despite the high efficacy and broad spectrum of the antimicrobials used in infectious keratitis, their insolubility in water, low precorneal residence time on the ocular surface, inadequate control of drug release and penetration, nasopharyngeal drainage, and toxicity hinders their performance [145]. To overcome such limitations, recent developments on drug-delivery systems are emerging.

Chhonker et al. developed amphotericin-B-loaded lecithin/chitosan nanoparticles with enhanced mucoadhesive properties for the prolonged ocular application [145]. The nanoparticles sized 161.9 to 230.5 nm improve drug bioavailability by approximately 2.04 fold and precorneal residence time by 3.36 fold in rabbit eyes [145]. Guo et al. developed self-assembled micelles of poly(ethylene glycol)-block-poly(glycidyl methacrylate) (PEG-b-PGMA) to deliver natamycin [146]. The sustained drug release from micelles allows reducing the frequency of natamycin application from 8 to only 3 times per day in rabbits with fungal keratitis. The use of contact lenses as drug carriers or sustained-release deposits has also been evaluated to improve antimicrobial efficacy. Huang et al. developed a hybrid hydrogel-based contact lens, loaded with voriconazole, comprised of quaternized chitosan, graphene oxide, and silver nanoparticles [147].

Another strategy employs carbon dots, which are small, highly fluorescent non-toxic element nanoparticles that measure less than 10 nm and are considered to replace metal-based quantum dots [148]. Zhao et al. demonstrated that nitrogen-doped carbon quantum dots sized 2–5 nm can destroy the cell structure of *Staphylococcus aureus* and methicillin-resistant *Staphylococcus aureus* (MRSA) [149].

There is a paucity of studies evaluating the efficacy of drug-delivery mechanisms to manage infectious keratitis in humans. Such mechanisms may enhance drug penetration, better compliance, and reduced toxicity, thus improving patient outcomes.

9.8 Surgical procedures

Surgical management must be considered to maintain the globe integrity in patients with unresponsive keratitis associated with severe stromal melt with impending perforation risk. Zhong et al. demonstrated that full-thickness conjunctival flap covering surgery with amniotic membrane transplantation might represent a viable option to save the eyeball for eyes with severe fungal keratitis without corneal perforation [150]. In their series, most eyes (15/17, 88%) achieved complete conjunctival re-epithelization. Seven of them achieved a mean best-corrected visual acuity of ~20/100, remaining disease-free at least one month after sclerokeratoplasty [150]. However, melting of the conjunctival flap, with subsequent endophthalmitis requiring evisceration, occurred in two eyes.

Therapeutic keratoplasty (TKP) should be reserved for patients who are not candidates for other therapies, and if possible, after quiescent infection [151]. In *Acanthamoeba* keratitis, TKP is recommended in cases of corneal perforation unresponsive to repeat gluing, severe corneal abscess, or significant cataract [113]. Because of the risk of rejection with large grafts in *Acanthamoeba* keratitis, corneal grafts must be kept to the minimum size required [113]. In cases of fungal keratitis, Selver et al. demonstrated that smaller grafts ($\leq$ 8 mm) were associated with lower rejection rates, but higher recurrence rates possibly related to incomplete removal of infected tissue [151, 152].

10. Conclusions

Despite significant technological development in contact lens materials resulting in remarkable improvement in safety and comfort, microbial keratitis continues to be a severe sight-threatening complication in contact lens wearers. Overnight extended contact lens wear and deficient lenses and case hygiene continue to be the primary risk factors for CLAIK worldwide; hence improvement in contact lens hygiene, education, and handling is necessary to reduce this potential complication.

The clinician must be able to promptly recognize the condition and identify the causative microorganism through corneal scraping, smear, and culture in case of severe keratitis, and treat the disease according to the suspected etiological agent; Empirical treatment must be initiated in every case and modified according to the clinical response and microbiology laboratory results.

Appendix

Fortified topical antibiotic formulations and mode of preparation

Tobramycin 14 mg/mL or gentamicin 14 mg/mL

1. Withdraw 2 mL of either drug from an injectable vial (40 mg/mL).
2. Add 2 mL to an ophthalmic solution (5 mg) of either drug to give a 14 mg/mL solution.
3. Refrigerate and shake prior to instillation.

Cefazolin 50 mg/mL or ceftazidime 50 mg/mL

1. Add 9.3 mL of lubricant eyedrops to a vial of either drug, 1 g (powder for injection).
2. Dissolve. Take 5 mL and add it to 5 mL of lubricant eyedrops.
3. Refrigerate and shake prior to instillation.

Amikacin 10–40 mg/mL

1. Dilute intravenous formulation (80 mg/2 mL ampules) with lubricant eyedrops or 0.9% sodium chloride for injection USP to the desired concentration.
2. Refrigerate and shake prior to instillation.

Vancomycin 15 mg/mL, 25 mg/mL, or 50 mg/mL

1. Add either 33 mL, 20 mL, or 10 mL of 0.9% sodium chloride for injection USP, or artificial tears, to a vial of 500 mg of vancomycin to produce a solution of 15, 25, or 50 mg/mL, respectively.
2. Refrigerate and shake prior to instillation.

Linezolid 2 mg/mL (for methicillin-resistant Staphylococcus aureus) 1. May be used directly from parenteral linezolid intravenous infusion available as 200 mg/100 mL.
Colistin 0.19% (for multiple drug-resistant *Pseudomonas aeruginosa*) 1. Add 1 million UI / 75 mg of parenteral colistimethate sodium powder to 10 ml of distilled water to obtain 7.5 mg/mL. 2. Withdraw 1 mL of the above solution and add to 3 mL of distilled water to obtain a 0.19% concentration
Trimethoprim (16 mg/mL) - sulfamethoxazole (80 mg/mL) 1. Commercial intravenous preparation may be used as topical solution without preparation.
Imipenem – cilastin (1%) 1. Add 10 mL of sterile water to parenteral imipenem (500 mg) – cilastin (500 mg) to create a 50 mg/mL solution. 2. Withdraw 1 mL of the above solution and add 4 mL of sterile water to make topical 1% imipenem to obtain 1 mg/mL 3. Storage in amber-colored bottles

Data retrieved from [153].

Author details

Jimena Alamillo-Velazquez, Raul E. Ruiz-Lozano, Julio C. Hernandez-Camarena and Alejandro Rodriguez-Garcia*
Tecnologico de Monterrey, School of Medicine and Health Sciences, Institute of Ophthalmology and Visual Sciences, Monterrey, Mexico

*Address all correspondence to: immuneye@gmail.com

References

[1] Forister JFY, Forister EF, Yeung KK, et al. Prevalence of contact lens-related complications: UCLA contact lens study. *Eye Contact Lens*. 2009;35(4):176-180. doi:10.1097/ICL.0b013e3181a7bda1

[2] Bourcier T, Thomas F, Borderie V, Chaumeil C, Laroche L. Bacterial keratitis: predisposing factors, clinical and microbiological review of 300 cases. *Br J Ophthalmol*. 2003;87(7): 834-838. doi:10.1136/bjo.87.7.834

[3] Edwards K, Keay L, Naduvilath T, Snibson G, Taylor H, Stapleton F. Characteristics of and risk factors for contact lens-related microbial keratitis in a tertiary referral hospital. *Eye Lond Engl*. 2009;23(1):153-160. doi:10.1038/sj.eye.6702953

[4] Fong C-F, Tseng C-H, Hu F-R, Wang I-J, Chen W-L, Hou Y-C. Clinical characteristics of microbial keratitis in a university hospital in Taiwan. *Am J Ophthalmol*. 2004;137(2):329-336. doi:10.1016/j.ajo.2003.09.001

[5] Erie JC, Nevitt MP, Hodge DO, Ballard DJ. Incidence of ulcerative keratitis in a defined population from 1950 through 1988. *Arch Ophthalmol Chic Ill 1960*. 1993;111(12):1665-1671. doi:10.1001/archopht.1993.01090120087027

[6] Upadhyay M, Karmacharya P, Koirala S, et al. The Bhaktapur eye study: ocular trauma and antibiotic prophylaxis for the prevention of corneal ulceration in Nepal. *Br J Ophthalmol*. 2001;85(4):388-392. doi:10.1136/bjo.85.4.388

[7] Hsiao C-H. Pediatric Microbial Keratitis in Taiwanese Children: A Review of Hospital Cases. *Arch Ophthalmol*. 2007;125(5):603. doi:10.1001/archopht.125.5.603

[8] Khor W-B, Prajna VN, Garg P, et al. The Asia Cornea Society Infectious Keratitis Study: A Prospective Multicenter Study of Infectious Keratitis in Asia. *Am J Ophthalmol*. 2018;195:161-170. doi:10.1016/j.ajo.2018.07.040

[9] Li W, Sun X, Wang Z, Zhang Y. A survey of contact lens-related complications in a tertiary hospital in China. *Contact Lens Anterior Eye J Br Contact Lens Assoc*. 2018;41(2):201-204. doi:10.1016/j.clae.2017.10.007

[10] Liesegang TJ. Contact lens-related microbial keratitis: Part I: Epidemiology. *Cornea*. 1997;16(2):125-131.

[11] Stapleton F. Contact lens-related microbial keratitis: what can epidemiologic studies tell us? *Eye Contact Lens*. 2003;29(1 Suppl):S85-89; discussion S115-118, S192-194. doi:10.1097/00140068-200301001-00024

[12] Stapleton F, Keay L, Edwards K, et al. The incidence of contact lens-related microbial keratitis in Australia. *Ophthalmology*. 2008; 115(10):1655-1662. doi:10.1016/j.ophtha.2008.04.002

[13] Stapleton F, Keay L, Edwards K, Holden B. The epidemiology of microbial keratitis with silicone hydrogel contact lenses. *Eye Contact Lens*. 2013;39(1):79-85. doi:10.1097/ICL.0b013e3182713919

[14] Watt K, Swarbrick HA. Microbial keratitis in overnight orthokeratology: review of the first 50 cases. *Eye Contact Lens*. 2005;31(5):201-208. doi:10.1097/01.icl.0000179705.23313.7e

[15] Steinemann TL, Pinninti U, Szczotka LB, Eiferman RA, Price FW. Ocular complications associated with the use of cosmetic contact lenses from unlicensed vendors. *Eye Contact Lens*. 2003;29(4):196-200. doi:10.1097/00140068-200310000-00002

[16] Sauer A, Bourcier T, French Study Group for Contact Lenses Related Microbial Keratitis. Microbial keratitis as a foreseeable complication of cosmetic contact lenses: a prospective study. *Acta Ophthalmol (Copenh)*. 2011;89(5):e439-442. doi:10.1111/j.1755-3768.2011.02120.x

[17] Spernovasilis N, Maraki S, Kokorakis E, et al. Antimicrobial susceptibility of isolated pathogens from patients with contact lens-related bacterial keratitis in Crete, Greece: A ten-year analysis. *Contact Lens Anterior Eye J Br Contact Lens Assoc*. Published online August 8, 2020:101355. doi:10.1016/j.clae.2020.07.006

[18] Stapleton F, Keay LJ, Sanfilippo PG, Katiyar S, Edwards KP, Naduvilath T. Relationship between climate, disease severity, and causative organism for contact lens-associated microbial keratitis in Australia. *Am J Ophthalmol*. 2007;144(5):690-698. doi:10.1016/j.ajo.2007.06.037

[19] Rattanatam T, Heng WJ, Rapuano CJ, Laibson PR, Cohen EJ. Trends in contact lens-related corneal ulcers. *Cornea*. 2001;20(3):290-294. doi:10.1097/00003226-200104000-00010

[20] Yildiz EH, Airiani S, Hammersmith KM, et al. Trends in contact lens-related corneal ulcers at a tertiary referral center. *Cornea*. 2012;31(10):1097-1102. doi:10.1097/ICO.0b013e318221cee0

[21] Mah-Sadorra JH, Yavuz SGA, Najjar DM, Laibson PR, Rapuano CJ, Cohen EJ. Trends in contact lens-related corneal ulcers. *Cornea*. 2005;24(1):51-58. doi:10.1097/01.ico.0000138839.29823.57

[22] Stapleton F, Naduvilath T, Keay L, et al. Risk factors and causative organisms in microbial keratitis in daily disposable contact lens wear. *PloS One*. 2017;12(8):e0181343. doi:10.1371/journal.pone.0181343

[23] Bottone EJ, Cho KW. Mycobacterium chelonae keratitis: elucidation of diagnosis through evaluation of smears of fluid from patient's contact lens care system. *Cornea*. 2005;24(3):356-358. doi:10.1097/01.ico.0000138858.95516.c5

[24] Allan BD, Dart JK. Strategies for the management of microbial keratitis. *Br J Ophthalmol*. 1995;79(8):777-786.

[25] Kaye R, Kaye A, Sueke H, et al. Recurrent bacterial keratitis. *Invest Ophthalmol Vis Sci*. 2013;54(6):4136-4139. doi:10.1167/iovs.13-12130

[26] Patel A, Hammersmith K. Contact lens-related microbial keratitis: recent outbreaks. *Curr Opin Ophthalmol*. 2008;19(4):302-306. doi:10.1097/ICU.0b013e3283045e74

[27] Khor W-B, Aung T, Saw S-M, et al. An Outbreak of Fusarium Keratitis Associated With Contact Lens Wear in Singapore. *JAMA*. 2006;295(24):2867. doi:10.1001/jama.295.24.2867

[28] Alfonso EC, Cantu-Dibildox J, Munir WM, et al. Insurgence of Fusarium keratitis associated with contact lens wear. *Arch Ophthalmol Chic Ill 1960*. 2006;124(7):941-947. doi:10.1001/archopht.124.7.ecs60039

[29] Bernal MD, Acharya NR, Lietman TM, Strauss EC, McLeod SD, Hwang DG. Outbreak of Fusarium keratitis in soft contact lens wearers in San Francisco. *Arch Ophthalmol Chic Ill 1960*. 2006;124(7):1051-1053. doi:10.1001/archopht.124.7.ecr60006

[30] Chang DC, Grant GB, O'Donnell K, et al. Multistate outbreak of Fusarium keratitis associated with use of a contact lens solution. *JAMA*. 2006;296(8):953-963. doi:10.1001/jama.296.8.953

[31] Zhang S, Ahearn DG, Noble-Wang JA, et al. Growth and survival of Fusarium solani-F. oxysporum complex on stressed multipurpose contact lens care solution films on plastic surfaces in situ and in vitro. *Cornea*. 2006;25(10):1210-1216. doi:10.1097/ICO.0b013e31802dd3a4

[32] Joslin CE, Tu EY, Shoff ME, et al. The association of contact lens solution use and Acanthamoeba keratitis. *Am J Ophthalmol*. 2007;144(2):169-180. doi:10.1016/j.ajo.2007.05.029

[33] Karaca I, Barut Selver O, Palamar M, Egrilmez S, Aydemir S, Yagci A. Contact Lens-Associated Microbial Keratitis in a Tertiary Eye Care Center in Turkey. *Eye Contact Lens*. 2020;46(2):110-115. doi:10.1097/ICL.0000000000000617

[34] Ahn M, Yoon K-C, Ryu S-K, Cho N-C, You I-C. Clinical aspects and prognosis of mixed microbial (bacterial and fungal) keratitis. *Cornea*. 2011;30(4):409-413. doi:10.1097/ico.0b013e3181f23704

[35] Keay L, Stapleton F. Development and evaluation of evidence-based guidelines on contact lens-related microbial keratitis. *Contact Lens Anterior Eye J Br Contact Lens Assoc*. 2008;31(1):3-12. doi:10.1016/j.clae.2007.10.003

[36] Dart JKG, Radford CF, Minassian D, Verma S, Stapleton F. Risk factors for microbial keratitis with contemporary contact lenses: a case-control study. *Ophthalmology*. 2008;115(10):1647-1654, 1654.e1-3. doi:10.1016/j.ophtha.2008.05.003

[37] Schein OD, Glynn RJ, Poggio EC, Seddon JM, Kenyon KR. The relative risk of ulcerative keratitis among users of daily-wear and extended-wear soft contact lenses. A case-control study. Microbial Keratitis Study Group. *N Engl J Med*. 1989;321(12):773-778. doi:10.1056/NEJM198909213211201

[38] Radford CF, Lehmann OJ, Dart JK. Acanthamoeba keratitis: multicentre survey in England 1992-6. National Acanthamoeba Keratitis Study Group. *Br J Ophthalmol*. 1998;82(12):1387-1392. doi:10.1136/bjo.82.12.1387

[39] Phillips SP. Defining and measuring gender: A social determinant of health whose time has come. *Int J Equity Health*. 2005;4:11. doi:10.1186/1475-9276-4-11

[40] Lim CHL, Carnt NA, Farook M, et al. Risk factors for contact lens-related microbial keratitis in Singapore. *Eye Lond Engl*. 2016;30(3):447-455. doi:10.1038/eye.2015.250

[41] Carnt N, Hoffman JJ, Verma S, et al. Acanthamoeba keratitis: confirmation of the UK outbreak and a prospective case-control study identifying contributing risk factors. *Br J Ophthalmol*. 2018;102(12):1621-1628. doi:10.1136/bjophthalmol-2018-312544

[42] Keay L, Edwards K, Naduvilath T, et al. Microbial Keratitis: Predisposing Factors and Morbidity. *Ophthalmology*. 2006;113(1):109-116. doi:10.1016/j.ophtha.2005.08.013

[43] Carnt NA, Willcox MDP, Hau S, et al. Association of Single Nucleotide Polymorphisms of Interleukins-1β, −6, and -12B with Contact Lens Keratitis Susceptibility and Severity. *Ophthalmology*. 2012;119(7):1320-1327. doi:10.1016/j.ophtha.2012.01.031

[44] Sankaridurg PR, Sharma S, Willcox M, et al. Bacterial colonization of disposable soft contact lenses is greater during corneal infiltrative events than during asymptomatic extended lens wear. *J Clin Microbiol*. 2000;38(12):4420-4424. doi:10.1128/JCM.38.12.4420-4424.2000

[45] Soumpasis I, Knapp L, Pitt T. A proof-of-concept model for the identification of the key events in the

infection process with specific reference to Pseudomonas aeruginosa in corneal infections. *Infect Ecol Epidemiol*. 2015;5:28750. doi:10.3402/iee.v5.28750

[46] Stapleton F, Tan J. Impact of Contact Lens Material, Design, and Fitting on Discomfort. *Eye Contact Lens*. 2017;43(1):32-39. doi:10.1097/ICL.0000000000000318

[47] Zaidi T, Mowrey-McKee M, Pier GB. Hypoxia increases corneal cell expression of CFTR leading to increased Pseudomonas aeruginosa binding, internalization, and initiation of inflammation. *Invest Ophthalmol Vis Sci*. 2004;45(11):4066-4074. doi:10.1167/iovs.04-0627

[48] Imayasu M, Petroll WM, Jester JV, Patel SK, Ohashi J, Cavanagh HD. The relation between contact lens oxygen transmissibility and binding of Pseudomonas aeruginosa to the cornea after overnight wear. *Ophthalmology*. 1994;101(2):371-388. doi:10.1016/s0161-6420(94)31326-1

[49] Ren DH, Yamamoto K, Ladage PM, et al. Adaptive effects of 30-night wear of hyper-O(2) transmissible contact lenses on bacterial binding and corneal epithelium: a 1-year clinical trial. *Ophthalmology*. 2002;109(1):27-39; discussion 39-40. doi:10.1016/s0161-6420(01)00867-3

[50] Cavanagh HD, Ladage PM, Li SL, et al. Effects of daily and overnight wear of a novel hyper oxygen-transmissible soft contact lens on bacterial binding and corneal epithelium: a 13-month clinical trial. *Ophthalmology*. 2002;109(11):1957-1969. doi:10.1016/s0161-6420(02)01278-2

[51] Wu YT, Zhu LS, Tam KPC, Evans DJ, Fleiszig SMJ. Pseudomonas aeruginosa Survival at Posterior Contact Lens Surfaces after Daily Wear. *Optom Vis Sci Off Publ Am Acad Optom*. 2015;92(6):659-664. doi:10.1097/OPX.0000000000000597

[52] McNamara NA, Polse KA, Brand RJ, Graham AD, Chan JS, McKenney CD. Tear mixing under a soft contact lens: effects of lens diameter. *Am J Ophthalmol*. 1999;127(6):659-665. doi:10.1016/s0002-9394(99)00051-3

[53] Paugh JR, Stapleton F, Keay L, Ho A. Tear Exchange under Hydrogel Contact Lenses: Methodological Considerations. *Invest Ophthalmol Vis Sci*. 2001;42(12):2813-2820.

[54] Fleiszig SMJ, Evans DJ. Pathogenesis of contact lens-associated microbial keratitis. *Optom Vis Sci Off Publ Am Acad Optom*. 2010;87(4):225-232. doi:10.1097/OPX.0b013e3181d408ee

[55] Stapleton F, Dart JK, Seal DV, Matheson M. Epidemiology of Pseudomonas aeruginosa keratitis in contact lens wearers. *Epidemiol Infect*. 1995;114(3):395-402.

[56] McLaughlin-Borlace L, Stapleton F, Matheson M, Dart JK. Bacterial biofilm on contact lenses and lens storage cases in wearers with microbial keratitis. *J Appl Microbiol*. 1998;84(5):827-838. doi:10.1046/j.1365-2672.1998.00418.x

[57] Anwar H, Dasgupta MK, Costerton JW. Testing the susceptibility of bacteria in biofilms to antibacterial agents. *Antimicrob Agents Chemother*. 1990;34(11):2043-2046.

[58] Szczotka-Flynn LB, Imamura Y, Chandra J, et al. Increased resistance of contact lens-related bacterial biofilms to antimicrobial activity of soft contact lens care solutions. *Cornea*. 2009;28(8):918-926. doi:10.1097/ICO.0b013e3181a81835

[59] Vijay AK, Sankaridurg P, Zhu H, Willcox MDP. Guinea pig models of acute keratitis responses. *Cornea*. 2009;28(10):1153-1159. doi:10.1097/ICO.0b013e3181a87a0b

[60] Willcox MDP, Naduvilath TJ, Vaddavalli PK, Holden BA, Ozkan J,

Zhu H. Corneal erosions, bacterial contamination of contact lenses, and microbial keratitis. *Eye Contact Lens*. 2010;36(6):340-345. doi:10.1097/ICL.0b013e3181f57b05

[61] Carnt NA, Evans VE, Naduvilath TJ, et al. Contact lens-related adverse events and the silicone hydrogel lenses and daily wear care system used. *Arch Ophthalmol Chic Ill 1960*. 2009;127(12):1616-1623. doi:10.1001/archophthalmol.2009.313

[62] Dumbleton K. Noninflammatory silicone hydrogel contact lens complications. *Eye Contact Lens*. 2003;29(1 Suppl):S186-189; discussion S190-191, S192-194. doi:10.1097/00140068-200301001-00051

[63] Poggio EC, Glynn RJ, Schein OD, et al. The incidence of ulcerative keratitis among users of daily-wear and extended-wear soft contact lenses. *N Engl J Med*. 1989;321(12):779-783. doi:10.1056/NEJM198909213211202

[64] Cheung N, Nagra P, Hammersmith K. Emerging trends in contact lens-related infections. *Curr Opin Ophthalmol*. 2016;27(4):327-332. doi:10.1097/ICU.0000000000000280

[65] Goodlaw E. Risk of infection from sleeping with contact lenses on: causes of risk. *Optom Vis Sci Off Publ Am Acad Optom*. 1996;73(3):156-158. doi:10.1097/00006324-199603000-00005

[66] Zimmerman AB, Nixon AD, Rueff EM. Contact lens associated microbial keratitis: practical considerations for the optometrist. *Clin Optom*. 2016;8:1-12. doi:10.2147/OPTO.S66424

[67] Das S, Sheorey H, Taylor HR, Vajpayee RB. Association between cultures of contact lens and corneal scraping in contact lens related microbial keratitis. *Arch Ophthalmol Chic Ill 1960*. 2007;125(9):1182-1185. doi:10.1001/archopht.125.9.1182

[68] Stapleton F, Carnt N. Contact lens-related microbial keratitis: how have epidemiology and genetics helped us with pathogenesis and prophylaxis. *Eye Lond Engl*. 2012;26(2):185-193. doi:10.1038/eye.2011.288

[69] Alipour F, Khaheshi S, Soleimanzadeh M, Heidarzadeh S, Heydarzadeh S. Contact Lens-related Complications: A Review. *J Ophthalmic Vis Res*. 2017;12(2):193-204. doi:10.4103/jovr.jovr_159_16

[70] Fonn D, Jones L. Hand hygiene is linked to microbial keratitis and corneal inflammatory events. *Contact Lens Anterior Eye J Br Contact Lens Assoc*. 2019;42(2):132-135. doi:10.1016/j.clae.2018.10.022

[71] Stellwagen A, MacGregor C, Kung R, Konstantopoulos A, Hossain P. Personal hygiene risk factors for contact lens-related microbial keratitis. *BMJ Open Ophthalmol*. 2020;5(1). doi:10.1136/bmjophth-2020-000476

[72] Keay L, Stapleton F, Schein O. Epidemiology of contact lens-related inflammation and microbial keratitis: a 20-year perspective. *Eye Contact Lens*. 2007;33(6 Pt 2):346-353, discussion 362-363. doi:10.1097/ICL.0b013e318157c49d

[73] Ladage PM, Yamamoto K, Ren DH, et al. Proliferation rate of rabbit corneal epithelium during overnight rigid contact lens wear. *Invest Ophthalmol Vis Sci*. 2001;42(12):2804-2812.

[74] Ladage PM, Jester JV, Petroll WM, Bergmanson JPG, Cavanagh HD. Vertical Movement of Epithelial Basal Cells toward the Corneal Surface during Use of Extended-Wear Contact Lenses. *Invest Ophthalmol Vis Sci*.

2003;44(3):1056-1063. doi:10.1167/iovs.02-0725

[75] Willcox MDP, Holden BA. Contact Lens Related Corneal Infections. *Biosci Rep*. 2001;21(4):445-461. doi:10.1023/A:1017991709846

[76] Holden BA, Sankaridurg PR, Sweeney DF, Stretton S, Naduvilath TJ, Rao GN. Microbial keratitis in prospective studies of extended wear with disposable hydrogel contact lenses. *Cornea*. 2005;24(2):156-161. doi:10.1097/01.ico.0000138844.90668.91

[77] Keay L, Edwards K, Stapleton F. Signs, symptoms, and comorbidities in contact lens-related microbial keratitis. *Optom Vis Sci Off Publ Am Acad Optom*. 2009;86(7):803-809. doi:10.1097/OPX.0b013e3181ae1b69

[78] Aasuri MK, Venkata N, Kumar VM. Differential diagnosis of microbial keratitis and contact lens-induced peripheral ulcer. *Eye Contact Lens*. 2003;29(1 Suppl):S60-62; discussion S83-84, S192-194. doi:10.1097/00140068-200301001-00017

[79] Dalmon C, Porco TC, Lietman TM, et al. The Clinical Differentiation of Bacterial and Fungal Keratitis: A Photographic Survey. *Invest Ophthalmol Vis Sci*. 2012;53(4):1787-1791. doi:10.1167/iovs.11-8478

[80] Eltis M. Contact-lens-related microbial keratitis: case report and review. *J Optom*. 2011;4(4):122-127. doi:10.1016/S1888-4296(11)70053-X

[81] Labetoulle M, Frau E, Offret H, Nordmann P, Naas T. Non-preserved 1% lidocaine solution has less antibacterial properties than currently available anaesthetic eye-drops. *Curr Eye Res*. 2002;25(2):91-97. doi:10.1076/ceyr.25.2.91.10159

[82] Lin A, Rhee MK, Akpek EK, et al. Bacterial Keratitis Preferred Practice Pattern®. *Ophthalmology*. 2019;126(1):P1-P55. doi:10.1016/j.ophtha.2018.10.018

[83] Sharma S, Kunimoto DY, Gopinathan U, Athmanathan S, Garg P, Rao GN. Evaluation of corneal scraping smear examination methods in the diagnosis of bacterial and fungal keratitis: a survey of eight years of laboratory experience. *Cornea*. 2002;21(7):643-647. doi:10.1097/00003226-200210000-00002

[84] Sharma S. Diagnosis of fungal keratitis: current options. *Expert Opin Med Diagn*. 2012;6(5):449-455. doi:10.1517/17530059.2012.679656

[85] Hong, Augustine. Bacterial Keratitis. In: *Cornea: Fundamentals, Diagnosis and Management*. Fifth Editiom. Elsevier; 2022:802-824.

[86] Mela EK, Giannelou IP, Koliopoulos JX, Gartaganis SP, John KX, Sotirios GP. Ulcerative keratitis in contact lens wearers. *Eye Contact Lens*. 2003;29(4):207-209. doi:10.1097/01.icl.0000078102.30635.A7

[87] Musa F, Tailor R, Gao A, Hutley E, Rauz S, Scott R a. H. Contact lens-related microbial keratitis in deployed British military personnel. *Br J Ophthalmol*. 2010;94(8):988-993. doi:10.1136/bjo.2009.161430

[88] Lam DSC, Houang E, Fan DSP, et al. Incidence and risk factors for microbial keratitis in Hong Kong: comparison with Europe and North America. *Eye Lond Engl*. 2002;16(5):608-618. doi:10.1038/sj.eye.6700151

[89] Martins EN, Farah ME, Alvarenga LS, Yu MCZ, Höflin-Lima AL. Infectious keratitis: correlation between corneal and contact lens cultures. *CLAO J Off Publ Contact*

Lens Assoc Ophthalmol Inc. 2002;28(3):146-148.

[90] Alexandrakis G, Haimovici R, Miller D, Alfonso EC. Corneal biopsy in the management of progressive microbial keratitis. *Am J Ophthalmol*. 2000;129(5):571-576. doi:10.1016/s0002-9394(99)00449-3

[91] Lee P, Green WR. Corneal Biopsy: Indications, Techniques, and a Report of a Series of 87 Cases. *Ophthalmology*. 1990;97(6):718-721. doi:10.1016/S0161-6420(90)32517-4

[92] Newton C, Moore MB, Kaufman HE. Corneal biopsy in chronic keratitis. *Arch Ophthalmol Chic Ill 1960*. 1987;105(4):577-578. doi:10.1001/archopht.1987.01060040147053

[93] Epstein SS. The phenomenon of microbial uncultivability. *Curr Opin Microbiol*. 2013;16(5):636-642. doi:10.1016/j.mib.2013.08.003

[94] Winand R, Bogaerts B, Hoffman S, et al. Targeting the 16S rRNA Gene for Bacterial Identification in Complex Mixed Samples: Comparative Evaluation of Second (Illumina) and Third (Oxford Nanopore Technologies) Generation Sequencing Technologies. *Int J Mol Sci*. 2019;21(1). doi:10.3390/ijms21010298

[95] Fleiszig SMJ, Kroken AR, Nieto V, et al. Contact lens-related corneal infection: Intrinsic resistance and its compromise. *Prog Retin Eye Res*. 2020;76:100804. doi:10.1016/j.preteyeres.2019.100804

[96] Gaudio PA, Gopinathan U, Sangwan V, Hughes TE. Polymerase chain reaction based detection of fungi in infected corneas. *Br J Ophthalmol*. 2002;86(7):755-760. doi:10.1136/bjo.86.7.755

[97] Turnbaugh PJ, Ley RE, Hamady M, Fraser-Liggett CM, Knight R, Gordon JI. The human microbiome project. *Nature*. 2007;449(7164):804-810. doi:10.1038/nature06244

[98] Low L, Fuentes-Utrilla P, Hodson J, et al. Evaluation of full-length nanopore 16S sequencing for detection of pathogens in microbial keratitis. *PeerJ*. 2021;9:e10778. doi:10.7717/peerj.10778

[99] Kim E, Chidambaram JD, Srinivasan M, et al. Prospective comparison of microbial culture and polymerase chain reaction in the diagnosis of corneal ulcer. *Am J Ophthalmol*. 2008;146(5):714-723, 723.e1. doi:10.1016/j.ajo.2008.06.009

[100] Borst A, Box ATA, Fluit AC. False-positive results and contamination in nucleic acid amplification assays: suggestions for a prevent and destroy strategy. *Eur J Clin Microbiol Infect Dis Off Publ Eur Soc Clin Microbiol*. 2004;23(4):289-299. doi:10.1007/s10096-004-1100-1

[101] Goh JWY, Harrison R, Hau S, Alexander CL, Tole DM, Avadhanam VS. Comparison of In Vivo Confocal Microscopy, PCR and Culture of Corneal Scrapes in the Diagnosis of Acanthamoeba Keratitis. *Cornea*. 2018;37(4):480-485. doi:10.1097/ICO.0000000000001497

[102] Ung L, Bispo PJM, Doan T, et al. Clinical metagenomics for infectious corneal ulcers: Rags to riches? *Ocul Surf*. 2020;18(1):1-12. doi:10.1016/j.jtos.2019.10.007

[103] Holm JB, Humphrys MS, Robinson CK, et al. Ultrahigh-Throughput Multiplexing and Sequencing of >500-Base-Pair Amplicon Regions on the Illumina HiSeq 2500 Platform. *mSystems*. 2019;4(1). doi:10.1128/mSystems.00029-19

[104] Johnson JS, Spakowicz DJ, Hong B-Y, et al. Evaluation of 16S rRNA gene sequencing for species and strain-level microbiome analysis. *Nat Commun*.

2019;10(1):5029. doi:10.1038/s41467-019-13036-1

[105] Chiu CY, Miller SA. Clinical metagenomics. *Nat Rev Genet*. 2019;20(6):341-355. doi:10.1038/s41576-019-0113-7

[106] Shigeyasu C, Yamada M, Aoki K, et al. Metagenomic analysis for detecting Fusarium solani in a case of fungal keratitis. *J Infect Chemother Off J Jpn Soc Chemother*. 2018;24(8):664-668. doi:10.1016/j.jiac.2017.12.019

[107] Kuo M-T, Chen J-L, Hsu S-L, Chen A, You H-L. An Omics Approach to Diagnosing or Investigating Fungal Keratitis. *Int J Mol Sci*. 2019;20(15). doi:10.3390/ijms20153631

[108] Cruzat A, Qazi Y, Hamrah P. In Vivo Confocal Microscopy of Corneal Nerves in Health and Disease. *Ocul Surf*. 2017;15(1):15-47. doi:10.1016/j.jtos.2016.09.004

[109] Ruiz-Lozano RE, Hernandez-Camarena JC, Loya-Garcia D, Merayo-Lloves J, Rodriguez-Garcia A. The molecular basis of neurotrophic keratopathy: Diagnostic and therapeutic implications. A review. *Ocul Surf*. 2021;19:224-240. doi:10.1016/j.jtos.2020.09.007

[110] Saliman NH, Morgan PB, MacDonald AS, Maldonado-Codina C. Subclinical Inflammation of the Ocular Surface in Soft Contact Lens Wear. *Cornea*. 2020;39(2):146-154. doi:10.1097/ICO.0000000000002192

[111] Carnt N, Samarawickrama C, White A, Stapleton F. The diagnosis and management of contact lens-related microbial keratitis. *Clin Exp Optom*. 2017;100(5):482-493. doi:10.1111/cxo.12581

[112] Chidambaram JD, Prajna NV, Palepu S, et al. In Vivo Confocal Microscopy Cellular Features of Host and Organism in Bacterial, Fungal, and Acanthamoeba Keratitis. *Am J Ophthalmol*. 2018;190:24-33. doi:10.1016/j.ajo.2018.03.010

[113] Maycock NJR, Jayaswal R. Update on Acanthamoeba Keratitis: Diagnosis, Treatment, and Outcomes. *Cornea*. 2016;35(5):713-720. doi:10.1097/ICO.0000000000000804

[114] Dahlgren MA, Lingappan A, Wilhelmus KR. The clinical diagnosis of microbial keratitis. *Am J Ophthalmol*. 2007;143(6):940-944. doi:10.1016/j.ajo.2007.02.030

[115] Carnt N, Robaei D, Watson SL, Minassian DC, Dart JKG. The Impact of Topical Corticosteroids Used in Conjunction with Antiamoebic Therapy on the Outcome of Acanthamoeba Keratitis. *Ophthalmology*. 2016;123(5):984-990. doi:10.1016/j.ophtha.2016.01.020

[116] Thomas PA, Leck AK, Myatt M. Characteristic clinical features as an aid to the diagnosis of suppurative keratitis caused by filamentous fungi. *Br J Ophthalmol*. 2005;89(12):1554-1558. doi:10.1136/bjo.2005.076315

[117] Sweeney DF, Jalbert I, Covey M, et al. Clinical characterization of corneal infiltrative events observed with soft contact lens wear. *Cornea*. 2003;22(5):435-442. doi:10.1097/00003226-200307000-00009

[118] Carnt N, Stapleton F. Silicone hydrogel lens-solution interaction and inflammation. *Eye Contact Lens*. 2013;39(1):37-41. doi:10.1097/ICL.0b013e31827d4ba1

[119] McDonald EM, Ram FSF, Patel DV, McGhee CNJ. Topical antibiotics for the management of bacterial keratitis: an evidence-based review of high quality randomised controlled trials. *Br J*

Ophthalmol. 2014;98(11):1470-1477. doi:10.1136/bjophthalmol-2013-304660

[120] Ray KJ, Srinivasan M, Mascarenhas J, et al. Early addition of topical corticosteroids in the treatment of bacterial keratitis. *JAMA Ophthalmol*. 2014;132(6):737-741. doi:10.1001/jamaophthalmol.2014.292

[121] Srinivasan M, Mascarenhas J, Rajaraman R, et al. The steroids for corneal ulcers trial (SCUT): secondary 12-month clinical outcomes of a randomized controlled trial. *Am J Ophthalmol*. 2014;157(2):327-333.e3. doi:10.1016/j.ajo.2013.09.025

[122] Austin A, Lietman T, Rose-Nussbaumer J. Update on the Management of Infectious Keratitis. *Ophthalmology*. 2017;124(11):1678-1689. doi:10.1016/j.ophtha.2017.05.012

[123] Qiu S, Zhao G-Q, Lin J, et al. Natamycin in the treatment of fungal keratitis: a systematic review and Meta-analysis. *Int J Ophthalmol*. 2015;8(3):597-602. doi:10.3980/j.issn.2222-3959.2015.03.29

[124] Ansari Z, Miller D, Galor A. Current Thoughts in Fungal Keratitis: Diagnosis and Treatment. *Curr Fungal Infect Rep*. 2013;7(3):209-218. doi:10.1007/s12281-013-0150-110.1007/s12281-013-0150-1

[125] Chang H-YP, Chodosh J. Diagnostic and therapeutic considerations in fungal keratitis. *Int Ophthalmol Clin*. 2011;51(4):33-42. doi:10.1097/IIO.0b013e31822d64dc

[126] Shapiro BL, Lalitha P, Loh AR, et al. Susceptibility testing and clinical outcome in fungal keratitis. *Br J Ophthalmol*. 2010;94(3):384-385. doi:10.1136/bjo.2009.158675

[127] Prajna NV, Krishnan T, Mascarenhas J, et al. The Mycotic Ulcer Treatment Trial. *JAMA Ophthalmol*. 2013;131(4):422-429.

[128] Prajna NV, Krishnan T, Rajaraman R, et al. Effect of Oral Voriconazole on Fungal Keratitis in the Mycotic Ulcer Treatment Trial II (MUTT II): A Randomized Clinical Trial. *JAMA Ophthalmol*. 2016;134(12):1365-1372. doi:10.1001/jamaophthalmol.2016.4096

[129] FlorCruz NV, Peczon IV, Evans JR. Medical interventions for fungal keratitis. *Cochrane Database Syst Rev*. 2012;(2):CD004241. doi:10.1002/14651858.CD004241.pub3

[130] Szentmáry N, Daas L, Shi L, et al. Acanthamoeba keratitis - Clinical signs, differential diagnosis and treatment. *J Curr Ophthalmol*. 2019;31(1):16-23. doi:10.1016/j.joco.2018.09.008

[131] Palioura S, Henry CR, Amescua G, Alfonso EC. Role of steroids in the treatment of bacterial keratitis. *Clin Ophthalmol Auckl NZ*. 2016;10:179-186. doi:10.2147/OPTH.S80411

[132] Wilhelmus KR. Indecision about corticosteroids for bacterial keratitis: an evidence-based update. *Ophthalmology*. 2002;109(5):835-842; quiz 843. doi:10.1016/s0161-6420(02)00963-6

[133] Wang JC, Su D, Lim L. Contact lens microbial keratitis and prior topical steroid use: a disaster in the making? *Ann Acad Med Singapore*. 2004;33(4):484-488.

[134] Herretes S, Wang X, Reyes JMG. Topical corticosteroids as adjunctive therapy for bacterial keratitis. *Cochrane Database Syst Rev*. 2014;(10):CD005430. doi:10.1002/14651858.CD005430.pub3

[135] Wouters KA, Verhoekx JS, van Rooij J, Wubbels R, van Goor AT. Topical corticosteroids in Acanthamoeba keratitis: Friend or foe? *Eur J Ophthalmol*. Published online November 13, 2020:1120672120973606. doi:10.1177/1120672120973606

[136] Fan F, Huang X, Yuan K, et al. Glucocorticoids May Exacerbate Fungal Keratitis by Increasing Fungal Aggressivity and Inhibiting the Formation of Neutrophil Extracellular Traps. *Curr Eye Res*. 2020;45(2):124-133. doi:10.1080/02713683.2019.1657464

[137] Bonzano C, Di Zazzo A, Barabino S, Coco G, Traverso CE. Collagen Cross-Linking in the Management of Microbial Keratitis. *Ocul Immunol Inflamm*. 2019;27(3):507-512. doi:10.1080/09273948.2017.1414856

[138] Hernandez-Camarena JC, Graue-Hernandez EO, Loya-García D, Ruiz-Lozano RE, Valdez-García JE. Correlation between corneal stromal demarcation line depth and topographic outcomes after two pulsed-light-accelerated crosslinking protocols. *Clin Ophthalmol Auckl NZ*. 2019;13:1665-1673. doi:10.2147/OPTH.S206103

[139] Price MO, Tenkman LR, Schrier A, Fairchild KM, Trokel SL, Price FW. Photoactivated riboflavin treatment of infectious keratitis using collagen cross-linking technology. *J Refract Surg Thorofare NJ 1995*. 2012;28(10):706-713. doi:10.3928/1081597X-20120921-06

[140] Said DG, Elalfy MS, Gatzioufas Z, et al. Collagen cross-linking with photoactivated riboflavin (PACK-CXL) for the treatment of advanced infectious keratitis with corneal melting. *Ophthalmology*. 2014;121(7):1377-1382. doi:10.1016/j.ophtha.2014.01.011

[141] Ting DSJ, Henein C, Said DG, Dua HS. Photoactivated chromophore for infectious keratitis - Corneal cross-linking (PACK-CXL): A systematic review and meta-analysis. *Ocul Surf*. 2019;17(4):624-634. doi:10.1016/j.jtos.2019.08.006

[142] Naranjo A, Pelaez D, Arrieta E, et al. Cellular and molecular assessment of rose bengal photodynamic antimicrobial therapy on keratocytes, corneal endothelium and limbal stem cell niche. *Exp Eye Res*. 2019;188:107808. doi:10.1016/j.exer.2019.107808

[143] Amescua G, Arboleda A, Nikpoor N, et al. Rose Bengal Photodynamic Antimicrobial Therapy: A Novel Treatment for Resistant Fusarium Keratitis. *Cornea*. 2017;36(9):1141-1144. doi:10.1097/ICO.0000000000001265

[144] Naranjo A, Arboleda A, Martinez JD, et al. Rose Bengal Photodynamic Antimicrobial Therapy for Patients With Progressive Infectious Keratitis: A Pilot Clinical Study. *Am J Ophthalmol*. 2019;208:387-396. doi:10.1016/j.ajo.2019.08.027

[145] Chhonker YS, Prasad YD, Chandasana H, et al. Amphotericin-B entrapped lecithin/chitosan nanoparticles for prolonged ocular application. *Int J Biol Macromol*. 2015;72:1451-1458. doi:10.1016/j.ijbiomac.2014.10.014

[146] Guo Y, Karimi F, Fu Q, G Qiao G, Zhang H. Reduced administration frequency for the treatment of fungal keratitis: a sustained natamycin release from a micellar solution. *Expert Opin Drug Deliv*. 2020;17(3):407-421. doi:10.1080/17425247.2020.1719995

[147] Huang J-F, Zhong J, Chen G-P, et al. A Hydrogel-Based Hybrid Theranostic Contact Lens for Fungal Keratitis. *ACS Nano*. 2016;10(7):6464-6473. doi:10.1021/acsnano.6b00601

[148] Ghosal K, Ghosh A. Carbon dots: The next generation platform for biomedical applications. *Mater Sci Eng C Mater Biol Appl*. 2019;96:887-903. doi:10.1016/j.msec.2018.11.060

[149] Zhao C, Wang X, Wu L, et al. Nitrogen-doped carbon quantum dots as an antimicrobial agent against Staphylococcus for the treatment of infected wounds. *Colloids Surf B*

Biointerfaces. 2019;179:17-27. doi:10.1016/j.colsurfb.2019.03.042

[150] Zhong J, Wang B, Li S, et al. Full-thickness conjunctival flap covering surgery combined with amniotic membrane transplantation for severe fungal keratitis. *Exp Ther Med*. 2018;15(3):2711-2718. doi:10.3892/etm.2018.5765

[151] Sha X-Y, Shi Q, Liu L, Zhong J-X. Update on the management of fungal keratitis. *Int Ophthalmol*. Published online April 30, 2021. doi:10.1007/s10792-021-01873-3

[152] Barut Selver O, Egrilmez S, Palamar M, Arici M, Hilmioglu Polat S, Yagci A. Therapeutic Corneal Transplant for Fungal Keratitis Refractory to Medical Therapy. *Exp Clin Transplant Off J Middle East Soc Organ Transplant*. 2015;13(4):355-359. doi:10.6002/ect.2014.0108

[153] Nixon, H. K. (2018). Preparation of fortified antimicrobial eye drops. *Kerala Journal of Ophthalmology*, *30*(2), 152.

Chapter 2

Recent Advances in the Diagnosis and Management of Herpetic Keratitis

Anna Nowińska

Abstract

The chapter is focused on one of the major cause of keratitis - Herpetic keratitis, its epidemiology, natural course, clinical forms, prognosis, diagnosis and treatment. The estimated global incidence of HSV keratitis is roughly 1,5 million, including 40,000 new cases of each year. Patients are usually affected in the early decades of live, therefore the disease has a severe impact on quality of life and quality of vision in young, productive adults. The author describes the detailed corneal characteristics, provides slit lamp photographs, optical coherence tomography scans and confocal microscopy results of different forms of the HSV keratitis: epithelial, stromal, necrotizing and endothelial. The chapter also discusses recent methods of diagnosis based on PCR testing as well as established and future methods of treatment based on the latest research results.

Keywords: HSV keratitis, Herpes simplex virus, confocal microscopy, optical coherence tomograpy

1. Introduction

Human herpesviruses, which include HSV-1 (Herpes simplex virus type-1), HSV-2 (Herpes simplex virus type-2), HZV (Herpes zoster virus), EBV (Epstein–Barr virus), CMV (Cytomegalovirus), HHV-6 (Human herpesvirus-6), HHV-7 (Human herpesvirus-7), HHV-8/KSHV (Human herpesvirus-8, Kaposi's sarcoma-associated herpesvirus) are the causative factor of various diseases, including mononucleosis, roseola, chickenpox and many forms of ocular involvement, such as conjunctivitis, blepharitis, keratitis, uveitis and retinitis. The common features of all human herpesviruses include a double-stranded DNA genome, a 20-faceted icosahedral capsid, a surrounding proteinaceous tegument, and an external glycoprotein-laden lipid envelope. All herpesviruses are able to achieve a state of the latency, where the virus remains inactive in cells and occasionally reactivates. Recurrence could be described as the most characteristic feature of corneal infections caused by HSV, subsequently leading to visual impairment and blindness. According to epidemiological data, HSV keratitis remains a leading infectious cause of blindness in the world. The estimated global incidence of HSV keratitis is roughly 1,5 million, including 40,000 new cases of each year. Additionally the recurrence rate is high. It was estimated as 9.6% at 1 year, 22.9% at 2 years, and 63.2% at 20 years after the first episode of documented HSV keratitis [1–4]. Also the worldwide seroprevalence rate is high and estimated above 50%, but recently it was reported declining in the United States [5].

IntechOpen

In this chapter we will focus on Herpes simplex virus 1 keratitis - the detailed corneal characteristics based on slit-lamp examination, optical coherence tomography scans and confocal microscopy results. The chapter also discusses recent methods of diagnosis based on PCR testing as well as established and future methods of treatment based on the latest research results.

2. Pathogenesis of the HSV keratitis

General pathogenesis of herpesvirus infections include: active viral replication, state of latency and reactivation. Primary infection, usually in the childhood could be asymptomatic, oral, but also could affect upper respiratory track or ocular surface in the form of the conjunctivitis or blepharoconiunctivitis. After a primary infection, HSV-1 begins a life-long latency in the trigeminal ganglia, where abundant viral RNAs are constantly produced. In order to establish latency, HSV-1 has evolved several mechanism to evade the host immune response. The process is complex based on HSV-1 several viral proteins targeting multiple steps of the cellular DNA-sensor-mediated antiviral signal pathway of the host. Moreover, it is believed, that viral protein activation varies between immediate period after infection and the late phase of infection. Inhibition of the type I interferon (IFN-I) activity has been described as the main pathogenetic pathway of downregulating the host immune response. Numerous mechanism including: inhibiting nuclear factor kappa-light-chain-enhancer of activated B cells (NF-κB) activation, modulating interferon regulatory factor 3 (IRF3), interferon regulatory factor 7 (IRF7) or stimulator of IFN genes (STING) function were identified. Recently a broad attention was brought to the HSV-1 immediate early (IE) protein infected-cell polypeptide 0 (ICP0), which is an E3 ubiquitin ligase, a nuclear phosphoprotein that was described to play an essential role in inhibition of IFN-I production through IRF7 protein expression reduction, thus promoting viral replication, latency, and reactivation. Certain triggering agents, physiological and environmental stress, including ultraviolet exposure, fever, injury, hormonal disruption or immunosuppression could cause viral reactivation in the tissues innervated by the trigeminal ganglion, causing different forms of the HSV keratitis: epithelial, stromal or endothelial. Epithelial keratitis is the most common form of HSV keratitis, but the recurrence infection may also affect other corneal layers. Recurrence varies in frequency between subjects and throughout the life and could cause irreversible corneal damage and decrease in visual acuity, ranging from superficial opacities to serious complications such as corneal perforation and endophthalmitis [6–10].

3. Diagnosis

The diagnosis of HSV keratitis is mainly based on the presence of typical unilateral corneal lesions on the slit lamp examination. However, the clinical diagnosis may be guided by modern imaging techniques, such as optical coherence tomography or confocal microscopy. Also, laboratory testing including polymerase chain reaction (PCR) and novel techniques based on multiplex dot hybridization (MDH) assay or immunochromatographic assay (ICGA) may serve as a potential guide in the diagnostic process.

3.1 Symptoms

Patients symptoms depend on the clinical form and stage of the disease. Primary infection may be asymptomatic. Recurrent infections symptoms include: foreign body sensation, ocular or ocular adnexa pain, lacrimation, photophobia, decreased vision and conjunctival hyperemia. Symptoms are usually not specific. Although, patient with recurrent keratitis are aware of the symptoms of the recurrent keratitis, which allows for the rapid referral and treatment. Patients with neutrotrophic keratitis due to HSV keratitis may experience only mild symptoms despite the advanced corneal involvement.

3.2 Slit lamp examination/clinical forms

Herpetic keratitis is usually classified by anatomical localization in regards to affected corneal layers. Although the inflammation process may overlaps different layers. Also, recurrent keratitis is not only limited to one layer and can subsequently affect different corneal parts [11, 12].

3.2.1 Epithelial keratitis

Epithelial keratitis is the result of the active HSV replication in corneal, epithelial cells. The most characteristic form is the dendritic ulcer containing small branches with terminal bulbs. The borders of the branches are raised above the corneal surface. The ulcer may be single or multiple. Several dendritic ulcers may form a geographic ulcer, especially in patients with immune system deficiency, treated with topical steroids or in the long course of the disease. Other forms of epithelial involvement include punctate keratitis or epithelial vesicles. On the slit lamp examination, epithelial defects stain with fluorescein and become evident with the use of a blue filter (450 nm) with or without additional yellow barrier filter between 1 and 3 min after the dye instillation. Other symptoms in epithelial keratitis may include: bulbar conjunctival and limbal hyperaemia, subepithelial stromal edema at the ulcer site and subepithelial infiltration of inflammation cells. Epithelial keratitis in the form of the dendritic ulcer may also be present in the stromal recurrent keratitis. However, if multiple recurrence occur, the neurotrophic ulcer is definitely more probable clinical form compared to the dendritic ulcer. Characteristic features of the different forms of the epithelial keratitis are presented in **Figure 1**.

3.2.2 Stromal keratitis

Stromal involvement in case of herpetic keratitis develops on an immune related basis. Inflammatory response to the HSV is connected with the activation and infiltration of myeloid-derived cells, CD4+ T-cell and NK cells. Stromal inflammation may lead to the reduced corneal transparency, persistent scar formation, may also cause an irreversible tissue pathology including vascularization and stromal necrosis. The inflammation process is often accompanied by stromal localized or extensive corneal edema and a mild anterior chamber reaction. Several recurrences may lead to the lack of the corneal innervation. Moreover, the severity of disease may increase with each subsequent episode, as inflammatory reaction becomes stronger despite no detectable viral activity.

Throughout the years multiple clinical forms in terms of stromal keratitis were described, being the source of confusion in diagnostic terminology, including: immune stromal, interstitial, necrotizing, nonnecrotizing, disciform, focal, multifocal, diffuse. This could contributed to misdiagnosis, especially in early phases of the disease and misapplications of therapy in clinical practice. For example, in Japan, "disciform" keratitis is considered a type of stromal keratitis. "Immune stromal" term also is misleading, suggesting, that other forms of HSV stromal keratitis do not involve immune reaction. That is why a simplified classification of the stromal keratitis was

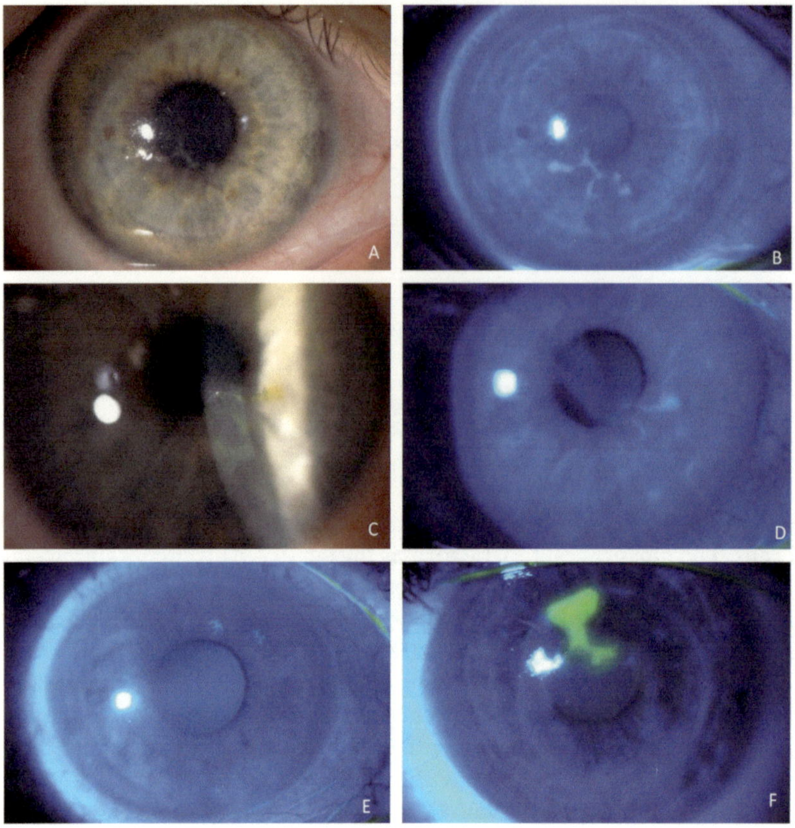

Figure 1.
Representative images of the slit-lamp photograph of the epithelial HSV keratitis. (A, B) Central, single dendritic ulcer before and after fluorescein installation. Branches with terminal bulbs visible. (C, D) Single dendritic ulcer with branches are raised above the corneal surface. Stromal haze accompanying the ulcer is noticeable. (E) Multiple, small dendritic ulcers visible under blue light after fluorescein installation. (F) Geographic, paracentral ulcer visible under blue light after fluorescein installation.

proposed, dividing the keratitis into two distinct forms: stromal with and without an overlying epithelial ulceration. Stromal keratitis without ulceration, is the more common form, historically described as "nonnecrotizing," "immune-stromal," and "interstitial." Stromal keratitis with ulceration is the effect of severe inflammation and relates to historical description of "necrotizing" keratitis. The form with the ulcer is more probably the result of stromal HSV reactivation, although the neurotrophic pathogenesis of the ulcer also cannot be ruled out. This terminology could be easily implemented in clinical practice and allows ophthalmologists to properly counsel patients regarding diagnosis, treatment and prognosis [12]. **Figure 2** contains clinical presentations of the range stromal keratitis. **Figure 3** present a clinical case of a patient diagnosed with stromal keratitis with ulceration throughout the treatment process.

Marginal keratitis is a special, rarely occurring form of stromal and epithelial keratitis. Clinically it is difficult to differentiate from other forms of marginal keratitis, thus laboratory testing may be helpful in establishing the final diagnosis. The lack of corneal sensitivity could also be used as a clinical clue in differential diagnosis.

3.2.3 Endothelitis

This form is believed to be a result of endothelial cells viral infection coexisting with immune reaction. Usually, the endothelitis is localized with a distinct area of

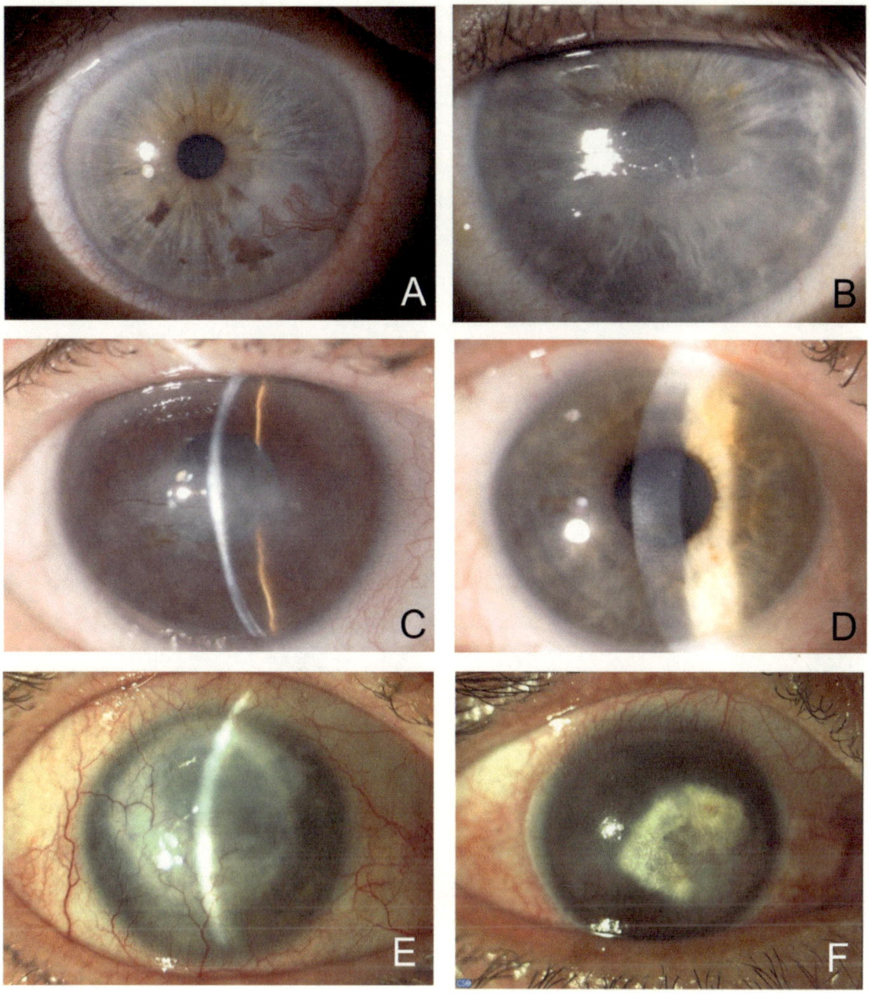

Figure 2.
Representative images of the slit-lamp photograph of eyes with the different involvement of the stromal keratitis or with corneal scars following HSV keratitis. (A) Paracentral stromal infiltration with profound, active limbal vascularization. (B) Epithelial, dendritic ulcer accompanied by active stromal keratitis with vascularization. (C) Central stromal scarring with deep, peripheral vascularization. (D) Stromal haze in the course of recurrent stromal HSV keratitis. (E) Excessive corneal scarring with significant, deep, peripheral vascularization. (F) Significant area of corneal scar accompanied by lipid keratopathy and deep vascularization.

the corneal edema. Therefore, it was historically described as disciform endothelial keratitis. Focal keratic precipitates, as well as Descemet membrane folds may be spotted in the affected area. Rarely, diffuse stromal edema, accompanied by trabeculitis with elevated intraocular pressure occurs. Various range of endothelitis is presented in **Figure 4**.

3.2.4 Neurotrophic ulcer/metaherpetic ulcer

This should be considered as a different entity, because there is no virus activation in case of neurotrophic ulcer. Also, the inflammation level compared to active HSV keratitis is lower. The most characteristic feature is the absence of corneal innervation and a non-healing corneal ulcer with smooth margins. As HSV keratitis alters the corneal nerves, the disease is one of the leading causes of neurotrophic keratopathy,

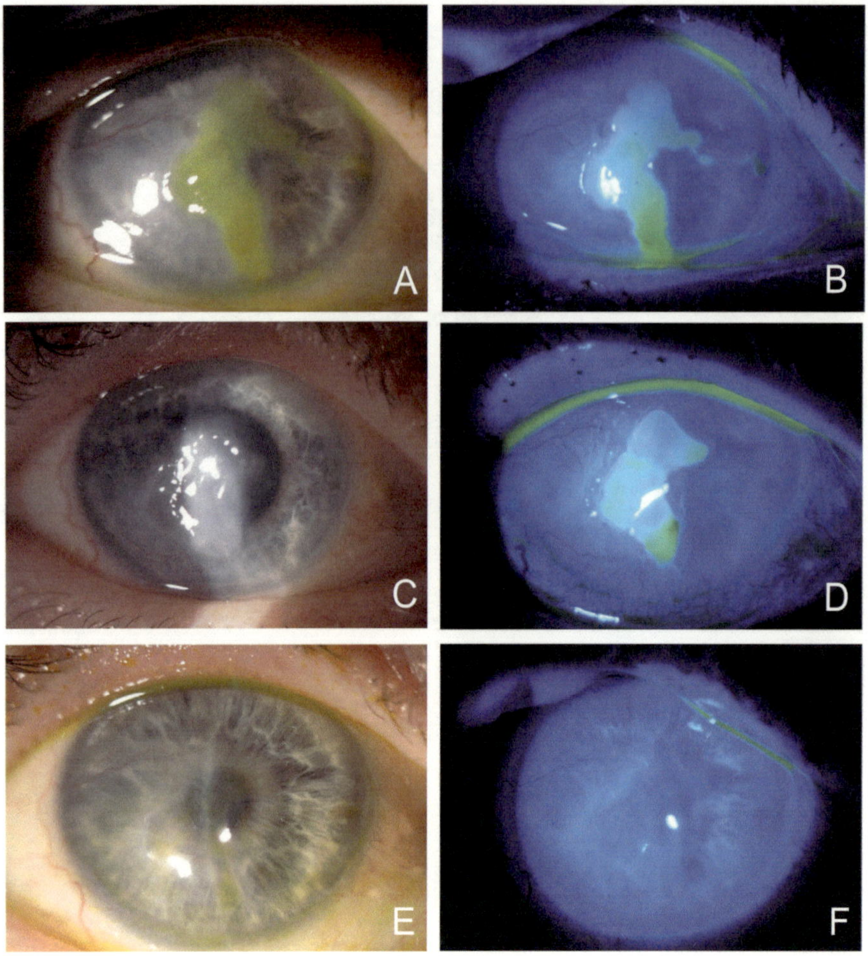

Figure 3.
Slit-lamp photographs presenting the follow up of a 65-year old patient with HSV stromal keratitis with ulcer. (A, B) Baseline, at diagnosis. Recurrent stromal keratitis with significant ulcer, stromal infiltration, vascularization and corneal thinning. Patient treated with the combination of antiviral medication (Oral acyclovir 800 mg, 5 times daily at baseline; topical 3% acyclovir ointment 4 times daily) combined with 0,1% dexamethasone (3 times daily) and preservative free lubricant eye drops (hourly). (C, D) At 1 month in the course of treatment. Significant decrease of the area of the ulcer. Remaining significant corneal infiltration with vascularization. Oral acyclovir dosage tapered gradually to 400 mg 4 times daily. Topical acyclovir discontinued. (E, F) At 3 months in the course of treatment. Ulcer healed completely. Punctate keratopathy visible under blue light. Decreased stromal infiltration, but stromal haze, thinning and vascularization visible. Oral acyclovir and 0,1% dexamethasone doses tapered very carefully within months to prevent active keratitis recurrence. Patient was recommended a frequent use of the preservative free eye lubricant drops.

among others, such severe dry eye disease, ocular burns or denervation post neurosurgical procedures. The pathogenesis is complex and include toxicity from antiviral medications, lack of nerve growth factors, the nerve damage as a result of recurrent keratitis. The neurotrophic keratitis is characterized by three stages of the severity: stage 1, punctate epithelial keratitis (PEK); stage 2, a nonhealing corneal persistent epithelial defect (PED); and stage 3 involving stromal involvement in the form of the neurotrophic ulceration. Possible accompanying signs are neovascularization, stromal haze and scarring. Consequently corneal poor ability to heal may result in corneal melting, prolonged ulceration, corneal perforation and endophthalmitis. A corneal sensitivity test is essential to confirm a diagnosis of neurotrophic keratitis. The test should be performed in regards to corneal location (central, peripheral), using a cotton-tipped swab or an esthesiometer. **Figure 5** presents forms of the neurotrophic keratitis.

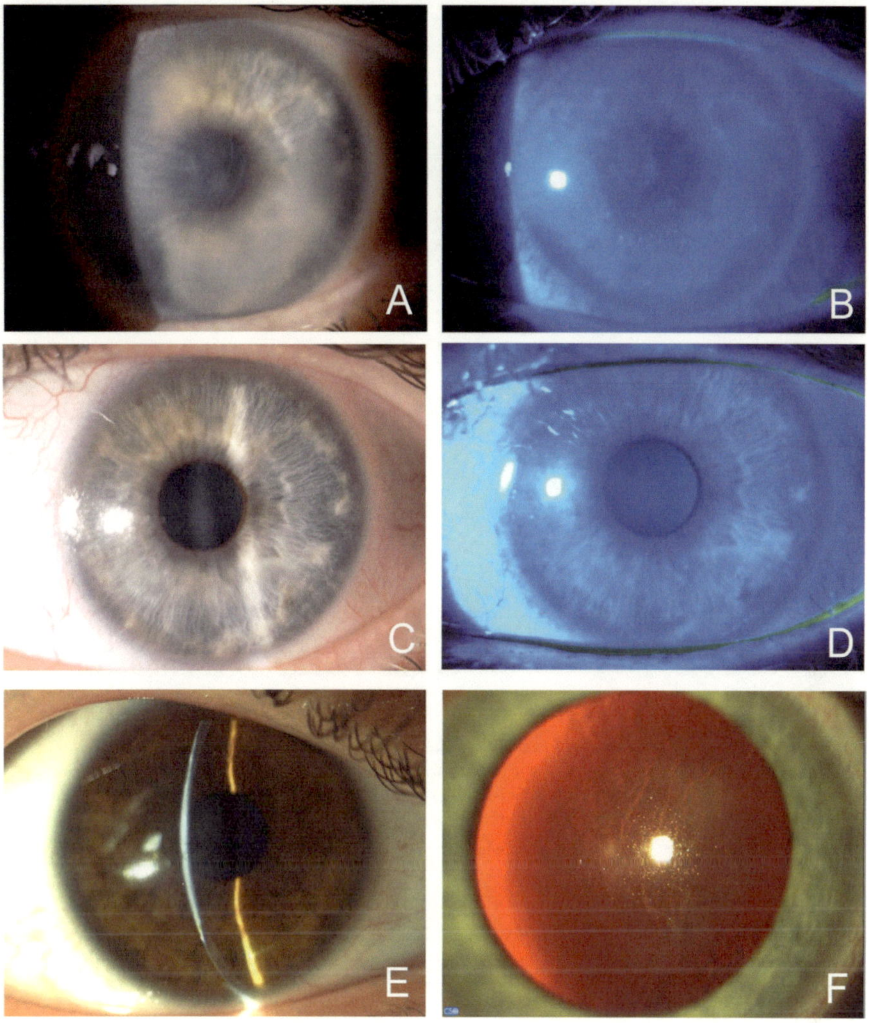

Figure 4.
Representative images of the slit-lamp photograph of the different forms of HSV endothelitis. (A, B, C, D) The slit lamp photographs of the eye of a 34-year old patient with recurrent, excessive endothelitis with significant corneal edema and Descemet folds. (A, B) At baseline. Diffuse corneal edema with Descemet folds and punctate keratopathy. Patient treated with the combination of antiviral medication (oral acyclovir 800 mg, 5 times daily at baseline combined with 0,1% dexamethasone (7 times daily) and preservative free lubricant eye drops (5 times daily). (C, D) At 2 months in the course of treatment. Significant decrease in stromal edema, with only subtle stromal haze. Improvement of the punctate epitheliopathy. (E) Distinct area of the corneal edema - disciform endothelial keratitis. (F) Distinct area of the corneal edema - disciform endothelial keratitis at retroillumination. Ghost, profound vessels visible.

3.3 Confocal microscopy

Confocal microscopy (IVCM - in vivo confocal microscopy) is the imaging technique developed to analyze corneal layers with the resolution of 1 μm. Imaging with confocal microscopy is used in clinical practice in differential diagnosis of microbial keratitis, corneal dystrophies and degenerations. The technique allows microscopic analysis of the cornea layer by layer and detailed assessment of keratocytes and inflammation cells. Features characteristic for HSV-1 keratitis depending on the stage and form include: microerosions, distortion of the superficial and basal epithelium, changes in superficial epithelial cell density, increase in epithelial cell size, squamous metaplasia, subepithelial infiltration of highly reflective dendritic

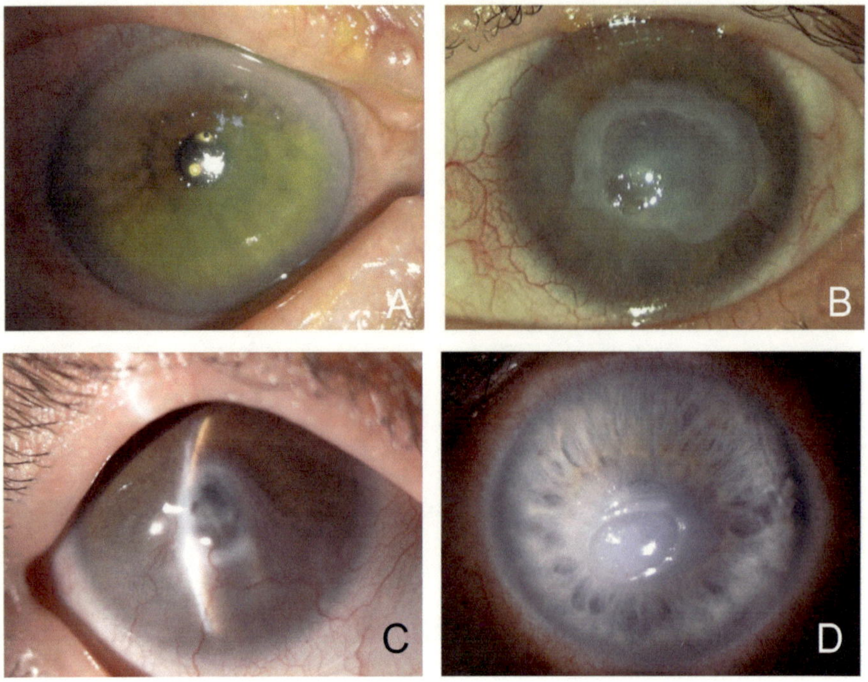

Figure 5.
Representative images of the slit-lamp photograph of the different forms of neurotrophic keratitis. (A) Neurotrophic keratitis stage 2. A nonhealing corneal persistent epithelial defect (PED) after fluorescein installation. (B) A single, central corneal ulcer with stromal infiltration and peripheral corneal vascularization. (C) Central corneal perforation in the course of the corneal thinning and scarring and vascularization. (D) Neurotrophic keratitis stage 3. Neurotrophic ulceration with elevated borders and significant stromal haze.

structures (correspondind to Langerhans cells), keratocytes activation, sub-basal nerve plexus alteration or absence, stromal fibrosis and endothelial precipitates. **Figure 6** presents the example of confocal microscopy results in case of patients with HSV keratitis. Confocal microscopy could guide in the disease diagnosis and monitoring the treatment results. In patients with stromal involvement the mean subbasal nerve density was proved to be significantly lower compared to healthy eyes. Also, in patients qualifying for surgical interventions, the technique has a potential role in assessing the sub-basal nerve plexus anatomy, helping the surgeons to procced with intervention decisions. The prognosis of patients with significantly altered corneal nerve plexus is poor after traditional transplant surgery [13–16].

3.4 Optical coherence tomography

Anterior eye segment imaging with 830 nm optical coherence tomography (AS OCT) was first demonstrated and published in 1994. Changing the light wavelength from 830 nm to 1310 nm allowed the direct transcleral anterior eye segment structures including trabecular-iris angle visualization in 2000. OCT provides in vivo anterior eye segment imaging with the axial resolution from 18 μm with time domain OCT (TD OCT) to 5 μm with spectral domain OCT (SD OCT) and to 5 μm with ultra high resolution spectral domain OCT. OCT is proven to provide reliable anterior eye segment morphology and morphometry results with high reproducibility and repeatability. Application of OCT in herpetic keratitis patients include: assisting in diagnosis of patients at active stage and assessing the scars in patients qualified for laser or surgical interventions. Active keratitis could be characterized

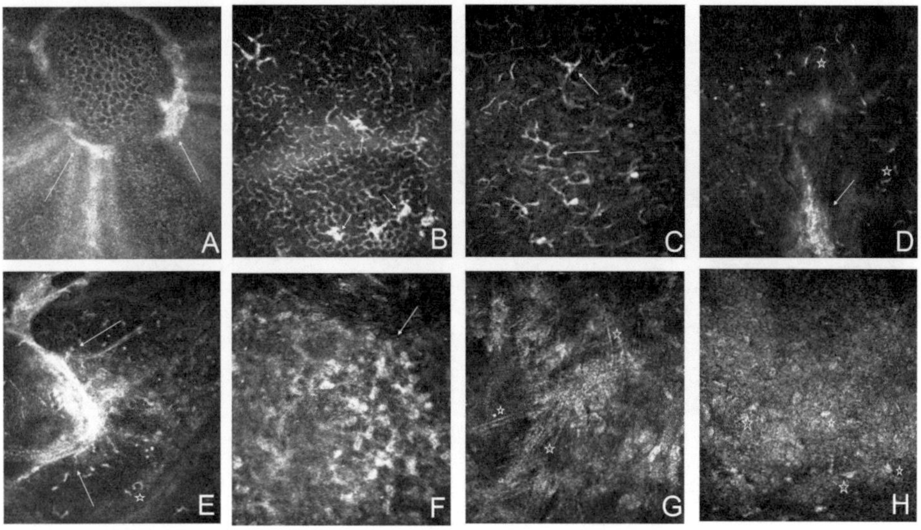

Figure 6.
Representative images of the confocal microscopy scans revealing significant features characteristic for HSV keratitis. (A) Epithelial, healed dendritic ulcer with noticeable fibrotic borders (arrows). (B) Multiple infiltration of small dendritic structures as the level of the epithelium. Clusters of inflammation cells (arrows). (C) Multiple infiltration of pronounced dendritic cells forming a lattice pattern (arrows) at the level of the basal epithelial cells. (D) Marked fibrosis at the level of the Bowman layer (arrow) with inflammation cells infiltration (stars). (E) Excessive fibrosis and inflammation cells infiltration forming clusters at the level of the Bowman layer (arrows). Dendritic structures visible (star). (F) Anterior stromal keratocytes activation with accompanying haze (arrow). (G) Stromal infiltration and haze accompanied by multiple crystalline structures due to the lipid degeneration (stars). (H) Multiple endothelial opacities. Examples marked with stars.

by the presence of the ulceration, stromal edema and inflammatory hyperreflective infiltrates. Corneas with inactive keratitis are characterized by stromal scarring and thinning, and epithelial remodeling [17–22]. Characteristic OCT features are presented in the **Figure** 7.

3.5 Laboratory testing

There are several laboratory techniques, which may help in the diagnostic process. Clinical samples for the analysis may be obtained through collection of tears, corneal epithelial cells, and conjunctival cells. Tear samples are usually obtained using Schirmer test. Epithelial or conjunctival cells may be collected through corneal scrapings, corneal impression membranes (CIM) or using conjunctival or corneal swab. The less invasive the technique the lesser probability of obtaining a clinically detectable material.

The isolation of the HSV from the cornea and performing a viral culture remains a conventional, gold standard technique, however the main disadvantages of this methods are low sensitivity and a time consuming process. Giemsa staining of the epithelial corneal cells may visualize multinucleated giant cells, resulting from coalescence of HSV infected epithelial cells and intranuclear HSV inclusions. Immunofluorescence assay (IFA) is one of the modern techniques developed to diagnose HSV keratitis. The principle of the method is to introduce antibodies, that bind to HSV antigens specifically to gain fluorescence based immunological detection of HSV-1 antigen through color visualization under microscopy. Disadvantages of the method include: required subjective interpretation by an experienced technician and the risk of obtaining false positives results due to cross-reactivity between other microorganisms.

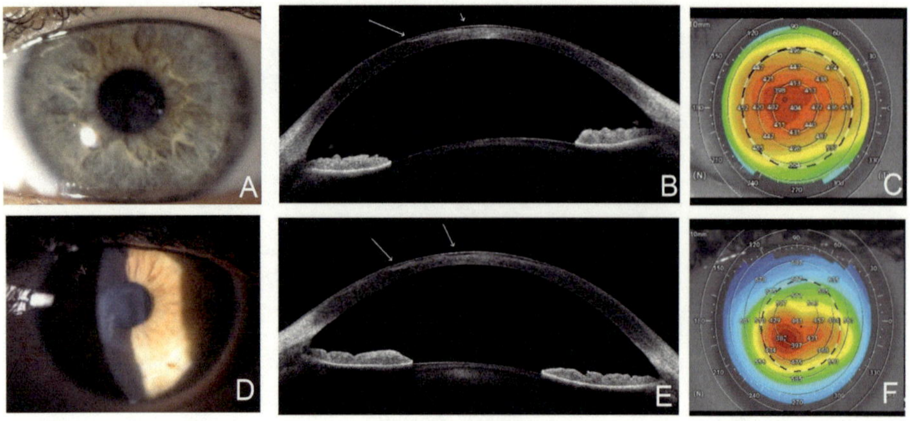

Figure 7.
Representative images of the anterior segment swept source optical coherence scans revealing significant features characteristic for HSV corneal scars. (A) Slit lamp photograph of the central post herpetic keratitis scar. (B) High resolution scan. Hyperreflective tissue within corneal stroma with irregular borders (arrows). (C) Pachymetry map. Marked paracentral corneal thinning to 398 μm. (D) Slit lamp photograph of the central post herpetic keratitis scar. (E) High resolution scan. Hyperreflective tissue within corneal stroma with irregular borders. Note the relatively smooth corneal surface and epithelial compensation over the irregular corneal stroma (arrows). (F) Pachymetry map. Marked irregular, paracentral corneal thinning to 382 μm.

Advanced diagnostic techniques include: Polymerase Chain Reaction (PCR) - conventional PCR, reverse transcriptase PCR (RT-PCR), real-time PCR (qPCR) and multiplex PCR. qPCR overcomes the disadvantages of conventional PCR by acquiring more rapid and sensitive results. Guda SJM. et al. assessed sensitivity and specificity of the conventional and real-time PCR compared to IFA performed on corneal scrapings. The sensitivity and specificity of conventional PCR was 100% and 76.9% and 100% and 28.2% of qPCR respectively. Satpathy et al. assessed and concluded, that specificity and positive predictive value (PPV) of PCR was higher in tear (90.6% and 37.5%). compared to cornea scrapings (71.3% and 30.3%). Moreover, Akbarian A. et al. reported, that conventional PCR with added internal amplification control (IAC) had higher sensitivity (100%) vs. culture method (66.66%), while the specificity was 100% for both diagnostic methods.

Also novel methods, such as multiplex dot hybridization (MDH) assay, immunochromatographic assay (ICGA, AmpliVue) or Infected cell protein 0 (ICP0) detection in tears are either tested or incorporated into a clinical practice. AmpliVue is a commercially available immunochromatographic assay, office-based diagnostic test characterized by a 64.7% positive detection rate. Sensitivity and specificity of AmpliVue was assessed as 84% and 100% respectively, based on true positives from culture and PCR combined. The MDH assay is a rapid technique, that involves a series of oligonucleotide probes specific for HSV genes. Compared to the real-time PCR, the MDH assay is characterized by very high values of sensitivity, specificity, positive predictive value (PPV), and negative predictive value (NPV) of 93.3%, 100%, 100% and 98.4%, respectively. The infected cell protein 0 (ICP0) is an acute phase protein during HSV infection and plays a significant role in the virus gene expression activation. ICP0 could be potentially defected in tears of affected subjects [23–28].

4. Differential diagnosis

Differential diagnosis is dependent on the corneal layer affected by the keratitis. Epithelial keratitis should be differentiated with epithelial regeneration line after traumatic epithelial defect, epithelial corneal dystrophies, such as epithelial basement membrane corneal dystrophy (EBMCD; map-finger-dot dystrophy, Cogan microcystic dystrophy), epitheliopathy associated with excessive contact lens wear or iatrogenic epitheliopathy after topical drops containing preservatives. Stromal involvement requires differentiation with other microbial keratitis (bacterial, fungal or amoebic), vaccinia virus keratitis (VACVK), Varicella Zoster virus keratitis, Thygeson superficial punctate keratopathy, stromal or Bowman layer corneal dystrophies, such as TGFBI corneal dystrophies. Marginal keratitis should be differentiated with other forms of marginal ulcers, such as staphylococcal marginal keratitis or related to atopic or autoimmune diseases, such as rheumatoid arthritis, systemic lupus or granulomatosis with polyangiitis (GPA). Also, neurotrophic keratitis may be initiated by multiple other causes, such as surgical and laser procedures, chemical burns, excessive contact lens wear and preservative-containing topical medicines, diabetes mellitus, multiple sclerosis and congenital or acquired abnormalities of the trigeminal nerve. Examples of the diseases, which require differential diagnosis with HSV keratitis are presented in **Figure 8**.

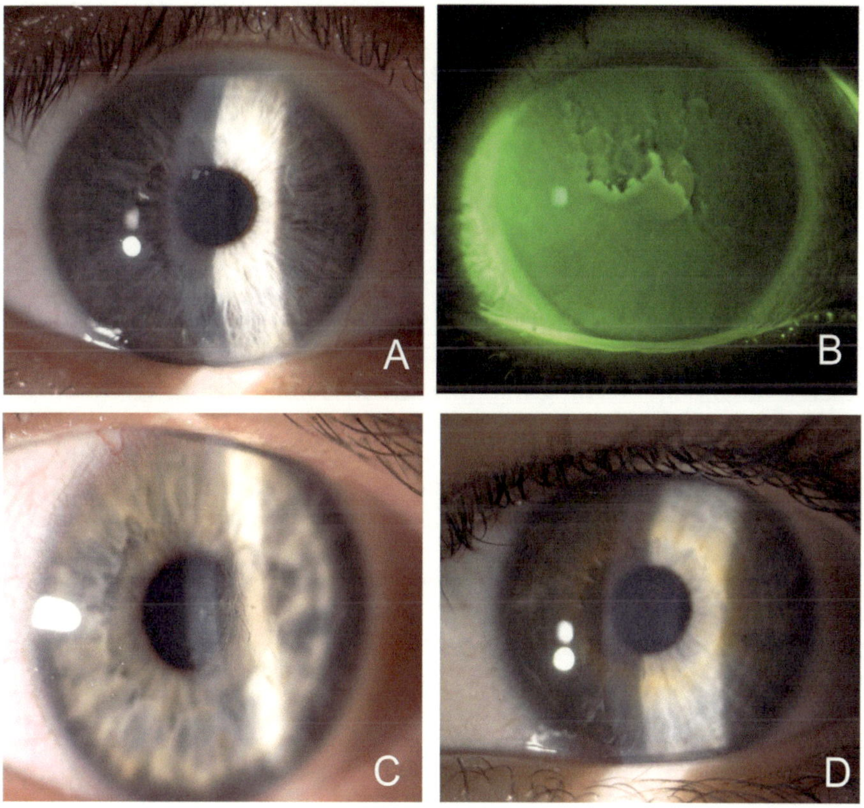

Figure 8.
Representative images of the slit-lamp photograph of the different forms of corneal diseases, which should be differentiated with HSV-keratitis. (A) Slit-lamp photograph of the epithelial basement membrane corneal dystrophy (EBMCD; map-finger-dot dystrophy, Cogan microcystic dystrophy). Superficial white dots visible. (B) The slit lamp photograph after fluorescein installation under blue light with additional yellow barrier filter of the patient 9A. An irregular area of the disrupted epithelium visible. (C) Slit-lamp photograph of the lattice corneal dystrophy (LCD). A dystrophy was confirmed by the TGFBI gene testing, which revealed a H626R mutation. (D) Slit-lamp photograph of the pediatric form of the lattice corneal dystrophy (LCD). Epithelial haze with multiple small, gray dots is visible. A dystrophy was confirmed by the TGFBI gene testing, which revealed a R124C mutation.

5. Management

Major advances in the treatment of HSV keratitis have been provided by the evidence-based results and conclusions of the Herpetic Eye Disease Study (HEDS) randomized clinical trials, which were multicenter, characterized by double-masking with placebo controls studies. Based on this knowledge, further treatment guidelines were proposed and published [12, 29–37]. Although the HEDS clinical trials directly addresses multiple clinical concerns, the studies have also several limitations. These include: inadequate sample size in case of HSV stromal keratitis with epithelial ulceration to determine the optimal course of therapy, relatively high rate of follow up failure within the study group. Also, the corticosteroid regimen was standardized and fixed in the study group, thus lacking the evidence of benefit of delivery of personalized care. Finally, the concerns regarding the dose and the optimal period of antiviral prophylaxis have not been resolved.

5.1 Active keratitis

Nowadays, the main treatment line of the active keratitis is a combination of the antiviral and corticosteroids drugs, depending on the epithelial and stromal involvement. The general rule to follow is to avoid corticosteroids in epithelial keratitis, because the entity of this form is virus activation and to treat with corticosteroids in stromal and endothelial keratitis without epithelial involvement, because those forms are strongly connected with the significant reaction of the immune system.

Antiviral drugs are used in two main forms: topical and oral. Topical anti HSV-1 drugs include: trifluridine solution (1%), ganciclovir gel (0.15%), and acyclovir ointment (3%). Oral anti HSV-1 drugs include: acyclovir, valacyclovir, and famciclovir. Historically, other systemic drugs were also used, such as idoxuridine, vidarabine, valganciclovir, foscarnet, and cidofovir, but they were withdrawn from the market or are relatively too toxic in combination with the achieved therapeutic effect.

Most common antiviral drug worldwide is acyclovir used either orally or topically or in combination. Common side effects of the prolonged oral acyclovir include nausea, vomiting, diarrhea, headache and weakness. Potentially serious, but very rare side effects include renal failure and hematology complications, such as: thrombotic thrombocytopenic purpura (TTP) and hemolytic uremic syndrome (HUS).

In recent years, there have been an increasing interest in valacyclovir, due to its proven improved bioavailability and steadier plasma concentration compared to acyclovir. Valacyclovir is considered a prodrug of acyclovir. The lower frequency of dosing (2 times daily versus 5 times daily) may be a strong benefit for some patients. However, there is a lack of strong evidence, that treatment with valaciclovir provides leads to better results and less ocular and systemic complications. Comparing to herpes zoster ophthalmicus, the authors of the systematic Cochrane report indicated uncertainty of the relative benefits and harms of valacyclovir over acyclovir [38]. All topical antiviral drugs are characterized by ocular surface toxicity, could cause allergic reactions, and punctal and nasolacrimal duct stenosis, therefore the prolonged usage of those formulas is not advised. Authors of the Cochrane systematic review on HSV keratitis treatment, published in 2015 also assessed other methods of HSV keratitis treatment, such as manual debridement of the corneal epithelium or experimental biologic agents. Manual debridement alone has been proved to be not effective. Also, topical treatment with interferon has only a modest benefit over placebo [39]. In case of epithelial keratitis, the mainstay of treatment is antiviral agents. Corticosteroids excessive usage may lead to geographical ulcers and delay healing of the epithelium. When stromal involvement is present, the mainstay of treatment is the use of corticosteroids with the combination of antiviral agents. The HEDS clinical trials have brought solid rationale for the treatment of the stromal keratitis with corticosteroids. Nowadays, there are several available topical corticosteroids formulas with different anti-inflammatory potency and different potential for adverse reactions: Dexamethasone 0,1%, Betamethasone at concentrations ranging from 0.01% to 0.1%, Prednisolone 1%, Loteprednol Etabonate 0.5%, Rimexolone 1%, Dexamethasone 0.1%, Hydrocortisone 0.335%, Fluorometholone 0,1%. The strongest anti-inflammatory effect is demonstrated by dexamethasone, the weakest by hydrocortisone. This should be taken into consideration, when choosing the medication depending on the level of the corneal inflammation. Moreover, steroid medication must be withdrawn gradually, tapering the doses generally over few weeks' time. During the drug withdrawal, instead of sudden discontinuation of the stronger corticosteroid, one may consider replacing it with a relatively weaker one to avoid a rebound increase in inflammation and a disease recurrence immediately after drug cessation. The recommended treatment for HSV stromal keratitis without ulceration should include a topical corticosteroid for at least a period exceeding ten weeks in conjunction with a prophylactic oral antiviral. A treatment period greater than ten weeks has been recommended, because of the high treatment failure rates six weeks after a ten-week prednisolone taper in the HEDS clinical trial. The most concerning side effects of topical steroids include: increase of the intraocular pressure, cataract and secondary infections (including bacterial, fungal, and also viral infections). Therefore, patients must be monitored carefully when treating with topical steroids.

5.2 Recurrence prevention

The HEDS study on recurrence rate clearly demonstrated that short-course oral during an active HSV epithelial keratitis does not prevent later stromal keratitis or iritis. On the other hand, a 12-month course of prophylactic oral acyclovir (400 mg) twice daily significantly decreased a recurrence rate of the stromal involvement. Although the HEDS study authors did not recommend a prolonged, beyond 12 months acyclovir prophylaxis, clinical practice recommendations and observations seem to postulate a positive role of a long-term prophylaxis, especially in patients with a high recurrence rate, significant corneal thinning at risk of corneal perforation, with comorbidities, such as atopy, autoimmune diseases or in immunocompromised patients. Also patients with history of HSV keratitis undergoing surgical procedures, such as corneal transplant, photorefractive procedures or cataract surgery may benefit from acyclovir prophylaxis, until the level of inflammation associate with the procedure and the risk of recurrence is decreased [12, 29–37].

One of the future treatment strategies is to enhance patient's immune system resistance to the infection through a vaccine against HSV-1. Nowadays there are no approved vaccine available, but there are ongoing studies regarding this subject. In the recently published study in 2020, the authors identified 15 viral-encoded proteins, which could serve as candidates for further testing for the HSV-1 vaccine [40].

5.3 Neurotrophic keratitis

There are several methods of treatment depending on the severity level of keratitis. First line therapy includes discontinuing potentially toxic topical medications, tear replacement products and oral supplementation with omega-3 fatty acids. The next step of treatment is immunomodulatory therapy including:

lifitegrast, cyclosporine and steroids at different frequency and concentrations, and also autologous serum eye drops at concentrations from 20–100%. Autologous serum eye drops are characterized by multiple benefits: biochemical characteristics, including pH, nutrient content, vitamins, fibronectin, growth factors such as epithelial growth factor (EGF) or nerve growth factor (NGF), are similar to that of human tears, the serum eye drops also inhibit the release of inflammatory cytokines and increase the number of goblet cells and mucin expression in the conjunctiva. Prolonged use of serum eye drops is proved to restore homeostasis of the ocular surface.

In the last few years, there have been an increasing interest in the implementation of the Nerve Growth Factor (NGF) in the sub-basal nerve plexus regeneration, leading to the complete healing of the neurotrophic ulcers. NGF is an endogenous protein involved in the differentiation and maintenance of all systemic neurons, while in corneal tissue it is established to play a role in corneal innervation, tear secretion mechanism, and corneal epithelial cell growth and stability. Cenegermin is a recombinant human Nerve Growth Factor (rhNGF) that is structurally identical to the human NGF protein made in ocular tissues, it was introduced in the ophthalmic solution at concentration of 0.002% (20 mcg/mL). Two controlled clinical trails in Europe (REPARO) and USA (NGF0214) provided strong evidence on its effectiveness. 72% and 65% of patients with neurotrophic keratitis receiving cenegermin were completely healed in Europe and USA trails respectively [41–44]. Matrix regenerating agent (ReGenerating Agent; RGTA), mimicking natural heparan sulfate within the corneal tissue, is also a recent topical agent showing promising results in the treatment. RGTA eye drops (Cacicol; Thea) are preservative-free, well-tolerated, proved to promote regeneration of damaged tissues and to enhance corneal tissue healing [45, 46].

Novel emerging treatment approaches also include thymosine β4, CODA001, topical insulin, Substance P and insulin-like growth factor 1 (IGF-1). Thymosine β4 and CODA001 are in the most advanced evaluation undergoing clinical trials. Thymosin beta 4 is a 43-amino acid peptide, a major constituent protein of macrophages, and platelets. Currently, third-phase, multi-center, randomized, double masked, placebo controlled clinical study is ongoing regarding its role in ocular surface healing. Insulin at 3 different concentrations. CODA001 is an antisense oligonucleotide (antisense deoxynucleotide oligomer) that modulates and downregulates the expression of the gap junction protein Cx43 (Connexin-43), which is increased in persistent epithelial defects [47].

Other procedures implemented at different severity levels of neurotrophic keratitis include: therapeutic contact lenses, lacrimal punctual occlusion, amniotic membrane contact lens or transplantation, partial or complete tarsorraphy, corneal transplant, conjunctival flap transplant or direct neurotization.

Amniotic membrane transplantation (AMT) is proved to provide many benefits in the treatment of neurotrophic keratitis. AMT inhibits the activity of inflammatory cells, extends the life of corneal epithelial stem cells and maintains their ability to regenerate epithelial cells, promotes healing of the corneal wounds, blocks the TGF-ß cytokine system activation and the transformation of fibroblasts into myofibroblasts, also creates a protective membrane covering the affected ocular surface tissues. In dry eye disease, it is used in case of serious complications, such as corneal ulcer or microperforation. An interesting solution to consider is a sutureless, adhesiveless amniotic membrane transplant (AMT; ProKera; Bio-Tissue, Inc.) implantation. It is a corneal–epithelial device that consists of a polycarbonate ring conformer containing cryopreserved amniotic membrane. Advantages of this design include: shorter surgical time and prevention of suture-related complications [48].

To summarize neurotrophic keratitis treatment: a stepwise approach should be implemented with careful exclusion of the active infection. Topical treatments should be the first line therapy over the surgical interventions.

5.4 Surgical interventions

Surgical interventions in active HSV keratitis are limited to the severe stromal involvement with the increased risk of corneal perforation. Those may include: application of cyanoacrylate glue, amniotic membrane transplantation or therapeutic keratoplasty.

Other indications for surgical procedures include inactive corneal scarring after keratitis or cataract formation mainly due to prolonged treatment with topical steroids. Superficial opacifications could be considered as an indication for phototherapeutic keratectomy (PTK), although the corneal thinning is usual after HSV keratitis and therefore it limits the use of this method. The PTK ablation should always be limited to anterior one-third of stromal layers and leave a minimum residual stromal bed thickness (RSBT) of 250 μm to avoid further corneal ectasia. Also, spontaneous reactivation of HSV keratitis is well known after PTK, because laser ablation stimulates viral shedding in tears and reactivates the virus [49, 50].

When an extensive scar with corneal thinning is present a deep anterior lamellar keratoplasty (DALK) or penetrating keratoplasty (PK) should be considered. DALK eliminates the risk of endothelial immunologic rejection, but due to advanced corneal scarring and thinning may be difficult to perform. An obligatory preoperative assessment before keratoplasty procedures include the corneal sensitivity analysis and the exclusion of the active viral infection with neovascularization. It is well established, that the presence of deep stromal vascularization exceeding 2 or more quadrants, creates a significant risk for a graft immunologic rejection and graft failure. Another factor, strongly connected to the increased risk of the graft failure is a herpetic infection recurrence. To address those issues, the combination of the antiviral prophylaxis with the prophylaxis of a immunologic rejection should be implemented. Antiviral prophylaxis includes the use of high-dose oral acyclovir as recommended by American Academy of Ophthalmology (AAO guidelines recommended 800 mg 3 times daily for at least 1 year) [37]. The prophylaxis of a immunologic rejection includes usually systemic steroids combined with topical therapy. Despite the prophylaxis, there is a relatively high rate of graft failure performed in eyes after herpetic keratitis reported in the literature: 26% at 3 years, 15% at 5 years and 53.7% at 8 years [51–53]. In the last years, there have been an increasing interest in keratorosthesis surgery, as a viable option allowing a long term restoration of vision in patients with high risk for corneal transplantation. Boston type I keratoprosthesis (BKPro) is the most commonly implanted keratoprosthesis worldwide. BKPro was first used in 1965 by Professor Claes H. Dohlman [54, 55]. The BKPro surgery is usually complex with the high incidence of intraocular complications. Also the rate of postoperative complications is high and includes: glaucoma, retroprosthetic membrane formation, keratolysis, endophthalmitis, vitreoretinal complications, such as retinal detachment, cystoid macular edema, uveitis and hypotony/phthisis. In the latest study of the long term BKPro outcomes published in 2020, the probability of maintaining or improving vision was 75,0% at 5 years and 66,7% at 10 years [56].

In summary, surgical intervention in HSV keratits is challenging and high-risk procedure, therefore a special attention should be brought when referring such patients.

6. Conclusions

HSV keratitis due to its multiform occurrence remains a challenging diagnostic in clinical practice. Modern imaging technique, such as optical coherence tomography or confocal microscopy as well as modern laboratory testing including multiplex dot hybridization (MDH) assay, immunochromatographic assay (ICGA, AmpliVue) are useful in guiding the diagnostic process.

Ocular surface homeostasis should be always considered when treating HSV keratitis, especially in the neurotrophic keratitis at different severity grades.

Conflict of interest

The author has no conflict of interest.

Author details

Anna Nowińska[1,2]

1 Chair and Clinical Department of Ophthalmology, Faculty of Medical Sciences in Zabrze, Medical University of Silesia in Katowice, Poland

2 Ophthalmology Department, Railway Hospital in Katowice, Poland

*Address all correspondence to: anna.nowinska@sum.edu.pl

References

[1] Davison AJ. Herpesvirus systematics. Vet Microbiol. 2010;143:52-69.

[2] Farooq AV, Shukla D. Herpes simplex epithelial and stromal keratitis: an epidemiologic update. Surv Ophthalmol. 2012;57:448-462

[3] Liesegang TJ. Herpes simplex virus epidemiology and ocular importance. Cornea. 2001; 20: 1-13.

[4] Liesegang TJ. Epidemiology of ocular herpes simplex: natural history in Rochester Minn, 1950 through 1982. Arch Ophthalmol. 1989; 107: 1160-1165.

[5] Chemaitelly H, Nagelkerke N, Omori R, and Abu-Raddad LJ. 2019. Characterizing herpes simplex virus type 1 and type 2 seroprevalence declines and epidemiological association in the United States. PloS one 14: e0214151.

[6] Taylor TJ, Brockman MA, McNamee EE, Knipe DM. Herpes simplex virus. Front Biosci. 2002;7:d752–d764.

[7] Labetoulle M, Maillet S, Efstathiou S, Dezelee S, Frau E, Lafay F. HSV1 latency sites after inoculation in the lip: assessment of their localization and connections to the eye. Investigative ophthalmology & visual science. 2003;44(1):217-225.

[8] Conrady CD, Jones H, Zheng M, Carr DJ. A Functional Type I Interferon Pathway Drives Resistance to Cornea Herpes Simplex Virus Type 1 Infection by Recruitment of Leukocytes. J Biomed Res. 2011;25(2):111-119.

[9] Zheng C. Evasion of Cytosolic DNA-Stimulated Innate Immune Responses by Herpes Simplex Virus 1. J Virol. 2018;92(6):e00099–e00017.

[10] Shahnazaryan D, Khalil R, Wynne C, Jefferies CA, Ní Gabhann-Dromgoole J, Murphy CC. Herpes simplex virus 1 targets IRF7 via ICP0 to limit type I IFN induction. Sci Rep. 2020;10(1):22216.

[11] Holland EJ, Schwartz GS. Classification of herpes simplex virus keratitis. Cornea. 1999 Mar;18(2):144-154.

[12] Chodosh J, Ung L. Adoption of Innovation in Herpes Simplex Virus Keratitis. Cornea. 2020 Nov;39 Suppl 1(1):S7-S18.

[13] Erie JC, McLaren JW, Patel SV. Confocal microscopy in ophthalmology. Am J Ophthalmol 2009;148:639-646.

[14] Rosenberg ME, Tervo TM, Müller LJ, Moilanen JA, Vesaluoma MH. In vivo confocal microscopy after herpes keratitis. Cornea. 2002 Apr;21(3):265-269.

[15] Martone G, Alegente M, Balestrazzi A, Nuti E, Traversi C, Pichierri P, Tosi GM. In vivo confocal microscopy in bilateral herpetic keratitis: a case report. Eur J Ophthalmol. 2008 Nov-Dec;18(6):994-997

[16] Mocan MC, Irkec M, Mikropoulos DG, Bozkurt B, Orhan M, Konstas AG. In vivo confocal microscopic evaluation of the inflammatory response in non-epithelial herpes simplex keratitis. Curr Eye Res. 2012 Dec;37(12):1099-1106.

[17] Izatt JA, Hee MR, Swanson EA, Lin CP, Huang D, Schuman JS, Puliafito CA, Fujimoto JG. Micrometer-scale resolution imaging of the anterior eye in vivo with optical coherence tomography. Arch Ophthalmol. 1994;112:1584-1589.

[18] Hoerauf H, Gordes RS, Scholz C, Wirbelauer C, Koch P, Engelhardt R,

Winkler J, Laqua H, Birngruber R. First experimental and clinical results with transscleral optical coherence tomography. Ophthalmic Surg Lasers. 2000;31(3):218-222.

[19] Wylegała E, Teper S, Nowińska AK, Milka M, Dobrowolski D. Anterior segment imaging: Fourier-domain optical coherence tomography versus time-domain optical coherence tomography. J Cataract Refract Surg. 2009;35(8):1410-1414.

[20] Rodriguez-Garcia A, Alfaro-Rangel R, Bustamante-Arias A, Hernandez-Camarena JC. In Vivo Corneal Microstructural Changes in Herpetic Stromal Keratitis: A Spectral Domain Optical Coherence Tomography Analysis. J Ophthalmic Vis Res. 2020 Aug 6;15(3):279-288.

[21] Soliman W, Nassr MA, Abdelazeem K, Al-Hussaini AK. Appearance of herpes simplex keratitis on anterior segment optical coherence tomography. Int Ophthalmol. 2019 Dec;39(12):2923-2928.

[22] Lu L, Palioura S. Management of Stromal Herpes Simplex Virus Keratitis With Epithelial Ulceration Using Optical Coherence Tomography-Generated Corneal Thickness Maps. Cornea. 2020 Dec;39(12):1566-1570

[23] Subhan S, Jose RJ, Duggirala A, Hari R, Krishna P, Reddy S, et al. Diagnosis of herpes simplex virus-1 keratitis: Comparison of Giemsa stain, immunofluorescence assay and polymerase chain reaction. Curr Eye Res. 2004;29:209-213.

[24] Guda SJM, Sontam B, Bagga B, Ranjith K, Sharma S, Joseph J. Evaluation of multiplex real-time polymerase chain reaction for the detection of herpes simplex virus-1 and 2 and varicella-zoster virus in corneal cells from normal subjects and patients with keratitis in India. Indian J Ophthalmol. 2019 Jul;67(7):1040-1046.

[25] Satpathy G, Behera HS, Sharma A, Mishra AK, Mishra D, Sharma N, Tandon R, Agarwal T, Titiyal JS. A 20-year experience of ocular herpes virus detection using immunofluorescence and polymerase chain reaction. Clin Exp Optom. 2018 Sep;101(5):648-651.

[26] Nakano S, Sugita S, Tomaru Y, Hono A, Nakamuro T, Kubota T, Takase H, Mochizuki M, Takahashi M, Shimizu N. Establishment of Multiplex Solid-Phase Strip PCR Test for Detection of 24 Ocular Infectious Disease Pathogens. Invest Ophthalmol Vis Sci. 2017 Mar 1;58(3):1553-1559.

[27] Akbarian A, Shahhosseiny MH, Vafaei S, et al. Designing novel and simple competitive internal amplification control for reliable PCR diagnosis of herpes simplex virus. Jundishapur J Microbiol. 2015;8(2):e16260.

[28] Poon SHL, Wong WHL, Lo ACY, Yuan H, Chen CF, Jhanji V, Chan YK, Shih KC. A systematic review on advances in diagnostics for herpes simplex keratitis. Surv Ophthalmol. 2020 Nov 10:S0039-6257(20)30138-7.

[29] Dawson CR, Jones DB, Kaufman HE, et al. Design and organization of the herpetic eye disease study (HEDS). Curr Eye Res. 1991;10(suppl): 105-110. 101.

[30] Wilhelmus KR, Gee L, Hauck WW, et al. Herpetic Eye Disease Study. A controlled trial of topical corticosteroids for herpes simplex stromal keratitis. Ophthalmology. 1994;101:1883-1895; discussion 1895-1886.

[31] Barron BA, Gee L, Hauck WW, et al. Herpetic Eye Disease Study. A controlled trial of oral acyclovir

for herpes simplex stromal keratitis. Ophthalmology. 1994;101:1871-1882.

[32] Herpetic Eye Disease Study Group. A controlled trial of oral acyclovir for iridocyclitis caused by herpes simplex virus. Arch Ophthalmol. 1996;114:1065-1072. .

[33] Herpetic Eye Disease Study Group. A controlled trial of oral acyclovir for the prevention of stromal keratitis or iritis in patients with herpes simplex virus epithelial keratitis. Arch Ophthalmol. 1997;115:703-712.

[34] Wilhelmus KR, Beck RW, Moke PS, et al. Acyclovir for the prevention of recurrent herpes simplex virus eye disease. Herpetic Eye Disease Study Group. N Engl J Med. 1998;339:300-306.

[35] Herpetic Eye Disease Study Group. Predictors of recurrent herpes simplex virus keratitis. Cornea. 2001;20:123-128.

[36] Guess S, Stone DU, Chodosh Evidence-based treatment of herpes simplex virus keratitis: a systematic review. J.Ocul Surf. 2007 Jul;5(3):240-250

[37] White ML, Chodosh J. Herpes Simplex Virus Keratitis: A Treatment Guideline. Hoskins Center for Quality Eye Care and American Academy of Ophthalmology Website; 2014. Available at: https:// www.aao.org/clinical-statement/herpes-simplex-virus-keratitistreatment-guideline.

[38] Schuster AK, Harder BC, Schlichtenbrede FC, Jarczok MN, Tesarz J. Valacyclovir versus acyclovir for the treatment of herpes zoster ophthalmicus in immunocompetent patients. Cochrane Database Syst Rev. 2016 Nov 14;11(11):CD011503.

[39] Wilhelmus KR. Antiviral treatment and other therapeutic interventions for herpes simplex virus epithelial keratitis. Cochrane Database Syst Rev. 2015;1:CD002898.

[40] Carr DJJ, Gmyrek GB, Filiberti A, et al. Distinguishing Features of High- and Low-Dose Vaccine against Ocular HSV-1 Infection Correlates with Recognition of Specific HSV-1-Encoded Proteins. Immunohorizons. 2020;4(10):608-626.

[41] Sacchetti M, Lambiase A. Diagnosis and management of neurotrophic keratitis. Clin Ophthalmol. 2014;8:571-579.

[42] Bonini S, Lambiase A, Rama P, et al. Phase II randomized, double-masked, vehicle-controlled trial of recombinant human nerve growth factor for neurotrophic keratitis. Ophthalmology. 2018;125(9):1332-1343.

[43] Mastropasqua L, Massaro-Giordano G, Nubile M, et al. Understanding the pathogenesis of neurotrophic keratitis: the role of corneal nerves. J Cell Physiol. 2017;232:717-724.

[44] Ahuja AS, Bowden FW 3rd, Robben JL. A Novel Treatment for Neurotrophic Corneal Ulcer Using Topical Cenegermin (OXERVATE™) Containing Recombinant Human Nerve Growth Factor. Cureus. 2020;12(11):e11724. Published 2020 Nov 27. doi:10.7759/cureus.11724

[45] Aifa A, Gueudry J, Portmann A, Delcampe A, Muraine M. Topical treatment with a new matrix therapy agent (RGTA) for the treatment of corneal neurotrophic ulcers. Invest Ophthalmol Vis Sci. 2012 Dec 13;53(13):8181-8185.

[46] Pereira S, Resende R, Coelho P, Sampaio F. Matrix Regenerating Agent (RGTA) in a Neurotrophic Corneal Ulcer. Cureus. 2020 Oct 26;12(10):e11167.

[47] Bremond-Gignac D, Daruich A, Robert MP, Chiambaretta F. Recent innovations with drugs in clinical trials for neurotrophic keratitis and refractory corneal ulcers. Expert Opin Investig Drugs. 2019 Nov;28(11):1013-1020.

[48] Pachigolla G, Prasher P, Di Pascuale MA, McCulley JP, McHenry JG, Mootha VV. Evaluation of the role of ProKera in the management of ocular surface and orbital disorders. Eye Contact Lens. 2009 Jul;35(4):172-175.

[49] Fagerholm P. Phototherapeutic keratectomy: 12 years of experience. Acta Ophthalmol Scand. 2003 Feb;81(1):19-32.

[50] Nagpal R, Maharana PK, Roop P, Murthy SI, Rapuano CJ, Titiyal JS, Vajpayee RB, Sharma N. Phototherapeutic keratectomy. Surv Ophthalmol. 2020 Jan-Feb;65(1):79-108.

[51] Garcia DD, Farjo Q, Musch DC, Sugar A. Effect of prophylactic oral acyclovir after penetrating keratoplasty for herpes simplex keratitis. Cornea. 2007;26(8):930-934.

[52] Halberstadt M, Machens M, Gahlenbek KA, Böhnke M, Garweg JG. The outcome of corneal grafting in patients with stromal keratitis of herpetic and non-herpetic origin. Br J Ophthalmol. 2002 Jun;86(6):646-652.

[53] Wu SQ, Zhou P, Zhang B, Qiu WY, Yao YF. Long-term comparison of full-bed deep lamellar keratoplasty with penetrating keratoplasty in treating corneal leucoma caused by herpes simplex keratitis. Am J Ophthalmol. 2012 Feb;153(2):291-299.e2.

[54] Dohlman CH, Webster RG, Biswas SK, et al. Collar-button prosthesis glued to a corneal graft. In: Polack, FM, ed. Cornea and External Diseases of the Eye. First InterAmerican Symposium. Springfield, IL: Charles C. Thomas, 1970:189-192.

[55] Dohlman CH, Schneider H, Doane, MG. Prosthokeratoplasty. Am J Ophthalmol. 1974;77(5):694-700.

[56] Kanu LN, Niparugs M, Nonpassopon M, et al. Predictive factors of Boston Type I Keratoprosthesis outcomes: A long-term analysis. Ocul Surf. 2020;18(4):613-619.

Chapter 3

Fungal Keratitis: Recent Advances in Diagnosis and Treatment

Suwarna Suman, Arushi Kumar, Indu Saxena and Manoj Kumar

Abstract

Fungal keratitis or fungal corneal ulcer is potentially blinding infection of cornea, is considered one of the major cause of ocular morbidity, particularly in developing countries. It is a common cause of infectious keratitis, especially in tropical and subtropical countries. Fungal keratitis is notoriously challenging to diagnosis and difficult to treat. Delay in diagnosis may result in irreversible sequelae of corneal fungal infections, which can be preventable. Fungal keratitis often have worse treatment outcomes than bacterial keratitis, Delayed diagnosis and scarcity of effective antifungal agents are the major factors for poor outcome. In the recent years considerable advancement in the diagnosis and treatment has been occurred. In this chapter, we will discuss the recent advances in diagnosis and management of fungal keratitis with a brief discussion on pathogenesis and future therapeutic models.

Keywords: infectious keratitis, fungal keratitis, confocal microscopy, polymerase chain reaction, metagenomics deep sequencing, voriconazole, posaconazole

1. Introduction

Infectious keratitis is an inflammation of the cornea caused by microorganism. It is most commonly associated with bacterial, fungal or viral microorganisms that invade into the corneal stroma, resulting in inflammation and destruction of these structures; ultimately leading to visual impairment and blindness. Fungal keratitis (FK) or keratomycosis is one of the most challenging to diagnose and difficult to treat. The prevalence of fungal keratitis is variable depending upon the geographic location. It is more common in tropical and subtropical areas and relatively rare in temperate countries. It is reported about 1–60% of all cases of microbial keratitis in various studies [1–3]. A recent review including 37 countries reported highest proportion in Vietnam (59.58%) followed by Paraguay (58%) [2–4]. The fungi that commonly cause infection of the cornea include Fusarium, Aspergillus, Curvularia, Bipolaris, and Candida [1, 2, 5].

Most of the currently available antifungal medications have limitations, such as poor bioavailability and limited ocular penetration, especially in cases with deep keratitis [6–8]. This results in slow resolution of fungal infections. In addition, fungi can penetrate deeper into corneal stroma and Descemet membrane, therefore more difficult to eradicate. Surgical excision of the infected cornea is required to control the infection in nonresponsive cases [9–12]. In recent years, considerable research is being continue in the field of management of fungal keratitis and several newer antifungal agents and drug delivery techniques are being evolved to overcome these limitations and improve outcome. In this chapter, we discuss the recent advances in diagnosis and treatment of fungal keratitis with a brief discussion on pathogenesis and future considerations.

2. New aspects of pathogenesis

Pathogenesis of FK has not been fully elucidated. Recent studies and advances have contributed in better understanding of the complicated process and host immune response.

2.1 Risk factors

The common risk factors for fungal keratitis are trauma with vegetative matter or objects contaminated with soil, contact lenses, ocular surface disease, lacrimal duct occlusion, fungal skin infections, long-term use of antibiotics or steroids locally or systemically [2, 13–17]. Other relatively rare risk factors include history of eye surgery, herpes simplex virus keratitis, eyelid abnormalities, etc. [18, 19].

Still in developing countries, the most common risk factor for fungal keratitis is ocular trauma but in developed countries, contact lens emerged as more common risk factor. This change has been occurred due to industrialization of farming and increase use of contact lens in developed world. In a large case series of 695 cases with fungal keratitis reported from 10 tertiary eye care centres across the United States over a 7-year period, 283 (40.71%) cases involved the use of contact lens [1]. Similarly Keay et al. in a multicentre case series of 733 cases from 11 tertiary care centres across the United States reported that 37% cases were associated with refractive contact lens wear, 25% were associated with ocular trauma, and 29% were associated with ocular surface disease [20].

In a study, the storage of the anti-microbial agent alexidine in its plastic containers at higher than room temperatures was found as the reason for decreased effectiveness [21]. This temperature difference in the plastic containers led to decreased concentration of the agent in solution (2.8 times less) and a corresponding higher concentration in the walls of its plastic containers (3.1 times higher) [22]. The lens type and its soaking time significantly influences the fungicidal activity of cleaning and storage solutions and poor compliance significantly increase the risk of contamination [23, 24].

2.2 Causative fungi

A review article found about 144 species of fungi from 92 genera as causative agents in keratitis, showing largest diversity; whereas 77 species from 42 genera of bacteria, 12 species from 4 genera of protozoa and only 4 types of viruses were implicated in infectious keratitis. However, in the majority of cases of FK the causative organism belong to a few genera: Fusarium, Aspergillus, and Candida [25]. Other fungi implicated in mycotic keratitis are Curvularia, Alternaria, and Penicillium [2, 13, 14]. The rarely reported fungal pathogens include Lasiodiplodia theobromae, Cylindrocarpon species, Metarhizium anisopliae, Paecilomyces species, and Pythium insidiosum [15, 26–29].

2.3 Host immune response

Fungal infections initiates with adhesion of fungal cells with epithelial surfaces. Fungi produce various surface proteins to contribute to the adhesion to the corneal epithelium, which has potential fungal binding sites such as laminins, fibronectins, and collagens [30, 31]. Alterations of the corneal surface due to trauma or other predisposing condition result in easy invasion of organisms deeper into underlying layers, which leads to an innate and adaptive immune-mediated inflammation, resulting in subsequent tissue necrosis of the surrounding area, consequently leads to further tissue damage, scarring, and opacification of the cornea.

2.3.1 Cytokines and innate immunity

The contact between fungi and host, result in expression of pattern recognition receptors (PRRs) on host epithelial and immune cells, which recognize the fungi. PPRs are Toll-like receptors (TLRs, including TLR2 and TLR4), C-type Lectin receptors (CLRs, including Dectin-1, Dectin-2 and Mincle). Dectin-1 recognizes β-glucan in fungal cell wall, while Dectin-2 and Mincle recognize mannan of cell wall [32]. *Candida albicans* and Aspergillus fumigatus encounter during fungal keratitis have been reported to be sensed by TLR [33–35]. Activated TLRs in corneal epithelium induce production of CXC chemokines and recruit neutrophils (are more than 90% of the infiltrating cells). Neutrophils are predominant source of mature interleukin-1β (IL-1β) and acidic mammalian chitinase (AMCase) in corneas, which can inhibit the hyphal growth [36, 37]. The increased expression and the activation of PPRs in response to *A. fumigatus* with resultant increased secretion of inflammatory cytokines (IL-1β, IL-6, IL-8, IL-17 and IL-23) in human corneal epithelial cells and neutrophils is reported [38]. Increased production of reactive oxygen species (ROS) in response to increased levels of IL-1β, TLR4, Dectin-1 and LOX-1, facilitates the fungal killing [39, 40].

Leal et al. found that neutrophils produced NADPH oxidase to control the growth of fungi. The antifungal activity of neutrophils depended on CD18, and inhibiting thioredoxin, an antioxidant increased the sensitivity of fungal hyphae to neutrophil-mediated killing in vitro [41]. The expression of PPRs, promote the production of pro-inflammatory cytokines, as well as the recruitment of neutrophils that can also cause serious inflammatory damages to cornea leading to opacification [32, 40, 42]. In fungal keratitis, the levels of pro-inflammatory IL-1β, IL-6, IL-8, IL-17, IL-23 and IFN-γ in aqueous humor were significantly higher in comparison to the non-keratitis control group [38]. A study among a Han Chinese population of patients with FK compared controls found a particular TLR4 allele that was associated with an increased risk of developing FK [43].

Fungi can produce enzymes that degrade physical barriers and facilitate tissue invasion. The mycotoxins produced from Fusarium species can inhibit immunity, break down tissues, and promote the fungal survival in host. Corneal epithelial cells can be destroyed by some cytosolic proteins and peptide toxins produced by fungi [44]. The protease and phospholipase activities detected in *A. flavus and F. solani* isolated from human eyes and their role in causation of ulceration in fungal keratitis, are reported in several studies [45, 46].

2.3.2 Autophagy

Autophagy is a lysosome-mediated degradation process, which regulates intracellular homeostasis of eukaryotes by mediating the degradation of proteins and organelles [47]. It can be activated in response to starvation, stress, hypoxia, tumor, and infection [48]. Autophagy is proved to be involved in immune responses, a previous study found that autophagy maintains the cellular and immune homeostasis during the *Candida albicans* infection [49]. Autophagy can regulate IL-1β release in human primary macrophage to resist the fungal infection [50].

A study by Li C et al. reported that the progression of FK caused by *A. fumigatus* result in increased expression of autophagy and the severity of *A. fumigatus* keratitis, aggravated with inhibition of autophagy. The induction of autophagy reduced the severity of keratitis via regulating the recruitment of PMNs, balancing the pro-inflammatory and anti-inflammatiory cytokines release, and possibly affecting the differentiation of neutrophils. Autophagy may become a novel target for the treatment of FK in future. Further studies may add our understanding regarding the protective role of autophagy in FK [51].

2.4 Fungal biofilm

Biofilm formation is one of the primary mechanisms through which fungi evade the immune response and establish infection. Clinical isolates of Fusarium, Candida and Aspergillus have been shown to form biofilms. A study reported that *F. solani* formed a biofilm in vitro by 24 h while other species (*Cladosporium sphaerospermum and Acremonium implicatum*) formed at 48 h. A time-dependent decrease in efficacy for all six antifungal agents (amphotericin B, voriconazole, itraconazole, fluconazole, terbinafine, and natamycin) is reported with increase in minimum inhibitory concentration (MIC) of all six antifungal agents tested with the development of biofilm [52]. This suggests that an ability to disrupt the biofilm may prove useful in increasing antifungal efficacy.

3. Recent advances in diagnosis

3.1 Clinical diagnosis

Fungal keratitis can be diagnosed based on characteristic clinical features. Patients with keratitis usually present with sudden onset of pain, photophobia, watering and discharge and reduced vision. In fungal keratitis, symptoms are much milder than the signs [53].

A fungal keratitis classically presents as a dry, raised lesion with crenate or feathery borders, presence of satellite lesions and a hypopyon. An immune ring of Wesseley may be visible due to deposition of immune complexes and inflammatory cells around the ulcer (**Figures 1–5**). However, a study reported that Clinicians could correctly distinguished the microbial kingdom for 54 (73%) of 74 culture-positive infections, including 41 (79%) of 52 bacterial keratitis, 5 (38%) of 13 fungal

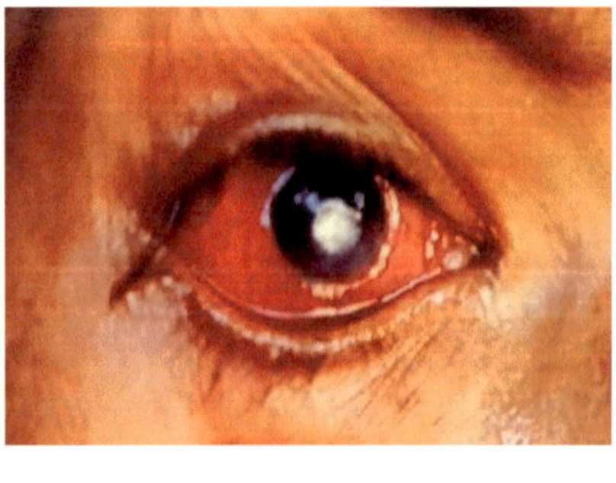

Figure 1.
Plaque-like ulcer with slightly defined margins, marked conjunctival injection and chemosis; fungal isolate-candida albicans.

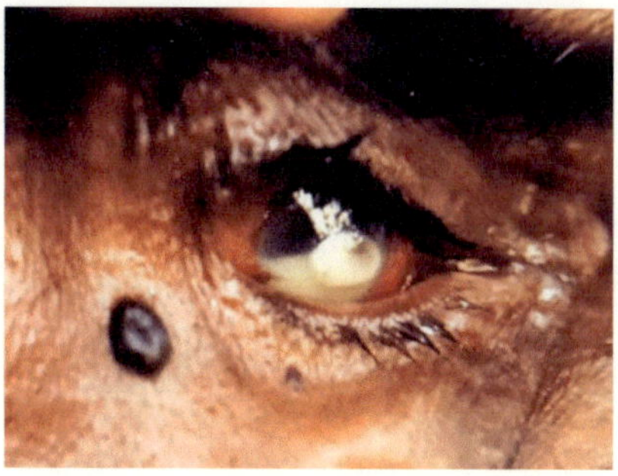

Figure 2.
A dry looking lesion with greyish white raised exudate appearing as plaque with hypopyon in a 56-year-old male with fugal keratitis from Aspergillus.

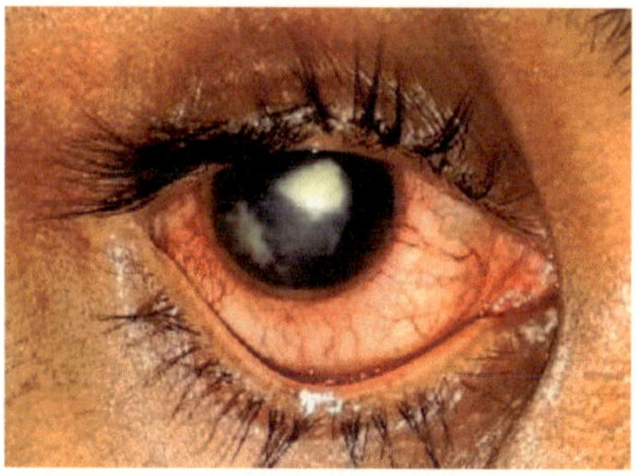

Figure 3.
A greyish white infiltrate with feathery borders and a satellite lesion in a case fungal keratitis caused by Fusarium.

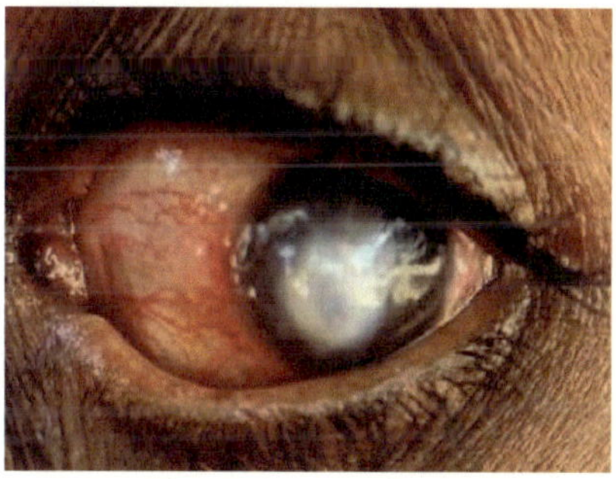

Figure 4.
Severe fungal keratitis with feathery edges in case Fusarium Keratitis.

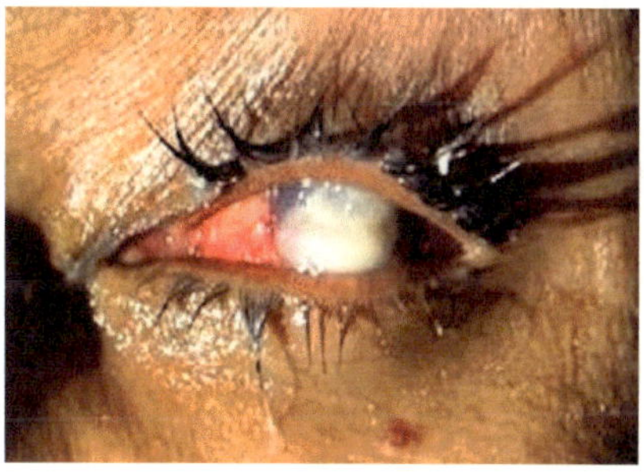

Figure 5.
Corneal thinning and necrosis in severe fungal keratitis caused by Fusarium in a 48-year-old male with history of topical steroid instillation.

keratitis, and 8 (89%) of 9 amoebic keratitis correctly [54]. In a photographic survey, clinician were able to distinguish between bacterial and fungal aetiologies 66% of the time. In 39 cases of fungal keratitis, the clinicians predicted genus in 27% of cases and species in 7.9% of cases [55].

3.1.1 Confocal microscopy

In vivo confocal microscopy (IVCM) of the cornea has been emerged as clinically useful non-invasive technique for early diagnosis of FK. It produces images from the cornea with a resolution of one micrometer (μm), which is enough for imaging of microorganisms larger than one μm, such as Acanthamoeba cysts and fungal hyphae [56]. This provides rapid and reliable diagnosis however, a clinical consensus in the interpretation of IVCM images is still lacking.

IVCM can directly visualize filamentous fungi within the whole cornea of patients. Confocal microscopy in vivo uses serial images to create optical sections through the full-thickness of the living cornea. It allows rapid identification of fungi and can be used to differentiate between fungal species.

Brasnu et al. diagnosed all the cases of suspected fungal keratitis (five out of five) caused by different fungal species using IVCM with sensitivity equal to the direct microscopy and culture [56]. They analyzed IVCM images of keratitis obtained using the Heidelberg Retina Tomograph (HRT) II confocal microscope (Heidelberg Engineering, Heidelberg, Germany) in five patients (four patients with *Fusarium soloni* and one patient with *Candida albicans* infection), and three donor corneas with Aspergillus fumigatus, *F. solani*, and *C albicans* infection. *F. soloni* hyphae seen as high contrast lines 3–5 microns (μm) in diameter, 200–300 μm in length, with a branching angle of 90° in IVCM images from patients as well as from the infected donor cornea. *A. fumigatus* hyphae seen as numerous high-contrast lines 200–300 μm in length and 3–5 μm in width, with the branching angle 45° in the infected donor cornea. *C albicans*-infected patient's cornea revealed numerous high-contrast elongated particles measuring 10–40 μm in length and 5–10 μm in width. *C albicans*-contaminated donor cornea revealed numerous characteristic high-contrast elongated particles measuring 10–40 μm in length and 5–10 in μm in width, consistent with Candida pseudofilaments [56].

The hyper-reflective elements seen on IVCM must be differentiated from the basal corneal epithelial nerves, which have a more regular branching pattern. Stromal nerves, on the other hand, are much larger in diameter (25–50 μm). There are now several studies reported the use of IVCM in diagnosis and monitoring of treatment of fungal keratitis with reported sensitivity of 80–94% [57–60].

IVCM is a noninvasive in vivo technique useful for early identification of fungal elements, monitoring and guidance of treatment, and determination of the depth of infection. The limitation of IVCM are that technique is extremely user-dependent, need a skilled operator and experienced viewer. The dense corneal infiltrates or scarring could preclude proper tissue penetration and visualization.

3.2 Laboratory diagnosis

Conventional methods for the diagnosis of fungal keratitis include staining of tissue scrapings with Gram-stain, 10% potassium hydroxide (KOH) wet mount, lactophenol cotton blue, Giemsa, or calcofluor white. Reported sensitivity of Gram staining is in the range of 36–50% [61]. KOH is a rapid and an inexpensive and one of the most commonly performed procedures for detection of fungi with a sensitivity of 61–94% and specificity of 91–97% for detecting fungus (**Figure 6**).

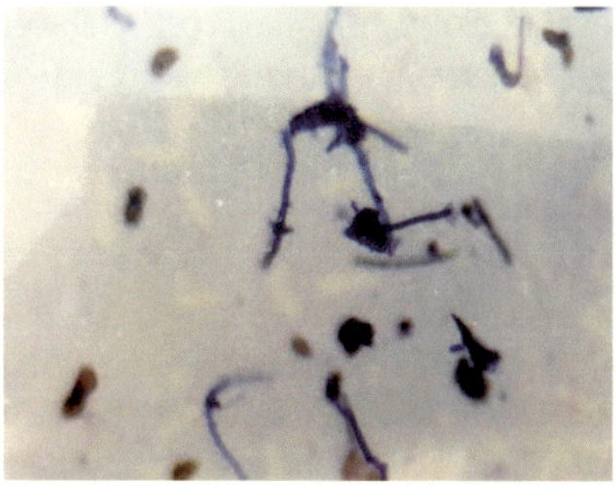

Figure 6.
Fungal hyphae in KOH wet mount counterstained with methylene blue.

Lactophenol cotton blue mounts had reported sensitivity of 85% and specificity of 90–91% [62]. Sabouraud dextrose agar medium is considered as a culture medium of choice for isolating fungi however it cause delay in diagnosis. Initial growth occurs within 72 hours in 83% of cultures and within 1 week in 97% of cultures [63]. Sometimes it may be necessary to wait for two weeks to confirm no growth in culture. Over the last decade, a number of newer methods have been devised for detection of fungi.

3.2.1 Polymerase chain reaction

Polymerase chain reaction (PCR) involves repeated cycles of denaturation, amplification, and replication, in which segments of deoxyribonucleic acid (DNA) are continuously multiplied. Specific DNA primers are employed to indicate the presence of the microorganism in question [64]. PCR has emerged as a sensitive and specific test for the diagnosis of fungal keratitis. Several techniques of PCR have been evolved and currently used for identification of fungi.

Traditional PCR by using single pair of primer to amplify the target genomic sequence is simple and efficient technique, but generation of nonspecific products can affect the results. In Nested PCR, two pairs of primers are used; one set of primer is an amplified sequence, and the other is complementary to the sequence amplified by the first one. It is more specific than traditional PCR; amplifies only the specific sequences looked for; but identify a set of fungal pathogens, not a single specific species.

In multiplex PCR Multiple primer, pairs are used. Advantage is Rapid amplification of multiple sequences, conserves template DNA, and minimizes expense; recognizes many pathogens at once. In real time PCR, one set of primers is used; amplified sequence is linked with a fluorescent probe, which emits light when bound to the amplified product. It is more specific, sensitive, and reproducible but not ideal for multiplexing [65–67].

PCR reported higher sensitivity in comparison to culture and stains for both bacteria and fungi [68, 69]. Zhao et al. reported significantly higher positive detection rate of PCR for fungal keratitis (84.5%) as compare to the positivity rate for culture (35.3%) and stain (64.7%) [69]. A higher sensitivity of PCR for infectious keratitis compared to culture (98% versus 47%), but a slightly lower specificity (83% versus 100%) is reported in this study [69].

The PCR is rapid test, it takes 4–8 h, and only a small clinical sample is needed for diagnosis [7]. The limitation of PCR is that it is expensive, not readily available and specificity is lower than culture. Extraction of artifacts and amplification of non-pathogenic DNA can lead to over diagnosis [66]. However, it can be used to detect fungal DNA in corneal scrape material, to start antifungal therapy at an early stage of the keratitis.

3.2.2 Metagenomic deep sequencing

Metagenomic deep sequencing (MDS) is a new technique for the diagnosis of FK; with next generation sequencing rapid and accurate diagnosis is possible. Next generation sequencing is high-throughput sequencing methods where billions of nucleic acid fragments can be sequenced simultaneously and independently. MDS is an unbiased approach that interrogates all genomes in a clinical sample and identify any organism whereas PCR is a targeted test the clinician must know the suspected causative organism.

It has been shown to enhance detection of common and unusual pathogens from the intraocular fluid of patients with infectious uveitis and other systemic infections [70–72]. A study by Seitzman et al. in a case series of nine patients of infectious keratitis diagnosed by conventional methods reported that MDS detected all the microorganisms identified by culture or PCR. MDS was able to identify parasitic, fungal, bacterial, and viral infections as a single assay. The pathogenic organisms ranged in size from smaller genomes (*herpes simplex virus-1* and *adenovirus*) to larger genomes (*Acanthamoeba* and *Aspergillus*). In one case, the MDS identified the organism not supposed to be a cause of infectious keratitis. The case was culture positive for Purpureocillium lilacinum was identified as the second most abundant organism and, the most abundant organism in the sample was Auricoccus indicus, which is not known to cause ocular infections and not even listed in the University of California San Francisco's mass spectrometry's database for identifiable organisms [73].

4. Recent advances in medical treatment

Polyenes (Amphotericin B and Natamycin) and azoles (fluconazole, itraconazole, ketoconazole, miconazole, voriconazole, and posaconazole) constitute two major classes of antifungal drugs used to treat ocular fungal infections including fungal keratitis. In Comparison to antibacterial agents, antifungals have a lower efficacy due to their mechanism of action (usually fungistatic, with dose dependent fungicidal action), lower tissue penetration, and the indolent nature of the fungal infection [74]. Still for the management of fungal keratitis, the traditional anti-fungal drugs like natamycin and fluconazole in topical and oral form are used most commonly. In recent years, other new drugs and drug delivery system to increase bioavailability of drugs have been evaluated. Anti-fungal agents are summarized in **Table 1**.

4.1 Natamycin

Natamycin is first antifungal agent approved for FK by Food and Drug Administration in the 1960s. After that, many antifungal agents have been evaluated, no single agent has emerged as the best and most cost effective agent [7]. Cochrane systematic review in 2008 and 2012, found no evidence that any single drug, or combination of drugs, is more effective in the management of fungal keratitis. The trials included in this review were of variable quality and were generally underpowered [75, 76].

Agent	Route of administration/ Dose	Indication	Limitations
Polyenes			
Amphotericin B	Topical 1.5-5 mg/ml *IS 5-10 μg *IC 5-10 μg/0.1 ml	First line therapy for Candida species. Good to moderate activity against filamentous fungi. Deep keratitis with partial response to topical therapy	Not commercially available. Side effects: cataract, transient iritis and corneal oedema
Natamycin	Topical 5% (50 mg/ ml) suspension	First choice for Fusarium, Good activity against Aspergillus, less effective against Candida species	Low corneal penetration
Azoles			
Imidazoles			
Econazole	Topical 2%	Effective against Fusarium, Aspergillus, and Candida species	Not commercially available for ophthalmic use
Miconazole	Topical 10 mg/ml *SC 1.2 to 10 mg	Effective against candida Adjuvant with topical therapy in patients with low compliance	Less effective than polyenes
Ketoconazole	Topical 1-2% Oral 200-400 mg/day	Broad spectrum As an adjuvant in deep keratitis	Less effective systemic toxicity (gastric intolerance, hepatotxicity)
Triazoles			
Fluconazole	Topical 0.2 % SC 2 mg/1 ml Oral 100-400 mg/ day oral	Effective against yeast, less effective against filamentous fungi Good intraocular penetration used as adjuvant with topical agents	Filamentous fungi exhibit resistance liver enzyme monitoring
Itraconazole	Topical 1% Oral 200-400 mg/day	Effective against Aspergillus, Candida, less effective against Fusarium As adjuvant with topical therapy in deep keratitis/ intraocular involvement by yeasts	Less effective than natamycin Lower bioavailability, and penetration into ocular tissues than other azoles
Voriconazole	Topical 1-2% IS 50 μg/0,1 m IC 50μg/0,1 m Oral 200 mg **BID	Broad spectrum, FK resistant to polyenes/ first-line triazoles. Deep keratitis and Intraocular involvement	Less effective than natamycin Side effects- blurred vision change in colour perception; liver enzyme monitoring during oral use
Posaconazole	Topical 100 mg/ml; 40 mg/ml Oral 200 mg **QID/ 400 mg BID	Broad spectrum, FK resistant to polyenes/first-line triazoles.	Limited information

Agent	Route of administration/ Dose	Indication	Limitations
Pyrimidines			
Flucytosine	Topical 10 mg/ml	Synergistic effect with topical Amphotericin B in FK due to yeasts	Narrow spectrum/ low penetration into ocular tissues
Echinocandins			
Capsofungin	Topical 0.5%	Yeasts resistant to polyenes and first-line triazoles	Limited information
Micafungin	Topical 0.1%	Yeasts resistant to polyenes and first-line triazoles	Limited information
Allyamine			
Terbinafine	Topical 0.5 % Oral 250 mg/day	Active against Aspergillus, Fusarium, Scedosporium and Candida.	Limited information

*IC: Intracameral, IS: Intrastromal, SC: Subconjunctival.
**BID: Twice a day, QID: for times a day.

Table 1.
Summary of antifungal agents used in Fungal Keratitis

Natamycin is a polyene antifungal drug, it binds preferentially to ergosterol on the fungal plasma membrane and causes localized membrane disruptions by altering membrane permeability. Natamycin is currently considered the most effective medication against Fusarium and Aspergillus [7]. Cochrane systematic review in 2015 found that there is evidence that natamycin is more effective than voriconazole in the treatment of fungal ulcers. However, the trials included in this review were of variable quality and were generally underpowered. Future research should evaluate treatment effects according to fungus species [77].

Several studies reported that fungal keratitis due to fusarium responded better to Natamycin as compare to itraconazole and voriconazole [77]. NTM is the treatment of choice for filamentous keratitis, especially that due to Fusarium species. However its poor penetration into corneal stroma, limits its use in deep stromal keratitis. In deep keratitis or with involvement of intraocular structures, natamycin should be associated with other antifungal agents using a different route of administration.

4.2 Amphotericin B

Amphotericin B is the first broad-spectrum antifungal agent, produced by the actinomycetes, *Streptomyces nodosus*. It acts by binding to ergosterol and by promoting oxidative action on cells, thus altering their metabolic functions. This binding also results in formation of pores or channels in the fungal cell membrane and increasing cell permeability. Its binding to cholesterol in human cells is responsible for its side effects. It is effective against *Aspergillus* and *Candida* species but less effective against *Fusarium* species [74]. It is administered as a topical solution in concentration of 1.5 to 5 mg/ml.

Amphotericin B has poor ocular penetration after intravenous administration and is toxic to human cells at a higher dose. Due to systemic (nephrotoxicity) and ocular toxicity (punctate epithelial erosions and greenish discoloration of the cornea), amphotericin B is not currently a first line agent in treating fungal keratitis.

In a study, Morand K, et al. compared the commercial 0.15% Amphotericin B with a liposomal formulation and found that the liposomal form was more stable and less toxic. The liposomal formulation also increased the potential amount of loaded drug by 3-fold compared with the conventional form [78].

4.3 Fluconazole

Fluconazole is a synthetic bistriazole available in oral, topical, and IV preparations. It has good intraocular penetration with low side effect. It shown to have excellent absorption from the gastrointestinal tract. Its plasma concentrations with oral use reach almost the same levels as with intravenous administration. Intraocular Penetration is effective, with aqueous concentrations similar to those in the plasma [74, 79]. Topical 0.2% fluconazole is effective against *Candida* keratitis with deep lesions. Oral fluconazole in a dose of 200 to 400 mg per day effective as an adjuvant with other topical antifungal agents.

4.4 Voriconazole

Voriconazole, a newer-generation triazole, with excellent ocular penetration and broad spectrum. Most of fungal isolates commonly implicated in keratitis were found to be susceptible to voriconazole.

Voriconazole has been reported to be effective in the treatment of fungal keratitis caused by different species and in cases not responding to other antifungal like natamycin and amphotericin [79–85]. Voriconazole has good intraocular penetration following oral administration. Advantage of oral administration is that it may provide steadier drug levels at the site of infection. Theil et al. compared aqueous samples after topical and oral voriconazole found that topical administration of voriconazole resulted in highly variable aqueous concentrations with troughs well below the minimum inhibitory concentration at which 90% of fungal isolates are inhibited (MIC90). Whereas, oral voriconazole provided relatively constant therapeutic concentration [84]. Many case reports reported successful treatment with topical voriconazole in conjunction oral or intravenous voriconazole [85, 86].

4.5 Posaconazole

Posaconazole is a new triazole, a synthetic structural analogue of itraconazole. It is available as an oral suspension (40 mg/ml), administered at a dose of 200 mg four times daily or 400 mg twice daily. Now also available as delayed release tablets (100 mg) and injection (18mg/ml). In vitro and in vivo studies showed that posaconazole has a broad spectrum against Candida spp., *Cryptococcus neoformans*, Aspergillus spp., and Fusarium spp. etc. and effective against most agents resistant to itraconazole and fluconazloe [87–91].

Evidence on its use in ocular infections is still limited, but initial results are encouraging. Sponsel et al. also describe a case of keratitis by *Fusarium solani* resistant to Amphotericin B and natamycin but successfully treated with topical drop (100 mg/ml prepared from an oral solution) associated with oral posaconazole 200 mg 4 times daily [89]. However, comparative controlled studies with first-line antifungal agents are still lacking. Altun et al. reported successful treatment with posaconazole in two cases with recalcitrant fugal keratitis that were resistant to conventional antifungal drugs (systemic and topical fluconazole or voriconazole and amphotericin B and topical natamycin were all ineffective) [90]. Posaconazole use resulted in rapid resolution of infection in these cases without significant toxicity. Posaconazole can be useful in cases of fungal keratitis that are resistant to standard antifungal therapy. However, the use of topical posaconazole as monotherapy needs to be evaluated as well as the optimum effective concentration has to be standardized. Two different concentration of the topical preparation is used in the above studies.

4.6 Echinocandins

Echinocandins (caspofungin and micafungin) are semisynthetic lipopeptides act by inhibiting the synthesis of glucan in the fungal cell wall causing osmotic imbalance and cell lysis. Matsumoto et al. have reported successful use of topical 0.2% micafungin in cases of refractory fungal keratitis [92]. In another study by Matsumoto et al. usiing topical micafungin 1 mg/ml reported found an efficacy comparable or superior to fluconazole in the treatment of keratitis by *Candida albicans* and *Candida parapsilosis* [93]. Topical caspofungin has been used in the cases of fungal keratitis refractory to voriconazole [94]. There are limited data on the use of echinocandins to treat fungal keratitis in humans.

5. Recent advances in surgical treatment

Surgical intervention may be an option for patients with refractory FK not responding to medical treatment and severe fungal infections. Penetrating keratoplasty is considered the most common surgical intervention for serious fungal keratitis and cases with perforation or impending perforation. Recent advances have added more options such as targeted drug delivery at the site of infection in the form of intrastromal injections, collagen cross-linking and rose Bengal aided photodynamic therapy.

5.1 Intrastromal voriconazole

The efficacy of topical, as well as systemic, voriconazole is well established. Intra stromal voriconazole has been found as an effective approach for targeted drug delivery in the management of deep FK not responding to standard topical therapy [95–97]. Targeted drug delivery overcomes the issue of poor bioavailability of drugs in cases of deep fungal keratitis. It provides a depot of drug, close to the infected area. However, risk of introducing a new infection, inadvertent anterior chamber entry while performing the procedure in a hazy cornea are associated.

5.2 Intracameral amphotericin B

Intracameral Amphotericin B is another approach for targeted drug delivery, indicated when medical treatment with topical and systemic antifungal has failed, especially in cases with deep mycosis, endothelial plaque and presence of hypopyon with inflammation of the anterior chamber. The concentration injected, ranges between 5 and 10 μg/0.1 ml [98, 99].

5.3 Penetrating Keratoplasty

Penetrating Keratoplasty (PK) is indicated for treatment of refractory or severe fungal keratitis, corneal thinning and perforation in FK [100]. A retrospective study including 52 eyes which underwent PK for corneal perforations secondary to FK, reported improved visual acuity in 46 eyes (88.5%) and clear grafts in 44 eyes (84.6%) at final follow-up [101]. The common complications of PK are graft rejection, recurrence of infection, and secondary glaucoma. Following PK, oral and topical antifungal medications are usually continued for 2 weeks and if pathology reports presence of fungus on the margin of the cornea sample, treatment continues for 6–8 weeks.

Cyclosporine has been recommended after PK in cases of fungal keratitis as it has been suggested to have dual antifungal and anti-immune properties [102]. However; evidences at present are limited, further studies are required to evaluate the risk and benefit of cyclosporine patients undergoing corneal transplant for fungal keratitis.

5.4 Amniotic membrane transplantation

Amniotic membrane transplantation (AMT) has emerged as an option to delay or prevent PK secondary to fungal keratitis. Amniotic membranes have been used to facilitate ocular surface reconstructions in other ocular surface conditions. AMT support re-epithelialization of tissue, and the active components present in the membrane like nerve growth factors are thought to reduce pain [103]. In a study, 23 culture-proven, acute fungal keratitis patients with non-healing corneal ulcers, or impending corneal perforation underwent AMT to prevent PK or to promote re-epithelialization. Following AMT, 25% of patients with persistent positive culture for fungus required PK. The final visual outcome was BCVA > 20/400. It improved in 17, did not changed in four and worsened in two patients [104].

In an inflamed eye, there is increased risk of infection to be introduced into the anterior chamber or vitreous after PK and the use of corticosteroids, to prevent corneal graft rejection, may increase the risk of recurrence of fungal infection. Delay in PK can avoid these complications.

5.5 Lamellar Keratoplasty

Lamellar keratoplasty (LK) is emerged as an alternate surgical procedure for fungal keratitis in which only diseased layers of the corneal surface are excised and replaced by donor cornea. In a study from China, reported the leading indication for LK in 2008 was infectious keratitis, and fungal keratitis constituted 67% of the infectious keratitis cases [105]. In another study, 55 antifungal refractory patients underwent LK with intensive topical and oral antifungal medication. In 93% of the patients, the fungal infection was eradicated. The remaining four patients were treated by a secondary PK. Visual acuity ranged from 20/20 to 20/63 with a few complications after 6–18 months follow-up [106].

5.6 Corneal collagen cross-linking (riboflavin with ultraviolet-A irradiation)

Corneal collagen cross-linking (CXL) has been found successful in halting the progression of keratoconus by using riboflavin and UV-A light. In recent years, role of CXL in infectious keratitis is investigated in several studies with conflicting results on the efficacy of CXL in infectious keratitis [107–113]. Specifically the term photoactivated chromophore cross-linking (PACK-CXL) is used for CXL to treat infectious keratitis [108].

CXL may act in cases of fungal keratitis by a direct antifungal effect and by halting the ongoing melting, thus helping to avoid emergency keratoplasty [109–111]. Said et al. found that although PACK-CXL did not shorten the time to corneal healing, it prevented corneal melting [107]. PACK-CXL is found to be useful in fungal keratitis [108–110]. Abbouda et al. reported halting of corneal melting with PACK-CXL in one case while the other developed perforation [112]. The safety of CXL is of concern because the ultraviolet (UV) -A could damage intraocular structures. Spoerl et al. analyzed the expected damage compared with acceptable damage thresholds. During standard CXL of a cornea with a 400-μm thickness, the irradiances of the UV light reaching the iris, lens, and retina are less than the damage thresholds, and only the microbes, the corneal endothelium, and the keratocytes are at risk [113]. Minor complications after CXL, like transient limbitis and a transient increase in the size of the hypopyon in the first 24 h after CXL reported to be regress subsequently [107].

5.7 Rose Bengal photodynamic therapy

Photodynamic therapy (PDT) has been used in treatment of choroidal neovascularization in age-related macular degeneration, corneal neovascularization and in infectious keratitis due to Acanthamoeba [114]. PDT involves the activation of photosensitizers using light of varying wavelengths. Rose Bengal photodynamic therapy (RB-PDT) involved a photochemical process using Rose Bengal, excited with green light (wavelength: 500–550 nm) to generate reactive oxygen species (ROS), which, react with various intracellular components to cause cell death. In an in vitro study, Arboleda et al. have demonstrated RB PDT to be successful in fungal keratitis [115].

In a pilot clinical study by Naranjo et al., RB-PDAT was performed in 18 patients with progressive infectious keratitis unresponsive to standard medical therapy. RB-PDAT was considered successful in 13 individuals, defined as control of infection without the need for a therapeutic PK [116]. Amescua G et al. in an vitro and in a case study evaluated the efficacy of rose bengal photodynamic antimicrobial therapy (PDAT). They found that Riboflavin CXL demonstrated no inhibition of fungal isolate growth, whereas rose bengal PDAT inhibited fungal isolate growth within the irradiation zone. In addition, a case with resistant fusarium keratitis was treated successfully [117].

6. Future perspective

6.1 New targets in immunology

In a study, the role of vitamin D receptor (VDR) in innate immunity being discovered, may be a new target of treatment that can be explored for FK [118]. Liposomes-encapsulated mannan extracts from *C. albicans* stimulate the production of antibodies protective against candidiasis in mice [119]. Probiotics, such as *L. rhamnosus*, *L. acidophilus*, *L. pyogenes*, *L. casei* GG and Bifidobacterium, reported to be protective from candidiasis by eliciting protective immune and non-immune responses in mice [120]. These experimental studies may further facilitate researches to develop fungal keratitis vaccine and use of probiotics in ocular surface for diseases prevention.

6.2 Ocular novel drug delivery system

Recently, many efforts have been made to improve topical ocular drug delivery by designing various novel drug delivery systems (NDDS), including liposomes, nanoparticles, nanoemulsions, nanosuspensions, micelles, nanofibers, etc.

Several in vitro and in vivo experimental studies have reported encouraging results with NDDS. In a study, the liposomal formulation of the antifungal drug voriconazole found to exhibit a sustained drug release profile, and an 8-fold increase in the amount of drug retained in the cornea after 1 hour of exposure compared with the conventional suspension formulation [121]. The nanoparticle formulation of amphotericin B showed a sustained and controlled drug release for up to 11 hours, while the conventional drug formulation (0.15%) released the entire drug in only 4 hours. Nanoparticle formulation has also shown better pharmacokinetic properties, including 1.5-fold increase in half-life compared to the conventional solution formulation [122]. The microemulsion formulations of fluconazole showed a controlled release profile, releasing 50–80% of the drug in 12 hours, compared to the conventional drug solution, which released almost the entire drug in the first 6 hours [123]. In future, these newer formulations can be very useful in management of fungal keratitis.

6.3 Antimicrobial peptides

Antimicrobial peptides (AMPs) have significant potential for use as antimicrobial agents for ocular or other infections [124]. AMPs, also known as host defense peptides, are naturally produced, small, cationic, amphiphilic peptides ranging in length from 12 to 50 amino acids. They are present on the surfaces of the eyes and in tears. More than 500 AMPs have been reported, including large molecules (RNases and S100A proteins); small peptides α and β defensins in human cationic antibacterial protein (CAP) 18, and α 37 amino acids; proteins like lysozyme and peptidoglycan recognition protein with significant bactericidal activity. The cations carried by AMPs can bind to the anion surface of the bacterial plasma membrane, causing the perforation of cell membrane and subsequently microbial death. AMPs also prevent microbial adhesion to and access into host cells and cause digestion of fungal cell wall by lysozyme [124, 125].

In vitro studies have shown AMPs Pc-C and Pc-E reduced binding of *Aspergillus fumigatus* to cells; CAP37 inhibits candida infection by fungicidal activity [124, 125]. Wu et al. evaluated in vivo application of synthetic β-sheet forming peptide (IKIK) 2-NH2 and (IRIK) 2-NH2 for treatment of FK in comparison with amphotericin B [126]. It was found that topical solutions of the designed peptides were safe, and as effective as the clinically-used Amphotercin B. Many other AMPs such as Clavanin A, Chitinase 3-like 1, and CXCL 10 and S100 proteins may have role in prevention of infection.

7. Conclusion

Early diagnosis and treatment of fungal keratitis remains a challenge. A better understanding of pathogenesis can broadened the approach to management. Recent advances in techniques such as in vivo confocal microscopy and the evolution of PCR and MDS can useful in rapid and accurate diagnosis. Newer antifungal agents and newer methods of targeted drug delivery system can be helpful in treating refractory cases and improving outcome. New evolving technique like PACK-CXL and RB-PDT can be useful as adjuvant therapy.

New researches are continue to investigate the new aspects of pathogenesis, to device the novel drug delivery system to overcome the poor ocular penetration of antifungal drugs and enhance their efficacy and evaluate newer antifungal drugs. In recent years focus on modifying the immune response to the infection, thereby reducing the corneal melting and scarring which lead to poor vision, may have the greatest potential to improve visual outcomes.

Conflict of interest

The authors declare no conflict of interest.

Author details

Suwarna Suman[1*], Arushi Kumar[2], Indu Saxena[3] and Manoj Kumar[4]

1 Department of Ophthalmology, All India Institute of Medical Sciences, Jodhpur, India

2 Dr. S.N. Medical College, Jodhpur, India

3 All India Institute of Medical Sciences Gorakhpur, India

4 M.V.A.S. Medical College, Basti, India

*Address all correspondence to: suwarnasuman@gmail.com

References

[1] Gower EW, Keay LJ, Oechsler RA, Iovieno A, Alfonso EC, Jones DB, *et al.* Trends in fungal keratitis in the United States, 2001 to 2007. Ophthalmology 2010;117:2263-7.

[2] Leck AK, Thomas PA, Hagan M, et al. Aetiology of suppurative corneal ulcers in Ghana and south India, and epidemiology of fungal keratitis. Br J Ophthalmol 2002;86(11): 1211-1215.

[3] Brown, L., Leck, A. K., Gichangi, M., Burton, M. J., & Denning, D. W. (2020). The global incidence and diagnosis of fungal keratitis. The Lancet Infectious Diseases. doi:10.1016/s1473-3099(20)30448-5

[4] Nhung PH, Thu TA, Ngoc LH, Ohkusu K, Ezaki T. Epidemiology of Fungal Keratitis in North Vietnam. J Clin Exp Ophthalmol 2012;3(7):238.

[5] Xie L, Zhong W, Shi W, Sun S. Spectrum of fungal keratitis in north China. Ophthalmology 2006;113(11):1943-1948

[6] Qiu S, Zhao GQ, Lin J, Wang X, Hu LT, Du ZD, *et al.* Natamycin in the treatment of fungal keratitis: A systematic review and Meta-analysis. Int J Ophthalmol 2015;8:597-602.

[7] Ansari Z, Miller D, Galor A. Current thoughts in fungal keratitis: Diagnosis and treatment. Curr Fungal Infect Rep 2013;7:209-18.

[8] Chang HY, Chodosh J. Diagnostic and therapeutic considerations in fungal keratitis. Int Ophthalmol Clin 2011;51:33-42.

[9] Xie L, Dong X, Shi W. Treatment of fungal keratitis by penetrating keratoplasty. Br J Ophthalmol 2001;85(9):1070-1074.

[10] Xie L, Shi W, Liu Z, Li S. Lamellar keratoplasty for the treatment of fungal keratitis. Cornea 2002;21(1):33-37.

[11] Thomas PA, Kaliamurthy J. Mycotic keratitis: epidemiology, diagnosis and management. Clin Microbiol Infect 2013;19(3): 210-220.

[12] O'Day DM, Head WS. Advances in the management of keratomycosis and Acanthamoeba keratitis. Cornea 2000;19(5):681-687

[13] R. Ursea, T.M.T. Feng, A.Z. Mccolgin, R.W. Snyder, Non-traumatic Alternaria keratomycosis in a rigid gas-permeable contact lens patient, British Journal of Ophthalmology, 94 (2010) 389-390.

[14] E.H. Yildiz, A. Haresh, K.M. Hammersmith, R.C. Eagle, C.J. Rapuano, E.J. Cohen, Alternaria and paecilomyces keratitis associated with soft contact lens wear, Cornea,29 (2010) 564.

[15] G. Li, J. Guo, R. Liu, W. Hu, L. Xu, J. Wang, S. Cai, H. Zhang, Y. Zhu, Lacrimal Duct Occlusion Is Associated with Infectious Keratitis, International Journal of Medical Sciences, 13 (2016) 800-805.

[16] K.W. Jin, H.S. Jeon, J.Y. Hyon, W.R. Wee, W. Suh, Y.J. Shin, A case of fungal keratitis and onychomycosis simultaneously infected by Trichophyton species, Bmc Ophthalmology, 14 (2014) 90.

[17] D.J. Galarreta, S.J. Tuft, A. Ramsay, J.K. Dart, Fungal keratitis in London: microbiological and clinical evaluation, Cornea, 26 (2007) 1082-1086

[18] R.S. Punia, R. Kundu, J. Chander, S.K. Arya, U. Handa, H. Mohan, Spectrum of fungal keratitis: clinicopathologic study of 44 cases, International Journal of Ophthalmology, 7 (2014) 114-117.

[19] J.W. Ho, M.M. Fernandez, R.A. Rebong, A.N. Carlson, T. Kim, N.A.

Afshari, Microbiological profiles of fungal keratitis: a 10-year study at a tertiary referral center, Journal of Ophthalmic Inflammation & Infection, 6 (2016) 1-4.

[20] Keay LJ, Gower EW, Iovieno A, Oechsler RA, Alfonso EC, Matoba A, *et al.* Clinical and microbiological characteristics of fungal keratitis in the United States, 2001-2007: A multicentre study. Ophthalmology 2011;118:920-6.

[21] Bullock JD, et al. Effects of time, temperature, and storage container on the growth of Fusarium species: implications for the worldwide fusarium keratitis epidemic of 2004-2006. Arch Ophthalmol. 2011;129(2):133-6.

[22] Bullock JD, et al. Mechanism of drug failure in fusarium keratitis, 2004-2006. N Engl J Med. 2014;370(1):88-9. This important article highlights the need for critical review of every aspect of clinical care, from device design and testing, implementation, and patient compliance to post-marketing surveillance.

[23] Clavet CR, et al. Impact of contact lens materials on multipurpose contact lens solution disinfection activity against *Fusarium solani*. Eye Contact Lens. 2012;38(6):379-84.

[24] Kuzman T, et al. Lens wearers non-compliance; is there an association with lens case contamination? Cont Lens AnteriorEye. 2014;37(2):99-105.

[25] Karsten E, Watson SL, Foster LJR. Diversity of microbial species implicated in keratitis: a review. Open Ophthalmol J. 2012;6:110.

[26] Lekhanont K, Nonpassopon M, Nimvorapun N, Santanirand P. Treatment With Intrastromal and Intracameral Voriconazole in 2 Eyes With Lasiodiplodia theobromae Keratitis: Medicine (Baltimore) Case Reports 2015;94:e541.

[27] Gaujoux T, Borsali E, Gavrilov JC, Touzeau O, Goldschmidt P, Despiau MC, *et al.* Fungal keratitis caused by *Cylindrocarpon lichenicola*. J Fr Ophtalmol 2012;35:356.e1-5.

[28] Motley WW, Melson AT, Mortensen JE. Pediatric Metarrhizium anisopliae keratitis. J AAPOS 2011;15:101-3.

[29] Yuan X, Wilhelmus KR, Matoba AY, Alexandrakis G, Miller D, Huang AJ. Pathogenesis and outcome of Paecilomyces keratitis. Am J Ophthalmol 2009;147:691-6.e3.

[30] Niu L, Liu X, Ma Z, Yin Y, Sun L, Yang L, Zheng Y. Fungal keratitis: Pathogenesis, diagnosis and prevention. Microb Pathog. 2020 Jan;138:103802. doi: 10.1016/j.micpath.2019.103802. Epub 2019 Oct 15. PMID: 31626916

[31] M.K. Hostetter, Adhesins and ligands involved in the interaction of Candida spp. with epithelial and endothelial surfaces, Clinical Microbiology Reviews, 7 (1994) 29-42.

[32] S.E. Hardison, G.D. Brown, C-type lectin receptors orchestrate antifungal immunity, Nat Immunol, 13 (2012) 817-822.

[33] J. Wu, Y. Zhang, Z. Xin, X. Wu, The crosstalk between TLR2 and NOD2 in Aspergillus fumigatus keratitis, Molecular immunology, 64 (2015) 235-243.

[34] Z. Jie, X.Y. Wu, F.S. Yu, Activation of Toll-like receptors 2 and 4 in Aspergillus fumigatus keratitis, Innate Immun, 15 (2009) 155-168.

[35] Jouault T, Ibata-Ombetta S, Takeuchi O, et al. *Candida albicans* phospholipomannan is sensed through Toll-like receptors. J Infect Dis. 2003; 188:165-172. [PubMed:12825186]

[36] Y. Sun, S. Abbondante, M. Karmakar, S. de Jesus Carrion, C. Che,

A.G. Hise, E. Pearlman, Neutrophil Caspase-11 Is Required for Cleavage of Caspase-1 and Secretion of IL-1beta in Aspergillus fumigatus Infection, J Immunol, 201 (2018) 2767-2775.

[37] S. de Jesus Carrion, S. Abbondante, H.L. Clark, M.E. Marshall, I. Mouyna, A. Beauvais, Y. Sun, P.R. Taylor, S.M. Leal, Jr., B. Armstrong, W. Carrera, J.P. Latge, E. Pearlman, Aspergillus fumigatus corneal infection is regulated by chitin synthases and by neutrophil-derived acidic mammalian chitinase, Eur J Immunol, 49 (2019) 918-927.

[38] P.R. Taylor, S. Roy, S.M. Leal, Jr., Y. Sun, S.J. Howell, B.A. Cobb, X. Li, E. Pearlman, Activation of neutrophils by autocrine IL-17A-IL-17RC interactions during fungal infection is regulated by IL-6, IL-23, RORgammat and dectin-2, Nat Immunol, 15 (2014) 143-151.

[39] X. Gao, G. Zhao, C. Li, J. Lin, N. Jiang, Q. Wang, L. Hu, Q. Xu, X. Peng, K. He, G. Zhu, LOX-1 and TLR4 affect each other and regulate the generation of ROS in *A. fumigatus* keratitis, Int Immunopharmacol, 40 (2016) 392-399.

[40] K. Yuan, G. Zhao, C. Che, C. Li, J. Lin, G. Zhu, K. He, Dectin-1 is essential for IL-1beta production through JNK activation and apoptosis in Aspergillus fumigatus keratitis, Int Immunopharmacol, 52 (2017) 168-175.

[41] Leal SM Jr, Vareechon C, Cowden S, et al. Fungal antioxidant pathways promote survival against neutrophils during infection. J Clin Invest. 2012; 122:2482-2498. [PubMed:22706306]

[42] Leal SM, Pearlman E. The role of cytokines and pathogen recognition molecules in fungal keratitis: insights from human disease and animal models. Cytokine. 2012;58(1):107-11.

[43] Wang N, et al. Association of TLR2 and TLR4 gene single nucleotide polymorphisms with fungal keratitis in Chinese Han population. Curr Eye Res. 2014;39(1):47-52.

[44] S.K. Raza, A.I. Mallet, S.A. Howell, P.A. Thomas, An in-vitro study of the sterol content and toxin production of Fusarium isolates from mycotic keratitis, Journal of Medical Microbiology, 41 (1994) 204-208.

[45] H. Sav, H.G. Ozdemir, R. Altınbas, N. Kiraz, M. Ilkit, S. Seyedmousavi, Virulence Attributes and Antifungal Susceptibility Profile of Opportunistic Fungi Isolated from Ophthalmic Infections, Mycopathologia, 181 (2016) 653-661.

[46] P.A. Thomas, Fungal infections of the cornea, Eye, 17 (2003) 852-862

[47] Mizushima N, Levine B, Cuervo AM, Klionsky DJ. Autophagy fights disease through cellular self-digestion. *Nature*. 2008;451:1069-1075.

[48] Feng Y, He D, Yao Z, Klionsky DJ. The machinery of macroautophagy. *Cell Res*. 2014;24:24-41.

[49] Kanayama M, Inoue M, Danzaki K, Hammer G, He YW, Shinohara ML. Autophagy enhances NFkappaB activity in specific tissue macrophages by sequestering A20 to boost antifungal immunity. *Nat Commun*. 2015;6:5779.

[50] Tam JM, Mansour MK, Khan NS, et al. Dectin-1-dependent LC3 recruitment to phagosomes enhances fungicidal activity in macrophages. *J Infect Dis*. 2014;210:1844-1854

[51] Li C, Li C, Lin J, et al. The role of autophagy in the innate immune response to fungal keratitis caused by *Aspergillus fumigatus* infection. *Invest Ophthalmol Vis Sci*. 2020;61(2):25.

[52] Zhang X, et al. Keratitis-associated fungi form biofilms with reduced antifungal drug susceptibility. Invest Ophthalmol VisSci. 2012;53(12):7774-8.

[53] Parsons' Diseases of the Eye. 21edition Elsevier,2015;201p

[54] Dahlgren MA, Lingappan A, Wilhelmus KR. The clinical diagnosis of microbial keratitis. Am JOphthalmol. 2007; 143:940-944. [PubMed: 17408586]

[55] Dalmon C, Porco TC, Lietman TM et al. The clinical differentiation of bacterial and fungal keratitis: a photographic survey. Invest Ophthalmol Vis Sci. 2012;53(4):1787-91.

[56] Brasnu E, Bourcier T, Dupas B, et al. In vivo confocal microscopy in fungal keratitis. Br J Ophthalmol 2007;91:588-91.

[57] Labbé A, Khammari C, Dupas B, Gabison E, Brasnu E, Labetoulle M, et al. Contribution of in vivo confocal microscopy to the diagnosis and management of infectious keratitis. Ocul Surf 2009;7:41-52.

[58] Takezawa Y, Shiraishi A, Noda E, Hara Y, Yamaguchi M, Uno T, et al. Effectiveness of in vivo confocal microscopy in detecting filamentous fungi during clinical course of fungal keratitis. Cornea 2010;29:1346-52.

[59] Kanavi MR, Javadi M, Yazdani S, Mirdehghanm S. Sensitivity and specificity of confocal scan in the diagnosis of infectious keratitis. Cornea 2007;26:782-6.

[60] Shi W, Li S, Liu M, Jin H, Xie L. Antifungal chemotherapy for fungal keratitis guided by in vivo confocal microscopy. Graefes Arch Clin Exp Ophthalmol 2008;246:581-6.

[61] McLeod SD, Kolahdouz-Isfahani A, Rostamian K, Flowers CW, Lee PP, McDonnell PJ. The role of smears, cultures, and antibiotic sensitivity testing in the management of suspected infectious keratitis. Ophthalmology. 1996; 103:23-28. [PubMed: 8628555]

[62] Zhang W, Yang H, Jiang L, Han L, Wang L. Use of potassium hydroxide, Giemsa and calcofluor white staining techniques in the microscopic evaluation of corneal scrapings for diagnosis of fungal keratitis. J Int Med Res. 2010; 38:1961-1967. [PubMed: 21226999]

[63] McGinnis, M. New York: Academic Press; 1980. Laboratory handbook of medical mycology.

[64] Waters DL, Shapter FM. The polymerase chain reaction (PCR): general methods. Methods Mol Biol. 2014;1099:65-75. doi: 10.1007/978-1-62703-715-0_7 pmid: 24243196

[65] Kourkoumpetis T K, Fuchs BB, Coleman JJ, Desalermos A, Mylonakis E. Polymerase Chain Reaction–Based Assays for the Diagnosis of Invasive Fungal Infections. Clinical Infectious Diseases 2012;54(9):1322-31

[66] P.A. Thomas, A.T. Philip, T. Joseph, G. Pitchairaj, PCR for the molecular diagnosis of mycotic keratitis, Expert Review of Molecular Diagnostics, 12 (2014) 703-718.

[67] D. He, J. Hao, S. Gao, X. Wan, W. Wang, Q. Shan, L. Wang, Etiological Analysis of Fungal Keratitis and Rapid Identification of Predominant Fungal Pathogens, Mycopathologia, 181 (2016) 75-82.

[68] Eleinen KG, Mohalhal AA, Elmekawy HE, Abdulbaki AM, Sherif AM, El-Sherif RH, et al. Polymerase chain reaction-guided diagnosis of infective keratitis - a hospital-based study. Curr Eye Res. 2012;37:1005-11.

[69] Zhao G, Zhai H, Yuan Q, Sun S, Liu T, Xie L. Rapid and sensitive diagnosis of fungal keratitis with direct PCR without template DNA extraction. Clin Microbiol Infect. 2014;20:O776-82. doi: 10.1111/1469-0691.12571 pmid: 24471925

[70] Doan T, Wilson MR, Crawford ED, et al. Illuminating uveitis: metagenomic deep sequencing identifies common and rare pathogens. Genome Med. 2016;8:90.

[71] Wilson MR, Naccache SN, Samayoa E, et al. Actionable diagnosis of neuroleptospirosis by next-generation sequencing. N Engl J Med. 2014;370:2408e2417.

[72] Graf EH, Simmon KE, Tardif KD, et al. Unbiased detection of respiratory viruses by use of RNA sequencing-based metagenomics: a systematic comparison to a commercial PCR panel. J Clin Microbiol. 2016;54:1000e1007.

[73] Seitzman GD, Hinterwirth A, Zhong, L, Cummings, S, Chen C, Driver, TH, Lee, MD, Doan T. Metagenomic Deep Sequencing for the Diagnosis of Corneal and External Disease Infections. Ophthalmology 2016;126 (12), 1724-26

[74] Bennett J. Agentes antimicrobianos, agentes antifúngicos. In: Brunton L, editor. Goodman & Gilman: as bases farmacológicas da terapêutica. 11a ed. Rio de Janeiro: McGraw-Hill; c2007. p. 1103-17.

[75] Florcruz NV, Peczon I Jr. Medical interventions for fungal keratitis. Cochrane database of systematic reviews. 2008:CD004241. [PubMed: 18254043]

[76] FlorCruz NV, Peczon IV, Evans JR.Medical interventions for fungal keratitis. *Cochrane Database of Systematic Reviews* 2012,Issue 2. Art. No.: CD004241.

[77] FlorCruz NV, Evans JR. Medical interventions for fungal keratitis. Cochrane Database Syst Rev. 2015:CD004241.

[78] Morand K, Bartoletti AC, Bochot A, Barratt G, Brandely ML, Chast F. Liposomal amphotericin B eye drops to treat fungal keratitis: physico-chemical and formulation stability. Int J Pharm 2007;344(1-2):150-3. doi: 10.1016/j.ijpharm.2007.04.028

[79] O'Day DM, Foulds G, Williams TE, Robinson RD, Allen RH, Head WS. Ocular uptake of fluconazole following oral administration. Arch Ophthalmol. 1990;108(7):1006-8.

[80] Anderson KL, Mitra S, Salouti R, et al. Fungal keratitis caused by Paecilomyces lilacinus associated with a retained intracorneal hair. *Cornea* 2004;23:516-21.

[81] Ozbek Z, Kang S, Sivalingam J, et al. Voriconazole in the management of Alternaria keratitis. *Cornea* 2006;25:242-4.

[82] Gracitelli C P B, Ferrar P V, Pereira CA P, Hirai F E., & Freitas de D. A case of recurrent keratitis caused by Paecilomyces lilacinus and treated by voriconazole. *Arquivos Brasileiros de Oftalmologia*. 2019; *82*(2), 152-154.

[83] Lee SJ, Lee JJ, Kim SD. Topical and oral voriconazole in the treatment of fungal keratitis. *Korean J Ophthalmol*. 2009;23(1):46-48.

[84] Thiel MA, Zinkernagel AS, Burhenne J, et al. Voriconazole concentration in human aqueous humor and plasma during topical or combined topical and systemic administration for fungal keratitis. Antimicrob Agents Chemother. 2007;51: 239-244.

[85] Hernandez Prats C, Llinares Tello F, Burgos San Jose A, et al. Voriconazole in fungal keratitis caused by Scedosporium apiospermum. Ann Pharmacother. 2004;38:414-417.

[86] Jones A, Muhtaseb M. Use of voriconazole in fungal keratitis. J Cataract Refract Surg. 2008;34:183-184.

[87] Cuenca-Estrella M, Gomez-Lopez A, Mellado E, Buitrago MJ, Monzon A, Rodriguez-Tudela JL. Head-to-head comparison of the activities of currently available antifungal agents against 3,378 Spanish clinical isolates of yeasts and filamentous fungi. Antimicrob Agents Chemother. 2006;50(3):917-21.

[88] Torres HA, Hachem RY, Chemaly RF, Kontoyiannis DP, Raad II. Posaconazole: a broad-spectrum triazole antifungal. Lancet Infect Dis. 2005;5(12):775-85.

[89] Sponsel WE, Graybill JR, Nevarez HL, Dang D. Ocular and systemic posaconazole(SCH-56592) treatment of invasive *Fusarium solani* keratitis and endophthalmitis. Br J Ophthalmol. 2002;86(7):829-30.

[90] Altun A, Kurna SA, Sengor T, Altun G, Olcaysu OO, Aki SF, *et al.* Effectiveness of posaconazole in recalcitrant fungal keratitis resistant to conventional antifungal drugs. Case Rep Ophthalmol Med 2014;2014:701653.

[91] Arnoldner MA, Kheirkhah A, Jakobiec FA, Durand ML, Hamrah P. Successful treatment of *Paecilomyces lilacinus* keratitis with oral posaconazole. Cornea 2014;33:747-9.

[92] Matsumoto Y, Dogru M, Goto E, Fujishima H, Tsubota K. Successful topical application of a new antifungal agent, micafungin, in the treatment of refractory fungal corneal ulcers: report of three cases andliterature review. Cornea. 2005;24(6):748-53.

[93] Matsumoto Y, Murat D, Kojima T, Shimazaki J, Tsubota K. The comparison of solitary topical micafungin or fluconazole application in the treatment of Candida fungal keratitis. Br J Ophthalmol. 2011;95(10):1406-9.

[94] Hurtado-Sarrió M, Duch-Samper A, Cisneros-Lanuza A, Díaz-Llopis M, Peman-Garcíia J, Vazquez-Polo A. Successful topical application of caspofungin in the treatment of fungal keratitis refractory to voriconazole. Arch Ophthalmol 2010;128:941-2.

[95] Tu EY, Hou J. Intrastromal antifungal injection with secondary lamellar interface infusion for late-onset infectious keratitis after DSAEK. Cornea 2014;33:990-3.

[96] Tu EY. Alternaria keratitis: Clinical presentation and resolution with topical fluconazole or intrastromal voriconazole and topical caspofungin. Cornea 2009;28:116-9.

[97] Haddad RS, El-Mollayess GM. Combination of intracameral and intrastromal voriconazole in the treatment of recalcitrant Acremonium fungal keratitis. Middle East Afr J Ophthalmol 2012;19:265-8.

[98] Yilmaz S, Ture M, Maden A. Efficacy of intracameral amphotericin B injection in the management of refractory keratomycosis and endophthalmitis. Cornea 2007;26:398-402.

[99] Yoon KC, Jeong IY, Im SK, Chae HJ, Yang SY. Therapeutic effect of intracameral amphotericin B injection in the treatment of fungal keratitis. Cornea 2007;26:814-8.

[100] Xie L, Dong X, Shi W. Treatment of fungal keratitis by penetrating keratoplasty. Br J Ophthalmol. 2001; 85:1070-1074. [PubMed: 11520759]

[101] Xie L, Zhai H, Shi W. Penetrating keratoplasty for corneal perforations in fungal keratitis. Cornea. 2007; 26:158-162. [PubMed: 17251805]

[102] Bell NP, Karp CL, Alfonso EC, Schiffman J, Miller D. Effects of methylprednisolone and cyclosporine A on fungal growth in vitro. Cornea. 1999; 18:306-313. [PubMed: 10336034]

[103] Tseng SC. Amniotic membrane transplantation for ocular surface reconstruction. Biosci Rep. 2001; 21:481-489. [PubMed: 11900323]

[104] Chen HC, Tan HY, Hsiao CH, Huang SC, Lin KK, Ma DH. Amniotic membrane transplantation for persistent corneal ulcers and perforations in acute fungal keratitis. Cornea. 2006; 25:564-572. [PubMed: 16783145]

[105] Qu LJ, Xie LX. Changing indications for lamellar keratoplasty in Shandong, 1993 –2008. Chin Med J (Engl). 2010; 123:3268-3271. [PubMed: 21163128]

[106] Xie L, Shi W, Liu Z, Li S. Lamellar keratoplasty for the treatment of fungal keratitis. Cornea. 2002; 21:33-37. [PubMed: 11805504]

[107] Said DG, Elalfy MS, Gatzioufas Z, El-Zakzouk ES, Hassan MA, Saif MY, et al. Collagen cross-linking with photoactivated riboflavin (PACK-CXL) for the treatment of advanced infectious keratitis with corneal melting. Ophthalmology 2014;121:1377-82.

[108] Tabibian D, Richoz O, Riat A, Schrenzel J, Hafezi F. Accelerated photoactivated chromophore for keratitis-corneal collagen cross-linking as a first-line and sole treatment in early fungal keratitis. J Refract Surg 2014;30:855-7.

[109] Iseli HP, Thiel MA, Hafezi F, Kampmeier J, Seiler T. Ultraviolet A/riboflavin corneal cross-linking for infectious keratitis associated with corneal melts. Cornea 2008;27:590-4.

[110] Li Z, Jhanji V, Tao X, Yu H, Chen W, Mu G. Riboflavin/ultraviolet light-mediated crosslinking for fungal keratitis. Br J Ophthalmol 2013;97:669-71.

[111] Saglk A, Uçakhan OO, Kanpolat A. Ultraviolet A and riboflavin therapy as an adjunct in corneal ulcer refractory to medical treatment. Eye Contact Lens 2013;39:413-5.

[112] Abbouda A, Estrada AV, Rodriguez AE, Alió JL. Anterior segment optical coherence tomography in evaluation of severe fungal keratitis infections treated by corneal crosslinking. Eur J Ophthalmol 2014;24:320-4.

[113] Spoerl E, Mrochen M, Sliney D, Trokel S, Seiler T. Safety of UVA-riboflavin cross-linking of the cornea. Cornea 2007;26:385-9.

[114] Szentmáry N, Goebels S, Bischoff M, Seitz B. Photodynamic therapy for infectious keratitis. Ophthalmologe 2012;109:165-70.

[115] Arboleda A, Miller D, Cabot F, Taneja M, Aguilar MC, Alawa K, et al. Assessment of rose bengal versus riboflavin photodynamic therapy for inhibition of fungal keratitis isolates. Am J Ophthalmol 2014;158:64-70.e2.

[116] Naranjo A, Arboleda A, Martinez JD, Durkee H, Aguilar MC, Relhan N,et al. Rose Bengal Photodynamic Antimicrobial Therapy for Patients With Progressive Infectious Keratitis: A Pilot Clinical Study. Am J Ophthalmol. 2019 Dec;208:387-396.

[117] Amescua G, Arboleda A, Nikpoor N, et al. Rose Bengal Photodynamic Antimicrobial Therapy: A Novel Treatment for Resistant Fusarium Keratitis. Cornea. 2017;36(9):1141-1144.

[118] Cong L, Xia YP, Zhao GQ, Lin J, Xu Q, Hu LT, Qu JQ, Peng XD. Expression of vitamin D receptor and cathelicidin in human corneal epithelium cells during *fusarium solani* infection. 2015;8 (5):866-871.

[119] Y. Han, ., M.A. Ulrich, J.E. Cutler, *Candida albicans* mannan extract-protein

conjugates induce a protective immune response against experimental candidiasis, Journal of Infectious Diseases, 179 (1999) 1477-1484.

[120] Rossoni R.D., de Barros P.P.,. de Alvarenga J.A, Ribeiro F.C., Velloso M.D.S. et al. Antifungal activity of clinical Lactobacillus strains against *Candida albicans* biofilms: identification of potential probiotic candidates to prevent oral candidiasis, Biofouling, 34 (2018) 212-225.

[121] de Sá FA, Taveira SF, Gelfuso GM, Lima EM, Gratieri T. Liposomal voriconazole (VOR) formulation for improved ocular delivery. Colloids Surf B Biointerfaces 2015;133:331-8. doi: 10.1016/j.colsurfb.2015.06.036

[122] Zhou W, Wang Y, Jian J, Song S. Self-aggregated nanoparticles based on amphiphilic poly(lactic acid)-grafted-chitosan copolymer for ocular delivery of amphotericin B. Int J Nanomedicine 2013;8:3715-28.

[123] Soliman OAE, Mohamed EA, Khatera NAA. Enhanced ocular bioavailability of fluconazole from niosomal gels and microemulsions: formulation, optimization, and in vitro-in vivo evaluation. Pharm Dev Technol 2019;24(1):48-62.

[124] Brandt CR. Peptide therapeutics for treating ocular surface infections. J Ocul Pharmacol Ther 2014;30:691-9.

[125] Pereira HA, Tsyshevskaya-Hoover I, Hinsley H, Logan S, Nguyen M, Nguyen TT, et al. Candidacidal activity of synthetic peptides based on the antimicrobial domain of the neutrophil-derived protein, CAP37. Med Mycol 2010;48:263-72

[126] Wu H, Ong ZY, Liu S, Li Y, Wiradharma N, Yang YY, et al. Synthetic ß-sheet forming peptide amphiphiles for treatment of fungal keratitis. Biomaterials 2015;43:44-9.

Section 2

Infectious Uveitis

Chapter 4

Ocular Toxoplasmosis: An Update on Diagnosis, Multimodal Imaging and Therapy

Terese Kamal Gerges

Abstract

Ocular toxoplasmosis remains to be the most common cause of infectious uveitis in immunocompetent individuals with highly variable prognosis. The transmission mode can be either congenital or acquired. A precise diagnosis of the disease is necessary to opt effective and rapid treatment. While ocular toxoplasmosis usually presents in the classic form, it may as well present in variable clinical spectrum. The diagnosis can be suspected by the ocular inflammatory clinical presentation as well as multimodal imaging. However, serologic tests including intraocular fluid testing may be needed. Treatment includes combination of systemic antiparasitic and anti-inflammatory drugs with variable effectivity. More recently, intravitreally antimicrobials may be used. The chapter aims to layout the different clinical presentations and complications of ocular toxoplasmosis. Diagnostic techniques and different antimicrobial combinations for treatment will also be discussed.

Keywords: ocular toxoplasmosis, clinical presentation, diagnosis, treatment

1. Introduction

Approximately 25 to 30% of the world's human population is infected by toxoplasma [1]. Ocular toxoplasmosis is one of the most common cause of posterior uveitis caused by an intracellular parasite, toxoplasma gondii [2, 3].

1952, Helenor Campbell Wilder (later Helenor Campbell Wilder Foerster) confirmed the growing suspicion that toxoplasma gondii was a cause of uveitis in otherwise healthy adults by identifying the presence of both trophozoites and brachyzoites in enucleated eyes, that suffered severe intraocular inflammation [4].

Retinitis is the most common manifestation of ocular toxoplasmosis with vitritis. Factors that may influence visual prognosis include severity of the inflammation, size of the lesion and site of the inflammation. Also, progression to complications such as a neovascularization, vitreomacular traction, retinal detachment, glaucoma and cataract renders worse visual prognosis. Multimodal imaging can assist in meticulously evaluating and studying the extent of intraocular damage imposed by toxoplasma inflammation. Laboratory testing of intraocular fluid has been widely studied and employed, including PCR testing and detection of intraocular antibodies using Goldmann-Witmer coefficient (GWC), to enable more precise diagnosis Ocular toxoplasmosis has a self-limiting nature, treatment can help rapid control of inflammation specially if the retinitis involves the posterior pole. Treatment includes different combinations of antimicrobials; none have can prevent

IntechOpen

recurrences, but some combinations have shown more effective reduction in the size of the retinal lesion in comparison to other combinations or no treatment [5].

2. Life cycle and mode of transmission

Toxoplasma exists in 3 infectious forms including sporozoites, which are contained within oocysts, tachyzoites and bradyzoites, which reside in tissue cysts. Oocysts are produced only in cat intestines and become infectious when defecated by cats. Tachyzoites are the fastest replicating form and responsible for systemic dissemination and active tissue infection in intermediate hosts. Tachyzoites can enter almost any type of host cell and multiply until the host cell is filled with parasites. Lysis of the host cell results in tachyzoite release followed by reentry into a new host cell. As a result of this cycle, multifocal tissue necrosis may occur. The host usually limits this phase of infection, then the parasite enters the dormant form, named bradyzoites, and gets isolated in tissue cysts. Cysts may contain hundreds of bradyzoites. These cysts usually cause no host reaction and may remain dormant throughout the life of the host [6].

The infection may be acquired or congenital by vertical transmission to the fetus. However, reports have supported the view that acquired infections might be a more important cause of ocular diseases than congenital [7–9].

Acquired infection occurs by consumption of raw meat containing cysts or ingestion of water or food contaminated by oocytes [9, 10]. Once the active parasite has invaded the body, it will spread via the blood stream, and due to a high affinity for cerebro- and retinovascular endothelial cells, can become established within the retina [10]. Following invasion of the parasite into the eye, the tachyzoite remains latent in the cyst under the control of the immune response of host [11–13]. In event of trigger of cyst rupture, the tachyzoite is converted to bradyzoite, and the inflammatory response is activated [5, 14].

3. Clinical presentation and phenotypes

Congenital- transplacental transmission occurs in 40–70%, while acquired ocular involvement was reported in 1–21% [15]. However, each entity has significantly different clinical manifestation. A study conduct in southern Brazil reported lower prevalence of ocular toxoplasmosis in children been 5.1% below the age of 13 and 21.3% above the age of 13, concluding that ocular toxoplasmosis is a sequela of postnatal rather than congenital infection [7].

3.1 Congenital ocular toxoplasmosis

Ocular lesions are the most frequent manifestations of congenital toxoplasmosis [16, 17]. Vertical transmission of toxoplasmosis occurs during primary infection in pregnant women, and generally the maternal disease goes unnoticed. When pregnant women become infected in the first trimester, the frequency of fetal infection goes up to 15–20%, in the second up to 25%, and in the third up to 65–70%. The most compromised fetuses are those who are infected earlier [1, 18, 19].

Besides retinochoroiditis, other ocular manifestations of congenital toxoplasmosis are described, such as microphthalmia, optic nerve atrophy, and abnormalities of the iris, cataract, and strabismus [17, 20–24].

However, typical presentation in the retina is an atrophic hyperpigmented scarred macular lesion that is described as 'wagon-wheel' lesion caused by congenital toxoplasmosis. It shows a central area composed of glial and pigmented material connected by pigmented strands to a peripheral ring of pigment at the edge of the lesion **Figure 1**. A study designed to detect ocular involvement in infants with congenital toxoplasma reported that ocular involvement occurred in 70.4% of the cases, with mean age of active lesion at 1.4 months. Bilateral involvement occurred in 15.7% of the patients, mainly involving the papillomacular bundle in 76.3%. The retinochoroiditis lesions were active in 15.7% of the eyes and had healed in 84.3% [25].

It is worth mentioning that new lesions continue to appear well after the age of 5 years, likely with severe visual impairments. Therefore, screening of women for toxoplasmosis before pregnancy is advisable [26].

A significant reduction in prevalence and severity of the disease has been attributed to prenatal and neonatal treatment maintained throughout the first year of life [27–29].

3.2 Acquired toxoplasma

Acquired ocular toxoplasmosis commonly manifests in the second through fourth decades [10, 30]. Approximately 10% of otherwise healthy individuals who contract the infection report nonspecific symptoms, such as fatigue, fever and myalgias. Cervical lymphadenopathy [31].

Though floaters with altered vision may be the most common symptom of toxoplasma retinitis, however, clinical presentation ranges a wide spectrum.

Anterior uveitis is a common finding, with mutton-fat keratic precipitates, fibrin, cells and flare, iris nodules and posterior synechiae [32]. Raised intraocular pressure has been reported in (30%–38%) of the cases [33, 34].

3.2.1 Typical toxoplasma retinitis

This usually manifests as active focal necrotizing retinitis, at the edge of an old, pigmented scar with overlying vitritis **Figure 2**. Bosch-Driessen et al. reported 72% of the patients had pre-existing retinochoroidal scars, indicating prior subclinical disease. The pigmented scar has been described to harbor the cysts that remain dormant until the cyst ruptures with release of organisms into the surrounding retina inducing adjacent retinitis [10].

Toxoplasma retinitis may occasionally manifest without an adjacent scar **Figure 3**. It is known that tissue cysts can exist in normal-appearing retina. The retina may be infected at the time of an initial systemic infection, but without clinically apparent lesions at the time [32].

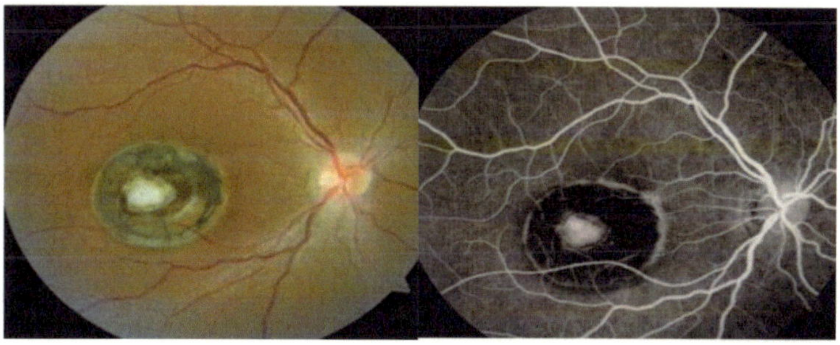

Figure 1.
Colored image (left) and fundus fluorescein angiography (right) of atrophic pigmented congenital toxoplasma 'wagon wheel' macular scar.

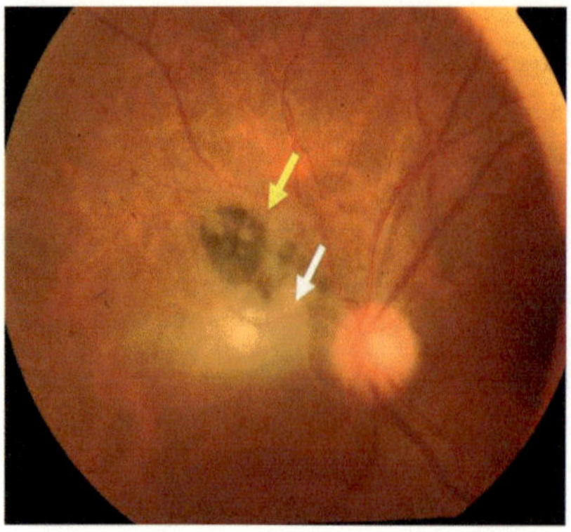

Figure 2.
Colored image of a supranasal peripapillary pigmented scar (yellow arrow) with adjacent area of active retinitis (white arrow)

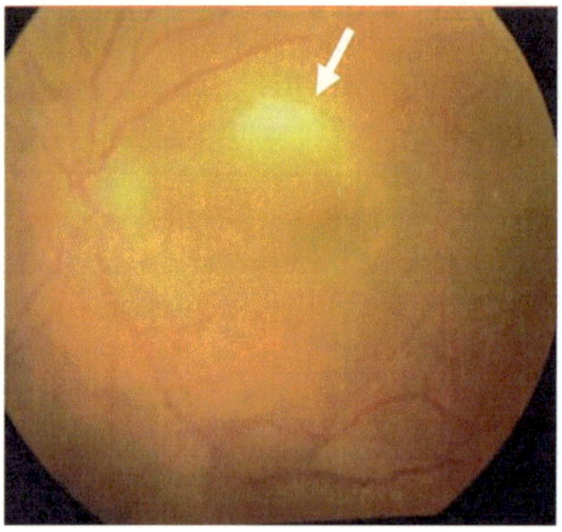

Figure 3.
Colored image of superior macular toxoplasma retinitis lesion (white arrow) without adjacent scar.

The focus of retinitis is of necrotizing nature and usually involves the full thickness of the retina, although occasional limited involvement of either inner or outer retina occurs, as described by Friedmann and Knox. Depending upon the thickness of involved retina, the overlying vitreous and underlying choroid are variably involved [30].

Large, full-thickness lesions tend to incite more severe vitritis, producing the classic 'headlight in the fog' sign. Optical coherence tomography (OCT) of active lesions can detect the level of retinal involvement, severity of choroiditis, as well as monitoring the regression of the lesion with treatment **Figures 4** and **5**. On regression of the retinitis, a pigmented scar that is smaller than the actual size of the retinitis forms.

Punctate outer retinal toxoplasma (PORT) was first described in 1985 by Doft and Gass [35]. They elucidated the outer variation of punctate toxoplasmosis that primarily affects the outer retinal layers of the macular area. This entity usually presents in younger, immunocompetent patients [35, 36]. These can be either a single or several deep retinal infiltrates that may extend as far as the inner plexiform layer (IPL). The underlying retinal pigment epithelium is interrupted with variable involvements of the Bruch's membrane and choroid. These lesions have been detected in the same eye with typical retinal toxoplasma lesions as in **Figures 6** and **7** or in eyes with no previous toxoplasma lesions [37]. PORT lesions resolve slowly, leaving an atrophic chorioretinal scar and frequently recur in adjacent areas of the macula [38].

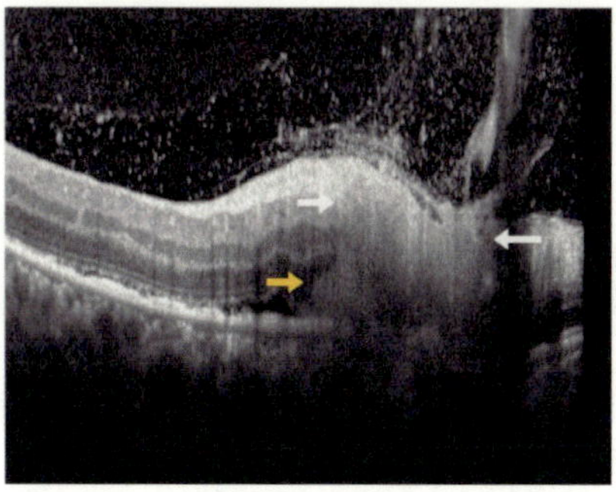

Figure 4.
OCT line scan through full thickness retinitis seen between the two white arrows with compete loss of architecture of inner retinal layers, with a small deep retinal infiltrate (orange arrow) and adjacent mild subretinal fluid. Dense localized overlying vitreous infiltration overlying the area of retinitis.

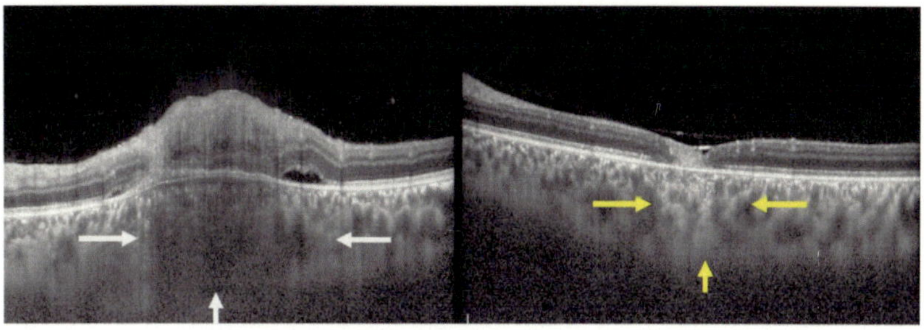

Figure 5.
OCT line scan through active toxoplasma retinitis seen between the white arrows in the photo on the left with underlying choroidal involvement exhibiting a hyporeflective elevated appearance. Healed lesion in the photo on the right between yellow arrows shows resolved retinitis with thinned retina, decreased thickness of the choroid with increased choroidal transmission.

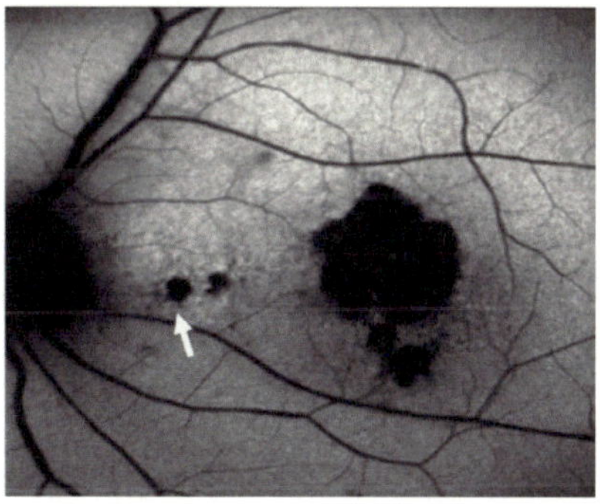

Figure 6.
Autofluorescence showing foveal hypoautofluorescent toxoplasma lesion with an active edge, and two nasal PORT lesions (white arrow).

3.2.2 Retinal vascular involvement of ocular toxoplasmosis

Inflammatory vascular involvement in acute toxoplasma retinochoroiditis constitutes an invariable clinical sign of the disease and was reported in (100%) of cases in a previous study [39].

During the acute phase of toxoplasmic retinochoroiditis, perivasculitis with arterial involvement in the form of multiple small periarterial plaques, previously

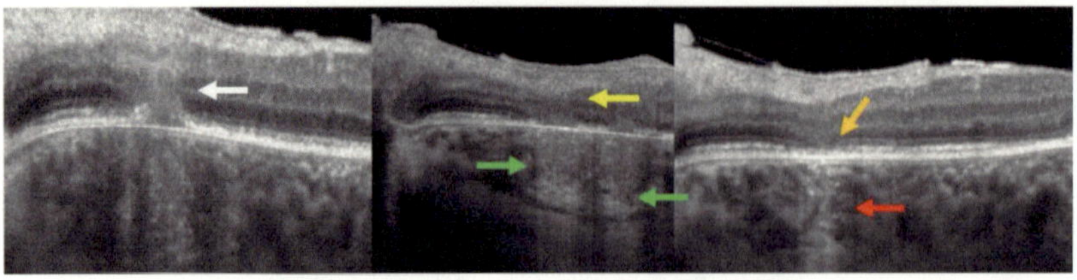

Figure 7.
Left image: *OCT of one of the PORT lesions in the active stage (white arrow) showing inflammatory nodular infiltrate breaking through the RPE and extending to the inner plexiform layer corresponding to the nasal PORT lesions in the autofluorescent image in* ***Figure 6****, both pointed on by white arrows. The underlying choroid shows thickening and loss of normal architecture.* ***Middle image:*** *As the lesion heals the infiltrate decreases in size (yellow arrow) and the choroid appears less thickened with incomplete recovery of the normal choroidal vasculature (green arrow).* ***Right image:*** *Complete recovery of the lesion with complete disappearance of the nodular infiltrate, leaving thinned depressed inner retinal layers (orange arrow) with partial recovery of the RPE and increased choroidal transmission with recovered choroidal vasculature (red arrow).*

described as Kyreiles plaques [40], may occur, whereas that of the vein may show scattered infiltration of the wall, sheathing, or both **Figure 8**. Obstruction of a branch of the central retinal artery and vein as well as choroidal vascular occlusion have also been reported to occur [41–45].

The pathogenesis of vasculitis, was previously explained to be, is secondary to a reaction between local antigens and circulating antibody, and the beads seen along the vessels represent cuffs of mononuclear cells [46, 47].

Inflammation of the retinal vessels can occur in close proximity to the area of retinitis. The intensity of the vascular involvement was reported to be more prominent were the vessel traverses the active lesion. Vasculitis may also present away from the actual focus of inflammation **Figure 9** and involve vessels in all four quadrants [39].

Occasionally, vascular occlusion may occur when thick focal retinitis engulfs the course of retinal vessels, leaving a permanent area of retinal ischemia [43] **Figure 10**. Retinal vascular occlusion has been reported to be 5% [39].

3.2.3 Optic nerve involvement in ocular toxoplasma

Optic nerve involvement may be due to parasitic invasion or reactive inflammation [48–51]. Eckert et al., reported optic nerve changes in 5% of the cases.

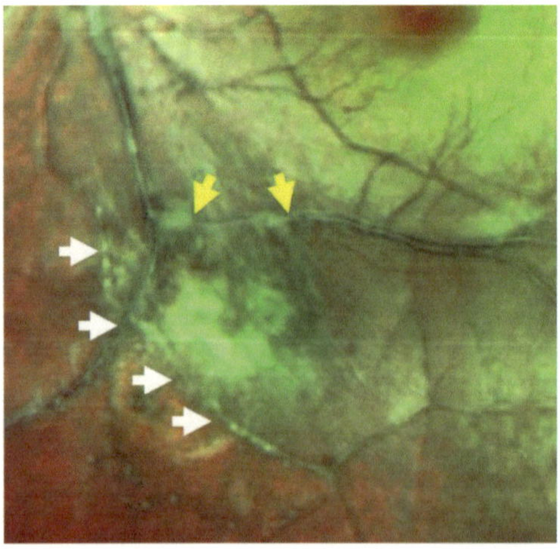

Figure 8.
Small Kyreilles plaques along the retinal artery (white arrow) adjacent to patch of toxoplasma retinitis with perivenular infiltrates (yellow arrow).

In 35% of the cases, retinitis was juxtapapillary **Figure 11**. In pure papillitis, the parasite affects the optic disc directly, causing a swollen papilla with sheathing of the peripapillary veins and there may be no concurrent active retinochoroiditis

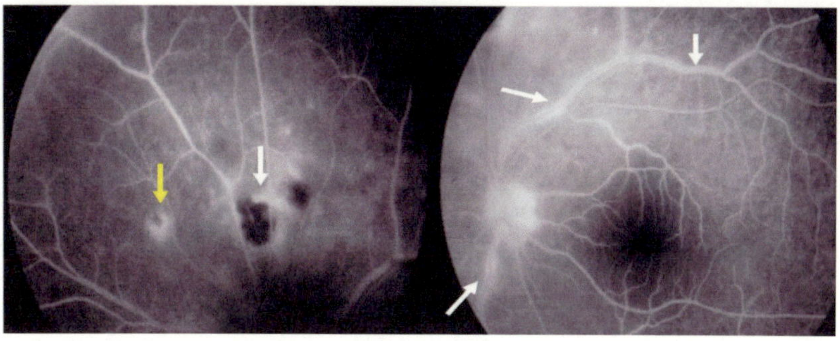

Figure 9.
Fundus fluorescein angiography (FFA) in the left image, exhibiting superior old hypofluorescent scar with adjacent active retinitis (white arrow) and supranasal active satellite lesion (yellow arrow). Perivenular leakage in the image on the right is evident supratemporally and infratemporally (white arrow) away from the actual foci of active retinitis.

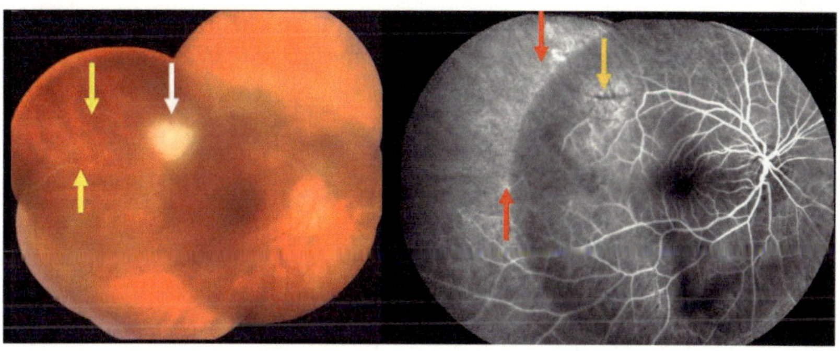

Figure 10.
Supratemporal thick toxoplasma retinitis along the supratemporal vessels (white arrow in the left side image) with occluded vessels distal to the lesion (yellow arrow). FFA performed after healing of the retinitis (right image), demonstrating an atrophic patch at previous site of retinitis (orange arrow) with occluded supratemporal vessels and a large area of retinal ischemia (red arrows).

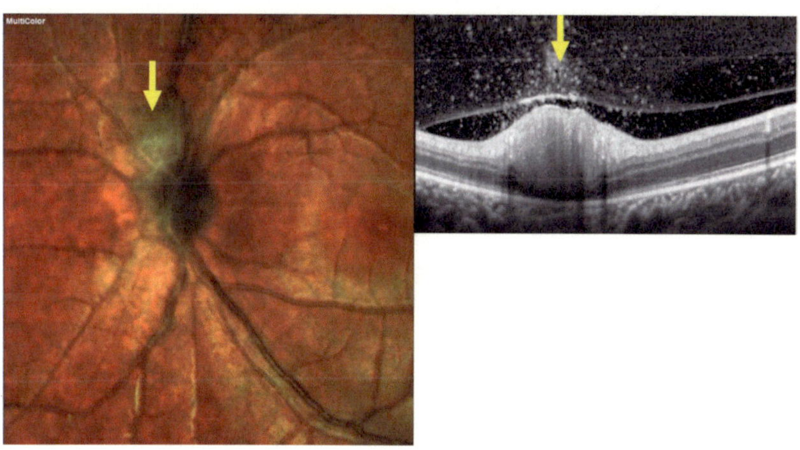

Figure 11.
Multicolored images (left side photo of superior peripapillary lesion (yellow arrow). OCT line scans through superior peripapillary lesion exhibiting almost full thickness retinitis with overlying localized dense vitritis (yellow arrow) in right side photo.

lesion [50]. Optic nerve involvement may induce severe visual field defects as well as loss of color vision [6]. Neuroretinitis has also been described as a unique presentation of ocular toxoplasmosis [51, 52].

3.2.4 Macular oedema in ocular toxoplasmosis

Macular oedema has been reported in 12% of toxoplasma cases [10]. Subretinal fluid accumulation (SRF) of variable severity, adjacent to area of retinochoroiditis involving the macula, has been described **Figure 12**. This was explained by. Khairallah, as the disrupted outer blood retinal barrier, secondary to the adjacent inflammatory process. Ultimately the fluid regresses as the retinitis heals [53].

Cystoid macular oedema (CME) may occur in active ocular toxoplasmosis with different phenotypes. Ouyang et al. reported that 7.5% of the cases presented with CME, while 2.5% presented with a huge outer retinal cyst (HORC). Interestingly, the same study reported that 3.5% of the cases showed cystoid degeneration in the inner retina next to the retinal vessels without other any retinal/choroidal abnormality in the macula [54].

HORC was described to be intraretinal cyst with a membranous structure bordering the outer border of that cyst **Figure 13**. Ouyang et al., hypothesized that this structure represents the tissue between ELM and the inner boundary of the RPE (i.e., photoreceptor layer), which further suggests that the lesion represents an intraretinal rather than a subretinal fluid accumulation. With regression of the fluid, the membranous structure resumes its anatomical location in the macular layer architecture [55].

3.2.5 Healing of toxoplasma retinocoroditis

Toxoplasma lesions healing starts to be appreciated as the vitritis regresses and the toxoplasma lesion starts to show more defined borders, because cicatrization occurs from the periphery towards the center, with variable pigmentary hyperplasia [32].

OCT is a sensitivity tool that has been used to study toxoplasma lesions in the active and healed stage [55, 56]. In the acute stage, retinal necrosis is detected by OCT as hypereflective disorganized thickening of the neurosensory retina. Underlying RPE clumping and disruption of the ELM and photoreceptors is seen. Choroidal inflammation may occasionally occur, and is detected by OCT appearing, hyporeflectivite thickening and, confined underneath area of retinitis. Overlying toxoplasma retinitis lesions, hyperreflective vitreous aggregates settling over inflamed retinal surface has also been reported [55].

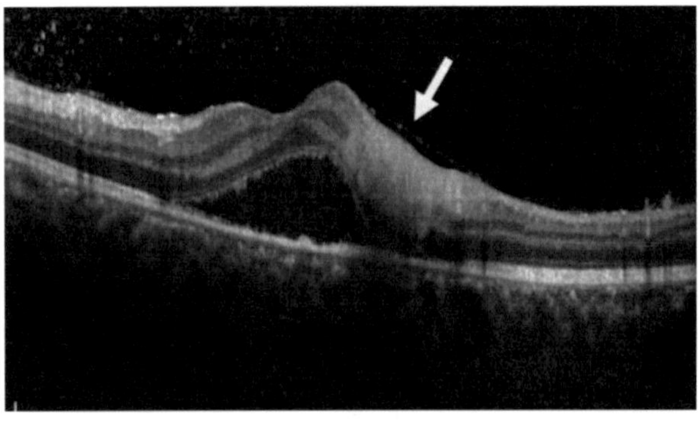

Figure 12.
Full thickness retinitis in OCT line scan indicated by the white arrow with adjacent foveal SRF.

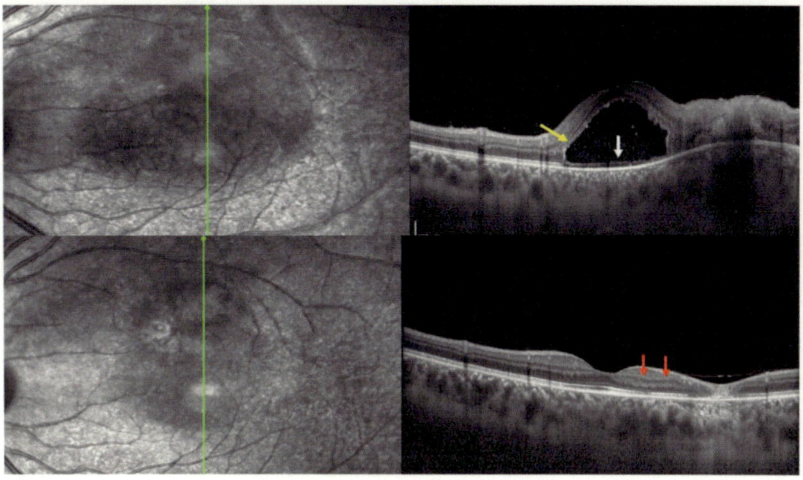

Figure 13.
***Photo on the top**: Superior parafoveal full thickness retinitis demonstrated by OCT line scan with adjacent large cystoid area within the outer plexiform layer (yellow arrow) and a thin membranous structure by the white arrow in the base of the cyst-. **Photo in the bottom** after resolution of the inflammation the cystoid space regresses, and the inner retinal layer resume the normal architecture (red arrow).*

As the retinitis starts to heal, the OCT scans show the hyperreflective area of retinitis, within the neurosensory retina starts to decrease in thickness with regressing of any adjacent SRF or CME. The RPE clumping starts to be more obvious and may show localized heaping which is likely the commencement of the pigmentary scar. As the hyperreflectivity of the retinitis recedes, degenerative cystoid spaces occasionally develop that resolves as healing reaches a final stage. The posterior hyaloid starts to get thicker, may exerts vitrocmacular traction, which occasionally may spontaneously be released, with the separation of the posterior hyaloid from the macular surface **Figure 14**.

Occasionally, when retinitis is severe and recalcitrant to treatment, upon eventually evolving into the healing stage, the retinal layers exhibit severe,

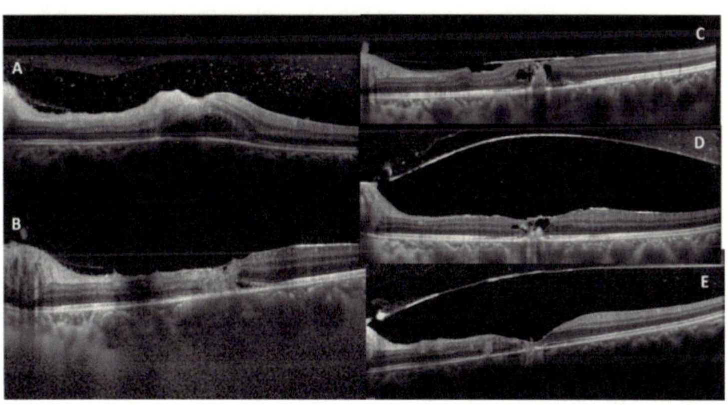

Figure 14.
OCT scan through the fovea demonstrating toxoplasma necrotizing retinitis evolving from the active stage into an atrophic healed scar tissue. A: Full thickness retinitis. B: The retinitis has resolved remarkably with evolution of small deep residual area foveally with overlying appearance of the thick posterior hyaloid. C: Decreased size of the residual deep hyperreflective material with adjacent degenerative cystoid spaces and vitreofovel tangential traction. D: As healing progresses, the posterior hyaloid detaches completely with release of the vitreofoveal traction. E: Complete resolution of the retinitis with atrophic appearance of the inner layers, resolved degenerative cyst and disrupted outer foveal layers.

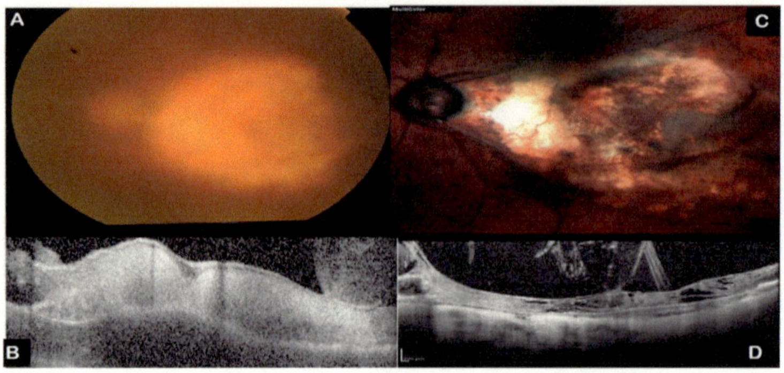

Figure 15.
55-year-old female patient with neglected toxoplasma retinitis a and B: Colored and OCT images respectively, exhibit large active retinitis involving all the macular area, with overlying dense vitritis. C and D multicolored and OCT images respectively, demonstrate photos after complete healing of the retinitis. D shows OCT image denoting complete disruption of the inner macular layers been replaced with laminated and split fibrosed tissue with focal area of traction parafoveally.

disorganization, thinning, with a fibrotic appearance, that may be laminated and splitted. Severe vitreomacular traction in such cases, can progress to retinal detachment **Figure 15**.

3.2.6 Ocular complications

Reported complications of ocular toxoplasmosis include isolated retinal tear (6%), retinal detachment, which is usually rhegmatogenous and/or tractional (6%), pre-retinal membrane (7%), choroidal neovascularization (<1%), vitreous hemorrhage (2%), optic atrophy (4%) and cataract (5%–13%) [10, 57].

3.2.7 Atypical toxoplasma retinitis in immunocompromised

Atypical manifestations include exceptionally large, multifocal, bilateral, diffuse retinal involvement or panophthalmitis. Elderly, AIDS, immunocompromised individual, or even rarely younger, immunocompetent patients as well [58] are likely to have specific defects in immune response that render them more at risk for atypical forms of toxoplasmosis [59]. This extensive toxoplasma retinitis presents similarly to necrotizing herpetic retinopathies, with large confluent full thickness areas of retinitis involving the peripheral retina and posterior pole. The thick, more densely yellow-white appearance of the lesion borders with a distinct, smooth contoured edge; and lack of hemorrhage, may distinguish these lesions from viral retinitis [60].

4. Recurrence and severity

4.1 Recurrence

Following an episode of toxoplasmic retinochoroiditis, the risk of recurrence is reportedly higher during the first year than during subsequent years: 29–32% of recurrences occur within 1 year, and 53–57% within 2 years [10, 32, 61].

Reasons for recurrences are not usually identified. They may arise from senescent changes in tissue cysts, with an accompanying release of parasites or antigens or as a result of trauma, hormonal fluctuations or even, transient immune responses of humoral or cellular nature [62]. Patients who are relatively young at the first presentation are at increased risk of recurrence compared to older patients who have been independently confirmed [63]. A larger retinal parasite load in younger patients is one explanation that Holland et al. offered for this observation [64]. In AIDS patients, recurrence is the rule in the absence of long-term antiparasitic therapy [65].

Pregnancy and cataract surgery have both been associated with an increased risk of reactivation [62, 66]. Bosch-Driessen and associates [10], reported that 9% of women with ocular toxoplasmosis developed recurrences during pregnancy. It has been hypothesized that this relationship is attributable to hormonal or immunological changes that occur during pregnancy [67].

4.2 Severity

There is substantial variation in the severity of intraocular toxoplasma inflammation, attributable to multiple host- and disease-related factors.

Individuals less than 60 years showed significantly higher incidence of having lesions less than1 disc area (DA) as compared to those above the age of 60, showing lesions more than 1DA in size with $P = 0.02$. The same study reported that larger lesions were associated with more severe vitreous humor inflammation [57]. Patients with AIDS develop extensive disease and frequently reactivate, if treatment is discontinued [68].

5. Diagnosis

Diagnosis of ocular toxoplasmosis starts at the point where the classic retinal manifestation is highly suggestive of the disease. However, in many instances the clinical findings cannot be sufficient to confirm a diagnosis, especially in the atypical form of presentation and thus laboratory investigations are necessary.

5.1 Serum serology

Ocular disease in the context of the presence of serum IgG and IgM antibodies against Toxoplasma gondii measured by screening tests such as the enzyme-linked immunosorbent assay (ELISA) or CLIA (Chemiluminescence immune assay) is compatible with acute or recent infection with toxoplasma supporting the diagnosis [69], yet can never be confirmatory, unless a definitive test like the dye test (Sabin-Feldman), IFAT (indirect fluorescent antibody test), immunoblot, and ISAGA (immunoglobulin-M immunosorbent agglutination assay) is performed. Nonetheless, these methods are performed only by specialized laboratories, they are complex and costly [70].

If retinitis develops within a year of an acquired systemic infection, anti-toxoplasma IgM should be detectable, but the variable rate of decline of this Ig isotype also limits the usefulness of such testing. The only exception is during pregnancy, when maternal IgM may herald acute infection of both the mother and foetus triggering urgent consultation with the obstetrician and neonatologist [71].

Since seropositivity is prevalent in most communities, the positive predictive value of IgG is low, and a positive IgG cannot be interpreted as indicative of active toxoplasmic infection. However, a rise in titer of specific IgG antibodies over a 3-week period has been used as an indicator of recent infection [72].

In immunosuppressed subjects, positive serological tests indicate infection, however, negative tests do not exclude previous or concurrent infections [73].

5.2 Goldman Witmer

Levels of antibodies in aqueous humor and their relationship to serum antibodies may help in establishing the diagnosis of ocular toxoplasmosis [74, 75]. The Goldmann-Witmer coefficient (GWC) has been proposed as a valuable index of intraocular antibody production in active toxoplasmic retinochoroiditis in the immunocompetent subject [76].

(GWC) is calculated as the proportion of specific immunoglobulin (Ig)G in ocular fluid versus serum samples. It is determined as follows (anti-Toxoplasma IgG in aqueous humor/total IgG in aqueous humor)/(anti-Toxoplasma IgG in serum/total IgG in serum). Although a ratio over one should indicate intraocular antibody production, this also occurs in healthy controls, and therefore a ratio of at least three is often preferred for certain diagnosis [77].

5.3 Polymerase chain reaction

The polymerase chain reaction (PCR) is an in-vitro method for exponentially replicating nucleic acids. PCR allows the detection and analysis of infinitesimal quantities of DNA. PCR of intraocular fluid has been extensively used to diagnosis infectious uveitis [78].

PCR testing of ocular sample can be useful in presumed toxoplasmosis in patients older than 50, in cases with inflammation (Tyndall ≥1/2+, panuveitis), area of retinochoroiditis>3 DA, and when ocular sampling performed within 1 week of presentation after onset of symptoms and up to 4 months [79, 80].

GWC testing is of better sensitivity than real time PCR, and is the preferred diagnostic procedure in ocular toxoplasmosis, especially if the testing is carried out in younger patients with quiet eyes and with smaller sized chorioretinal lesions [79].

Real time PCR confirmed the clinical diagnosis of toxoplasmosis in 62.5% of the cases, while the GWC confirmed in 87.5% [79]. Other studies reported that for 25 patients who suffered from ocular toxoplasmosis, the GWC was positive in 90%, while PCR testing was positive in just 36% [80]. Also, Labalette et al., noted the aqueous PCR was positive in 60% when lesions were larger than three-disc areas, but in only 25% when lesions were smaller. Overall, GWC was more likely positive than PCR (i.e., 89% vs. 44%) in this group [81]. Also, the rates of positive PCR are high in aqueous humor, obtained from HIV-infected or elderly subjects presenting toxoplasma retinitis [82].

6. Management

No drug has been proven to cure infection [5], therefore, the aim of antibiotic treatment is to reduce the duration and severity of symptoms of acute intraocular inflammation, the risk of permanent visual impairment (by reducing the size of the eventual retinochoroidal scar), and the risk of recurrent episodes [83].

6.1 Indication for treatment

In immunocompetent individuals, toxoplasma retinochoroiditis typically resolves over a period of 1 to 2 months [84].

Previous reports indicated that toxoplasma treatment was employed if dense vitritis developed, retinitis is located close to the optic nerve, papillomacular area, or close proximity of lesions to major retinal vessels or if decreased vision occurs [5]. However, Holland reported the results of a survey from1991 to 2001, where members of the AUS showed a shift in management over 10 years, were in favor of treatment of both mild and severe disease [85].

Treatment of active ocular toxoplasmosis in immunocompromised individuals regardless of the severity is the recommended practice with less debate [85].

6.2 Medical treatment

6.2.1 Systemic treatment

Several antimicrobial drug combinations are used to treat ocular toxoplasmosis.

6.2.1.1 Antiparasitic

Classic therapy is a combination of pyrimethamine 25 mg–50 mg daily orally with folinic acid 5 mg every other day and sulfadiazine 1 g four times daily orally with systemic corticosteroid [84]. Pyrimethamine side effects include gastrointestinal and dermatological manifestations as well as hematological adverse events, including leukopenia and thrombocytopenia, that mandate monitoring of the blood picture regularly throughout the treatment course. 26% of the patients on this regimen were reported to discontinue treatment due to complications from the drugs [5].

The alternate treatment regimen is trimethoprim-sulfamethoxazole 160 mg–800 mg twice daily orally with systemic corticosteroid, which is a well-tolerated combination although sulfonamide-related reactions may occur. The common side effects include mild gastrointestinal symptoms and mild maculopapular rash. However, this regimen is relatively well tolerated with side effects requiring discontinuation in 4% of patients [5].

Both pyrimethamine and sulfadiazine, as well as trimethoprim-sulfamethoxazole, have a similar mechanism of action, inhibiting tetrahydrofolate synthesis, thereby impacting nucleic acid synthesis of toxoplasma gondii. No reported difference in treatment results was reported when the classic or alternate treatment was used, however, treatment with classic therapy showed a greater reduction in the size of the retinal lesion than patients receiving other treatments or no treatment [5]. Other reports comparing these two regiments showed different results and concluded that drug efficacies in terms of reduction in retinal lesion size and improvement in visual acuity were similar. Reduction in the size of the lesion was comparable between the two treatment groups been 59% for trimethoprim-sulfamethoxazole and 61% for classic therapy, and there was no significant difference in post-treatment visual acuity. Therefore, trimethoprim/sulfamethoxazole seems to be an acceptable alternative for the treatment of ocular toxoplasmosis [86, 87].

Clindamycin 300 mg orally four times daily [84], is often added to triple therapy, which is then referred to as 'quadruple therapy'. Animal studies showed that clindamycin reduced numbers of tissue cysts [86]. However, experience has shown that it does not prevent recurrent disease in human beings [88]. Pseudomembranous colitis is a well-recognized potential complication of clindamycin, as well as diarrhea. Clindamycin continues to be the most popular supplemental agent for treatment of patients with severe or persistent disease.

Opremcak and associates reported a series of 16 patients who were treated for toxoplasmic retinochoroiditis with trimethoprim (160 mg)/sulfamethoxazole (800 mg). Four were treated with trimethoprim/sulfamethoxazole alone, four were treated with trimethoprim/sulfamethoxazole and clindamycin, and eight were treated with trimethoprim/ sulfamethoxazole, clindamycin and oral prednisone. They concluded that trimethoprim/sulfamethoxazole accelerated the rate of resolution of toxoplasmic retinochoroiditis and improved the visual outcomes of their patients, although the study was uncontrolled [89].

Atovaquone 750 mg three/four times daily orally or azithromycin 250 mg daily orally are two antiparasitic agents used for treatment of toxoplasma. However, these agents do not appear to prevent recurrent toxoplasmic retinochoroiditis in the human host convincing activity against encysted parasites in experiment systems [90, 91]. Atovaquone was well tolerated but reactivation was reported by Winterhalter et al., in 44% of the cases within an interval averaging 39 months. [92]. Azithromycin in treatment of ocular toxoplasmosis has shown regression of the retinitis within 1 month in 64% of the patients, however, 27% experienced recurrence within the first year of follow-up, thus debating the effectiveness in decreasing recurrences [91]. The effective potency of this drug with no reported side effects that needed stopping the drug while used in treatment of ocular toxoplasma has been reported [92].

6.2.1.2 Oral steroids

Recent research suggests that there is widespread variation for se of steroids in clinical practice for treating ocular toxoplasmosis. In a cross-sectional survey of uveitis specialists, 17% used oral corticosteroids in the treatment of ocular toxoplasmosis in immunocompetent patients, regardless of clinical findings. The other clinicians used corticosteroids for specific indications, such as severe vitreous inflammatory reaction (71%), decreased vision (59%), proximity of the lesions to the fovea or optic disc (35%), and for large lesions (5%) [93].

Oral corticosteroids are used during the active phase to reduce the retinal inflammation and thus further collateral tissue damage and also to prevent blood-retinal barrier breakdown. Furthermore, it can also reduce toxoplasma scarring. Steroids are usually started from 1 to 3 days after starting antiparasitic agent and continued for approximately 1 month. Indications for stopping therapy earlier include substantial improvement in the lesion appearance ("hardening" of lesion margins), substantial reduction of inflammatory reactions, marked improvement in vision, and adverse drug effects. Occasionally, antiparasitic agents are continued at least 2 days after stopping corticosteroids [84]. Oral corticosteroids are not used in immunocompromised individuals to treat ocular toxoplasma, thereby reducing the risk of further suppression of host defenses. Clinical series have shown that the signs of ocular toxoplasmosis, including inflammatory signs, can respond rapidly to antiparasitic therapy alone in immunocompromised patients [68, 94, 95].

6.2.2 Prophylactic treatment

Trimethoprim and sulfamethoxazole may be used in the prevention of recurrent attacks of ocular toxoplasmosis. Silveira et al. found that trimethoprim-sulfamethoxazole (160 mg–800 mg), taken orally every 3 days for 20 months, significantly reduced the risk of recurrent toxoplasmic retinochoroiditis from 23.8% in untreated control subjects to 6.6% [96].

The investigators suggested a role for such preventive treatment in patients with a history of frequent and severe recurrences or with toxoplasmic scars adjacent to the fovea where any reactivation can result in profound vision loss.

The rationale behind prophylactic treatment is the fact that recurrence rates decrease with duration of infection, even without treatment. If the frequency of recurrences decreases over time, it may be useful immediately after acquired infections to suppress recurrences during the period of greatest risk [96].

Recurrences of toxoplasmic retinochoroiditis may occur following LASIK and phacoemulsification with posterior chamber intraocular lens implantation [64, 97]. It is therefore recommended that prophylactic treatment be given to patients 2 days prior to surgery and to be continued for a period of 1 week.

6.2.3 Intravitreal treatment

Intravitreal clindamycin (1 mg) and dexamethasone (400 μg) have been used, injections can be repeated at 2-week intervals, based on a 5.6-day half-life of intravitreal clindamycin.

Soheilian et al. reported the results of treating patients with ocular toxoplasmosis involving or threatening macula or optic nerve, or adjacent to a large vessel and/or associated with severe vitritis with intravitreal treatment versus oral treatment using pyrimethamine and sulfadiazine plus prednisolone [98].

The mean number of injections in the intravitreal clindamycin was 1.6. Mean reduction in lesion size, increase in visual acuity and decrease in vitreous inflammation were not significantly different between groups, however, significantly reduction in size of lesions in IgM-positive patients who received classic treatment versus those who received intravitreal treatment was reported. This can be explained by the fact that a patient with acquired toxoplasmosis confronts a systemic infection that is treated better with systemic therapy.

The authors stressed that intravitreal clindamycin is a better alternative for pregnant and pediatric patients. Furthermore, the results of this study cannot be generalized to immunocompromised patients, monocular cases, and eyes with lesions inside the fovea (500 um). However, acquired toxoplasmosis confront systemic infection and, therefore, may benefit from systemic therapyas well, rather than just intravitreal injections [99].

6.2.4 Treatment of ocular toxoplasmosis during pregnancy

Bosch-Driessen and associates, reported that seven (9%) of 82 women with ocular toxoplasmosis developed recurrences during pregnancy [10]. Some reported, recurrent toxoplasma retinochoroiditis in a pregnant woman poses minimal risk to the fetus, and treatment is not indicated for the sole purpose of preventing vertical transmission [100]. However, other studies stressed that infection by toxoplasma will need treatment using spiramycin 1 g orally every 8 hours if a seronegative pregnant patient gets infected up to 18 weeks into the pregnancy or within the 6 months prior to pregnancy [71]. Intravitreal clindamycin can be a reasonable choice of treatment in pregnant mothers.

6.3 Surgical management

Vitreoretinal surgery may be indicated in cases of persistent vitreous opacities, tractional or rhegmatogenous retinal detachment. In the setting of severe refractory vitritis precluding fundus examination, pars plana vitrectomy may be used for both diagnostic and therapeutic purposes [85].

Retinal detachment was reported in 11.4% of the cases. 75% underwent pars plana vitrectomy and 25% underwent laser retinopexy. 50% presented with recurrent RD requiring scleral buckle. At final follow-up, all patients who underwent surgical repair had attached retinas; with severe vision loss of 20/200 or worse [101].

Cataract surgery with intraocular lens implantation is often indicated in cases of significant lens opacification, after resolution of inflammation.

7. Conclusion

Ocular toxoplasmosis presents in a myriad of manifestations in the eye with variable complications and can be vision depleting. Multimodal imaging is useful in carefully monitoring treatment response, detecting, regression or progression of toxoplasma lesions and also show complications such as vitreomacular traction, CNVs or even subtle SRF, that cannot be clinically detected early. Molecular biological advances have improved the ability for diagnosis. Though current treatment modalities are effective in healing active disease yet does not effectively prevent recurrence. Further studies could be dedicated to developing antimicrobials that can help eradicate the disease.

Acknowledgements

Al Watany Eye Hospital Cairo Egypt, the hospital I have worked at and learnt a lot over the years. The hospital is very supportive of research work and all the images included in this chapter were either captured in the hospital or were in the patient's electronic medical record. Retinal imaging team WEH dedicated hard work.

Conflict of interest

I have no financial disclosures or conflict of interest.

Thanks

'Special thanks to my dear Mother **Laila**, who has been my supportive backbone and has been ever encouraging, all the way through'.

Author details

Terese Kamal Gerges
Al Watany Eye Hospital, Cairo, Egypt

*Address all correspondence to:teresekamal@yahoo.com

References

[1] Montoya J, Liesenfeld O. Toxoplasmosis. Lancet. 2004; 363:1965-1976.

[2] Holland GN. Ocular toxoplasmosis: a global reassessment: Part I: epidemiology and course of disease. Am J Ophthalmol 2003; 136:973-988.

[3] Rothova A. Ocular manifestations of toxoplasmosis. Curr Opin Ophthalmol.2003;14:384-8.

[4] Wilder HC. Toxoplasma chorioretinitis in adults. Arch Ophthalmol 1952;48: 127-36.

[5] Rothova A, Meenken C, Buitenhuis HJ, et al. Therapy for ocular toxoplasmosis. Am J Ophthalmol.1993; 115:517-23. [PubMed: 8470726]

[6] Ozgonul C and. Besirli C G. : Recent Developments in the Diagnosis and Treatment of Ocular Toxoplasmosis; Ophthalmic Res 2017;57:1-12

[7] Glasner PD, Silveira C, Kruszon-Moran D, Martins MC, Júnior MB, Silveira S, Camargo ME, Nussenblatt RB, Kaslow RA, Júnior RB. An unusually high prevalence of ocular toxoplasmosis in southern Brazil. Am J Ophthalmol 1992; 114: 136-144.

[8] Holland GN. Ocular toxoplasmosis: new directions for clinical investigation. Ocul Immunol Inflamm 2000; 8: 1-7.

[9] Atmaca LS, Simsek T, Batioglu F. Clinical features and prognosis in ocular toxoplasmosis. Jpn J Ophthalmol 2003; 48: 386-391.

[10] Bosch-Driessen LE, Berendschot TT, Ongkosuwito JV, Rothova A. Ocular toxoplasmosis: clinical features and prognosis of 154 patients. Ophthalmology. 2002; 109:869-78.

[11] Jones JL, Kruszon-Moran D, Wilson M, McQuillan G, Navin T, McAuley JB. Toxoplasma gondii infection in the United States: seroprevalence and risk factors. Am J Epidemiol. 2001; 154:357-65.

[12] Moorthy RS, Smith RE, Rao NA. Progressive ocular toxoplasmosis in patients with acquired immunodeficiency syndrome. Am J Ophthalmol 1993; 115:742-7

[13] Chen KC, Jung JJ, Engelbert M. Single acquisition of the vitreous, retina and choroid with swept-source optical coherence tomography in acute toxoplasmosis. Retin Cases Brief Rep. 2016; 10:217-20.

[14] Rothova A. Ocular involvement in toxoplasmosis. Br J Ophthalmol. 1993; 77:371.

[15] Akstein RB, Wilson LA, Teutsch SM. Acquired toxoplasmosis. Ophthalmology 1982; 89:1299-302.

[16] Mets MB, Holfels E, Boyer KM, Swisher CN, Roizen N, Stein M et al. Ey3 manifestations of congenital toxoplasmosis. Am J Ophthalmol 1996;122: 309-324.

[17] Meenken C, Assies J, van Nieuwenhuizen O, Holwerda-van der Maat WG, van Schooneveld MJ, Delleman WJ et al. Long-term ocular and neurological involvement in severe congenital toxoplasmosis. Br J Ophthalmol 1995; 79: 581-584.

[18] Dunn D, Wallon M, Peyron F, Petersen E, Peckham C, Gilbert R. Mother-to-child transmission of toxoplasmosis: risk estimates for clinical counseling. Lancet 1999; 353: 1829-1833.

[19] Gilbert RE. Toxoplasmosis. In: Newel ML, McIntyre J (eds). Congenital and Perinatal Infections. Cambridge University Press: Cambridge, 2000, p 305.

[20] Peyron F, Wallon M, Bernardoux C. Long-term follow-up of patients with congenital ocular toxoplasmosis. N Engl J Med 1996; 334: 993-994.

[21] Orefice F, Pinheiro SRA, Ferreira CD. Calcificac¸o˜es no planocoro'ide –retina de pacientes com leso˜es cicatrizadas de toxoplasmose conge^nita diagnosticadas pela tomografia computadorizada. Rev Bras Oftalmol 1989; 48: 49-53.

[22] Bahia MD, Ore'fice F, Andrade CMQ. Ana'lise clı'nica das leso˜es d retinocoroidite em crianc¸as portadoras de toxoplasmose conge^nita. Rev Bras Oftalmol 1992; 51: 265-271.

[23] Vutova K, Peicheva Z, Popova A, Markova V, Mincheva N, Todorov T. Congenital toxoplasmosis: eye manifestations in infants and children. Ann Trop Paediatr 2002; 22: 213-218.

[24] Kodjikian L, Wallon M, Fleury J, Denis P, Binquet C, Peyron F et al. Ocular manifestations in congenital toxoplasmosis. Graefes Arch Clin Exp Ophthalmol 2006; 244: 14-21

[25] Melamed J, Eckert GU, Spadoni VS, Lago EG and Uberti F: Ocular manifestations of congenital toxoplasmosis: Eye 2010;24, 528-534

[26] Koppe JG, Loewer Sieger DH, de Roever Bonnet H. Results of 20-year follow-up of congenital toxoplasmosis. Lancet 1986; 1: 254-255.

[27] Mc Auley J, Boyer KM, Patel D, Mets M, Swisher C, Roizen N et al. Early and longitudinal evaluations of treated infants and children and untreated historical patients with congenital toxoplasmosis: the Chicago collaborative treatment trial. Clin Infect Dis 1994; 18: 38-72.

[28] Bre'zin AP, Thulliez P, Couvreur J, Nobre´ R, McLeod R, Mets MB. Ophthalmic outcomes after prenatal and postnatal treatment of congenital toxoplasmosis. Am J Ophthalmol 2003; 135: 779-784.

[29] McLeod R, Boyer K, Karrison T, Kasza K, Swisher C , Roizen N et al. Outcome of treatment for congenital toxoplasmosis, 1981-2004: The National Collaborative Chicago-based, Congenital Toxoplasmosis Study. Clin Infect Dis 2006; 42: 1383-1394.

[30] Friedmann CT, Knox DL. Variations in recurrent active toxoplasmic retinochoroiditis. Arch Ophthalmol. 1969; 81:481-93. [PubMed: 5777756]

[31] Montoya JG, Liesenfeld O. Toxoplasmosis. Lancet. 2004; 363:1965-76. [PubMed: 15194258]

[32] Bonfioli AA, Orefice F. Toxoplasmosis. Seminars in ophthalmology 2005; 20: 129-141.

[33] Westfall AC, Lauer AK, Suhler EB, Rosenbaum JT. Toxoplasmosis retinochoroiditis and elevated intraocular pressure: a retrospective study. J Glaucoma. 2005; 14:3-10

[34] Holland GN, Muccioli C , Silveira C, Weisz JM, Belfort R Junior and O'Connor GR. Intraocular Inflammatory Reactions Without Focal Necrotizing Retinochoroiditis in Patients with Acquired Systemic Toxoplasmosis. Am J Ophthamol. 1999; 128:413-420. PMID: 10577581

[35] Doft BH, Gass JDM. Punctate outer retinal toxoplasmosis. Arch Ophthalmol. 1985;103(9): 1332-1336.

[36] Doft BH, Gass JD. Outer retinal layer toxoplasmosis. Graefes Arch Clin Exp Ophthalmol. 1986; 224:78-82. [PubMed: 3943742]

[37] Fujiwara T, Machida S, Hasegawa Y and Tazawa Y. Punctae outer retinal toxoplasmosis with multiple choroidal neovascularization. Journal of Retina

and Vitreous Disease 2006: 29: (3); 360-362.

[38] Eduardo Cunha de Souza, MD; Antonio M. B. Casella, MD. Clinical and Tomographic Features of Macular Punctate Outer Retinal Toxoplasmosis Arch Ophthalmol. 2009;127(10):1390-1394.

[39] Theodossiadis P, Kokolakis S, Ladas I, Kollia AC, Chatzoulis D, Theodossiadis G. Retinal vascular involvement in acute toxoplasmic retinochoroiditis. Int Ophthalmol. 1995; 19:19-24. [PubMed: 8537191]

[40] Kyrieleis W. Ueber atypische gefaesstuberkulose der netzhaut (Periarteritis 'nodosa' tuberculosa). Arch Augenheilkd 1933; 107: 182-90

[41] Gass JDM. Stereoscopic Atlas of macular disease: diagnosis and treatment. St Louis, CV Mosby Co, pp 464-466, 1987.

[42] Pakalin S, Arnaud B. Arterial occlusion associated with toxoplasmic chorioretinitis. J Fr Ophthalmol 1990; 13 (11-12): 554-6

[43] Braunstein RA, Gass JDM. Branch artery obstruction caused by acute toxoplasmosis. Arch Ophthalmo11980; 98: 512-3.

[44] Morgan CM, Gragoudas E. Branch ~ retinal artery occlusion associated with recurrent toxoplasmic retinochoroiditis. Arch Ophthalmo11987; 105: 130.

[45] Williamson TH, Meyer PA. Br J Ophthalmol (letter) 1991;75: 253.

[46] O'Connor GR. The influence of hypersensitivity on the pathogenesis of ocular toxoplasmosis. Trans Am Ophthalmol Soc 1970; 68: 501-47.

[47] O'Connor GR. Ocular toxoplasmosis. Jpn J Ophthalmo11975i 19: 1-24.

[48] Borruat FX, Kapoor R, Sanders MD. Simultaneous retinal and optic nerve lesions in toxoplasmosis: the advantages of magnetic resonance imaging. Br J Ophthalmol. 1993; 77:450-2.[PubMed: 8343477]

[49] Song A, Scott IU, Davis JL, Lam BL. Atypical anterior optic neuropathy caused by toxoplasmosis.Am J Ophthalmol. 2002; 133:162-4. [PubMed: 11755864]

[50] Eckert GU, Melamed J, Menegaz B. Optic nerve changes in ocular toxoplasmosis. Eye (Lond).2007; 21:746-51. [PubMed: 16575416]

[51] Roach ES, Zimmerman CF, Troost BT, Weaver RG. Optic neuritis due to acquired toxoplasmosis. Pediatr Neurol. 1985; 1:114-6. [PubMed: 3880394]

[52] Fish RH, Hoskins JC, Kline LB. Toxoplasmosis neuroretinitis. Ophthalmology 1993; 100:1177-1182.

[53] Khairallah M, Yahia SB, Zaouali S et al. Acute choroidal ischemia associated with toxoplasmic retinochoroiditis. Retina 2007; 27:947-951.

[54] Ouyang Y, Pleyer U, Shao Q, Keane PA, Stu¨ biger N, et al. (2014) Evaluation of Cystoid Change Phenotypes in Ocular Toxoplasmosis Using Optical Coherence Tomography. PLoS ONE 9(2): e86626. DOI: 10.1371/journal.pone.0086626

[55] Park HJ, Lee S and Lee EK. Morphological characteristics of ocular toxoplasmosis and its regression pattern on swept-source optical coherence tomography angiography: a case report. BMC Ophthalmology 2019; 19:199 DOI:10.1186/s12886-019-1209-8

[56] Ammar F, Mahjoub A, Abdesslam N, Knani L, Ghorbel M, Mahjoub H. Spectral optical coherence tomography findings in patients with

ocular toxoplasmosis: A case series study. Annals of Medicine and Surgery 54 (2020) 125-128. DOI; 10.1016/j.amsu.2020.04.008

[57] Dodds EM, Holland GN, Stanford MR, et al. Intraocular inflammation associated with ocular toxoplasmosis: relationships at initial examination. Am J Ophthalmol. 2008; 146:856-65. e2. [PubMed: 19027421]

[58] Moshfeghi DM, Lowder CY, Dodds EM, et al. Diagnostic approaches to severe, atypical toxoplasmosis mimicking acute retinal necrosis. Ophthalmology 2004; 111:716-725

[59] Johnson MW, Greven CM, Jaffe GJ, et al. Atypical, severe toxoplasmic retinochoroiditis in elderly patients. Ophthalmology 1997; 104:48-57.

[60] Elkins BS, Holland GN, Opremcak EM, et al. Ocular toxoplasmosis misdiagnosed as cytomegalovirus retinopathy in immunocompromised patients. Ophthalmology 1994;101: 499-507.

[61] Amaro MH, Muccioli C, Abreu MT et al. Remote hypofluorescent dots in recurrent ocular toxoplasmosis on indocyanine green angiography. Arq Bras Oftalmol 2007:70:901-904

[62] Holland GN. Ocular toxoplasmosis: a global reassessment. Part II: disease manifestations and management. Am. J. Ophthalmol. 2004; 137, 1-17. DOI: 10.1016/j.ajo.2003.10.032

[63] Garweg JG, Scherrer JN, Halberstadt M. Recurrence characteristics in European patients with ocular toxoplasmosis. Br J Ophthalmol. 2008; 92:1253-6. [PubMed: 18211930]

[64] Holland GN, Crespi CM, ten Dam-van Loon N, et al. Analysis of recurrence patterns associated with toxoplasmic retinochoroiditis. Am J Ophthalmol. 2008; 145:1007-13. [PubMed: 18343351]

[65] Pivetti-Pezzi P, Accorinti M, Tamburi S, Ciapparoni V, Abdulaziz MA. Clinical features of toxoplasmic retinochoroiditis in patients with acquired immunodeficiency syndrome. Ann Ophthalmol. 1994; 26:73-84. [PubMed: 7944160]

[66] Bosch-Driessen LH, Plaisier MB, Stilma JS, Van der Lelij A, Rothova A. Reactivations of ocular toxoplasmosis after cataract extraction. Ophthalmology. 2002; 109:41-5. [PubMed: 11772577]

[67] O'Connor GR. Factors related to the initiation and recurrence of uveitis: XL Edward Jackson Memorial Lecture. Am J Ophthalmol 1983; 96:577-599.

[68] Holland GN, Engstrom R, Glasgow BJ, et al. Ocular toxoplasmosis in patients with the acquired immunodeficiency syndrome. Am J Ophthalmol 1988; 106:653-667.

[69] Liesenfeld O, Press C, Montoya JG et al. Falsepositive results in immunoglobulin M (IgM) toxoplasma antibody tests and importance of confirmatory testing: the Platelia Toxo IgM test. J Clin Microbiol 1997; 35:174-178

[70] Montoya JG, Remington JS. Management of Toxoplasma gondii infection during pregnancy. Clin Infect Dis. 2008; 47:554-66. [PubMed: 18624630]

[71] Villard, O., Cimon, B., L'ollivier, C., Fricker-Hidalgo, H., Godineau, N., Houze, S., & Candolfi, E. (2016). Serological diagnosis of Toxoplasma gondii infection: recommendations from the French National Reference Center for Toxoplasmosis. Diagnostic Microbiology and Infectious Disease, 84(1), 22-33.

[72] Ronday MJ, Luyendijk L, Baarsma GS, Bollemeijer JG, Van der Lelij A, Rothova A. Presumed acquired ocular toxoplasmosis. Arch Ophthalmol. 1995; 113:1524-9. [PubMed: 7487620]

[73] Pinon JM, Foudrinier F, Mougeot G et al (1995) Evaluation of risk and diagnostic value of quantitative assays for anti-Toxoplasma gondii immunoglobulin A (IgA), IgE, and IgM and analytical study of specifi c IgG in immunodefi cient patients. J Clin Microbiol 1995; 33:878-884.

[74] Garweg JG. Determinants of immunodiagnostic success in human ocular toxoplasmosis. Parasite Immunol 2005; 27:61-68

[75] Oliveira AA, Oréfi ce F, Nascimento E. The aqueous humor antibodies coeffi cient: part I. Arq Bras Oftalmol .1988;51:237-238

[76] Desmonts G Definitive serological diagnosis of ocular toxoplasmosis. Arch Ophthalmol.1966; 76:839-851

[77] De Boer JH, Luyendijk L, Rothova A, Kijlstra A. Analysis of ocular fluids for local antibody production in uveitis. Br J Ophthalmol. 1995; 79:610-6. [PubMed: 7626580]

[78] Russell N. Van Gelder Henry J. Kaplan Application of the polymerase chain reaction to the diagnosis of uveitis Ocular Immunology and Inflammation –1998, Vol. 6, No. 2, pp. 129-134

[79] Errera M, Goldschmidt P, Batellier L, Degorge S, Héron E, Laroche L. Real-time polymerase chain reaction and intraocular antibody production for the diagnosis of viral versus toxoplasmic infectious posterior uveitis Graefes Arch Clin Exp Ophthalmol 2011; 249:1837-1846

[80] Westeneng AC, Rothova A, De Boer JH, de Groot-Mijnes JD. Infectious uveitis in immunocompromised patients and the diagnostic value of polymerase chain reaction and Goldmann– Witmer coefficient in aqueous analysis. Am J Ophthalmol 2007; 144:781-785.

[81] Labalette P, Delhaes L, Margaron F, Fortier B, Rouland JF. Ocular toxoplasmosis after the fifth decade. Am J Ophthalmol. 2002; 133:506-15. [PubMed: 11931784]

[82] Rothova A, de Boer JH, Ten Dam-van Loon NH, et al. Usefulness of aqueous humor analysis for the diagnosis of posterior uveitis. Ophthalmology. 2008; 115:306-11

[83] Rothova A, Buitenhuis HJ, Meenken C, et al. Therapy of ocular toxoplasmosis. Int Ophthalmol 1989; 13:415-9.

[84] Holland GN, Lewis KG. An update on current practices in the management of ocular toxoplasmosis. Am J Ophthalmol. 2002; 134:102-14. [PubMed: 12095816]

[85] Smith JR, Cunningham ET Jr. Atypical presentations of ocular toxoplasmosis. Curr Opin Ophthalmol. 2002; 13:387-92.

[86] Soheilian M, Sadoughi MM, Ghajarnia M, et al. Prospective randomized trial of trimethoprim/sulfamethoxazole versus pyrimethamine and sulfadiazine in the treatment of ocular toxoplasmosis.Ophthalmology. 2005; 112:1876-82.

[87] McMaster PR, Powers KG, Finerty JF, Lunde MN. The effect of two chlorinated lincomycin analogues against acute toxoplasmosis in mice. Am J Trop Med Hyg 1973; 22:14-17.

[88] Lakhanpal V, Schocket SS, Nirankari VS. Clindamycin in the treatment of toxoplasmic retinochoroiditis. Am J Ophthalmol 1983; 95:605-613.

[89] Opremcak EM, Scales DK, Sharpe MR. Trimethoprimsulfamethoxazole therapy for ocular toxoplasmosis. Ophthalmology 1992; 99:920-925.

[90] Pearson PA, Piracha AR, Sen HA, Jaffe GJ. Atova-quone for the treatment of toxoplasma retinochoroiditis in immunocompetent patients. Ophthalmology. 1999; 106:148-53. [PubMed: 9917796]

[91] Rothova A, Bosch-Driessen LE, van Loon NH, Treffers WF. Azithromycin for ocular toxoplasmosis. Br J Ophthalmol. 1998; 82:1306-8

[92] Winterhalter S, Severing K, Stammen J, Maier AK, Godehardt E, Joussen AM. Does atovaquone prolong the disease-free interval of toxoplasmic retinochoroiditis? Graefes Arch Clin Exp Ophthalmol. 2010; 248:1187-92.

[93] Bosch-Driessen LH, Verbraak FD, Suttorp-Schulten MS, et al. A prospective, randomized trial of pyrimethamine and azithromycin vs pyrimethamine and sulfadiazine for the treatment of ocular toxoplasmosis. Am J Ophthalmol. 2002; 134:34-40. [PubMed: 12095805]

[94] Gagliuso DJ, Teich SA, Friedman AH, Orellana J. Ocular toxoplasmosis in AIDS patients. Trans Am Ophthalmol Soc 1990; 88:63-86.

[95] Cochereau-Massin I, Lehoang P, Lautier-Frau M, et al. Ocular toxoplasmosis in human immunodeficiency virus infected patients. Am J Ophthalmol 1992; 114:130-135.

[96] Jasper S, Vedula SS, John SS, Horo S, Sepah YJ, Nguyen QD. Corticosteroids as adjuvant therapy for ocular toxoplasmosis. Cochrane Database of Systematic Reviews 2017, Issue 1. DOI: 10.1002/14651858.CD007417.

[97] Silveira C, Belfort R Jr, Muccioli C, et al. The effect of long-term intermittent trimethoprim/ sulfamethoxazole treatment on recurrences of toxoplasmic retinochoroiditis. Am J Ophthalmol. 2002; 134:41-6.

[98] Soheilian M, Ramezani A, Azimzadeh A, et al. Randomized trial of intravitreal clindamycin and dexamethasone versus pyrimethamine, sulfadiazine, and prednisolone in treatment of ocular toxoplasmosis. Ophthalmology. 2011; 118:134-41.

[99] Barbara A, Shehadeh-Masha'our R, Sartani G, Garzozi HJ. Reactivation of ocular toxoplasmosis after LASIK. J Refract Surg. 2005;21(6):759-761.

[100] Holland, GN.; O'Connor, GR.; Belfort, R., Junior; Remington, JS. Toxoplasmosis. In: Pepose, JS.;Holland, GN.; Wilhelmus, KR., editors. Ocular Infection & Immunity. St. Louis: Mosby; 1996. p.1183-223.

[101] Ambar F, Steven Y , Eric SB, Justine SR and Christina F J. Retinal Detachment associated with ocular toxoplasmosis. Retina: 2015; 35: 2, 358-363

Section 3

Endophthalmitis

Chapter 5

Acute Postoperative Infectious Endophthalmitis: Advances in Diagnosis and Treatment

Sergio E. Hernandez-Da Mota,
Jose Luis Guerrero-Naranjo, Jose Dalma-Weiszhausz,
Raul Velez-Montoya and Jesus H. Gonzalez-Cortes

Abstract

Acute postoperative infectious endophthalmitis remains one of the most dreaded complications of ophthalmic surgery. One of the keys to success in treating this complication is to make an early clinical diagnosis and, if possible, an etiologic diagnosis that can guide treatment with antibiotic therapy. Different antibiotic therapy modalities have emerged over the years that have made it possible to treat even resistant strains of various microorganisms that cause endophthalmitis. Another relevant advance made in the etiological diagnosis of endophthalmitis is the advent of molecular biology techniques, such as the real-time polymerase chain reaction, which can detect minimal amounts of the genetic material of the causative microorganism present in the vitreous in a short period of time, thus improving treatment outcomes with better-guided therapy with intravitreal antibiotics. Aside from advances in postoperative diagnosis methods, the surgical treatment of endophthalmitis has had significant improvements in vitrectomy techniques, and in many cases, it has been proposed as the first-line treatment concomitantly with intravitreal antibiotic therapy. Moreover, there is increasing evidence that prophylaxis with intracameral antibiotic therapy further decreases postoperative endophthalmitis incidence.

Keywords: Acute postoperative endophthalmitis, vitrectomy, intravitreal antibiotics, polymerase chain reaction

1. Introduction

Acute postoperative infectious endophthalmitis (APIE) is an uncommon complication of eye surgery. It generally causes severe inflammation, which could significantly damage the ocular tissues and often has a poor prognosis, especially if it is not diagnosed and treated promptly [1–4].

APIE etiology is varied, being bacterial, the most frequent cause [3, 4]. Different ways to corroborate the microbiological diagnosis, such as a Gram staining on a smear and culture, have been described [2, 4]. Nonetheless, the use of molecular biology methods like the polymerase chain reaction (PCR) and other novel diagnostic tests has increased the speed and accuracy of etiologic diagnosis [2].

For several decades, intravitreal antibiotics injection (IAI) has been one of APIE treatment's mainstays [3, 4]. In recent years, the application of new antibiotic classes has been described, especially to treat APIE caused by resistant strains of the most prevalent causative pathogens [5]. Moreover, vitrectomy has become a crucial adjunctive therapeutic modality for infectious endophthalmitis [3–7]. Thanks to development in instrumentation and vitrectomy systems, visual results in APIE patients have consistently improved in recent years [6, 7].

2. Epidemiology

The incidence of APIE after cataract surgery has decreased considerably in the era of small incision surgery. In some reports, the incidence of APIE ranges from 0.12% to 1–3% [6, 7]. In patients undergoing trabeculectomy, the risk of developing endophthalmitis at five years is 1.1%, and the cumulative risk at 20 years can be as high as 20% [2–6, 8, 9]. The rate of endophthalmitis after endothelial keratoplasty and penetrating keratoplasty has been reported in up to 0.2% and 0.7%, respectively [10]. Regarding vitrectomy, the incidence of endophthalmitis tends to be relatively low. Some publications indicate an incidence of 0.05 to 0.06% [6]. Incidence of APIE following intravitreal injection of anti-VEGF agents is also infrequent. In one series of 10,164 injections only 3 cases of endophthalmitis were reported (0.030%) [1].

3. Risk factors

Multiple factors increase the likelihood of APIE in patients undergoing intraocular surgery. Some intraoperative complications such as posterior capsular rupture with or without vitreous loss, hypotony with aqueous humor filtration, especially in cases of clear corneal wounds and increased manipulation of intraocular tissues, are some factors that may raise the possibility of developing infectious endophthalmitis [3, 4, 11, 12].

The presence of inflammatory-infectious processes on the ocular surface or adnexa, such as conjunctivitis, keratitis, blepharitis, and dacryocystitis also, increases the incidence of endophthalmitis [4]. Additional systemic factors include advanced age [12] and chronic systemic debilitating diseases, such as diabetes mellitus (DM), malignancies, congenital or acquired immunodeficiencies and immunosuppression [3, 4, 12]. Patients with DM represent significant changes in the conjunctival flora, representing an important subgroup of patients who might develop endophthalmitis [3, 4].

APIE risk factors after anti-VEGF intravitreal injections, include not wearing a face mask, not using povidone prior to the injection and speaking while performing the injection [12].

A systematic review and meta-analysis [11] of the risk factors for APIE following cataract surgery, reported that there is a significant association between male gender and APIE. The overall OR for male gender was 1.43 (95% CI 1.29, 1.58). There was a significant association between extra- or intracapsular cataract extraction and APIE (OR 2.19, 95% CI 1.40, 3.42) compared with phacoemulsification. Furthermore, intracameral cefuroxime had a protective effect against APIE compared with topical antibiotics alone (OR 5.48, 95% CI 3.79, 7.92).

Analysis of the included retrospective studies in the meta-analysis showed that posterior capsular rupture was also a significant risk factor of APIE (OR 6.33, 95%

CI 4.22, 9.49), and a significant increase in risk of APIE with other intraoperative complications (OR 4.95, 95% CI 2.31, 10.63) was observed, as well.

4. Etiology

Multiple microorganisms may cause APIE [3, 4]. Bacterial pathogens are the most common [4]. Gram-positive cocci are responsible for 65–80% of APIE cases, mainly *Staphylococcus spp.* [12, 13].

Staphylococci belong to the *Micrococcaceae* family and have a diameter of between 0.2 and 12 microns [3, 14, 15]. The most common staphylococci species that cause endophthalmitis are coagulase-negative Staphylococci and *Staphylococcus aureus*.

Among all Staphylococci, *Staphylococcus epidermidis*, a coagulase-negative staphylococci, has emerged as the main cause of APIE [4, 13]. These bacteria have the property of producing an exopolysaccharide, which can be a factor that hampers phagocytosis and induces antibiotic resistance, including methicillin and beta-lactam antibiotics. However, these microorganisms are almost always susceptible to vancomycin [3].

Staphylococcus aureus is a non-spore-forming facultative aerobic microorganism that colonizes human skin. It produces different enzymes such as catalase, coagulase, beta-lactamase, many of which, are related to its pathogenicity [14, 15]. *Staphylococcus aureus* is the second most common bacteria isolated in cases of APIE [3, 13].

Other causes of APIE include Streptococci, Gram-positive bacilli, Gram-negative cocci, and Gram-negative bacilli [4].

Streptococci are facultative Gram-positive, aerobic microorganisms or obligate anaerobes and produce various toxins that increase their virulence. They are also sensitive to vancomycin [3].

Gram-positive bacilli causative agents of endophthalmitis include bacteria from the Bacillus genus. The most common intraocular Gram-positive bacilli pathogen is *Bacillus cereus* [3, 4]. Bacillus is a spore-forming rod that is Gram-positive or Gram-variable. It produces extracellular products, including toxins that induce severe inflammation when injected into the eye. Bacillus infection risk factors include foreign bodies, immunosuppression from malignant tumors, corticosteroid use, penetrating and perforating trauma, as well as acquired immunodeficiency syndrome. The infection is quite virulent and may significantly damage the eye in less than 24 hours. Systemically, it may induce fever and leukocytosis [3]. Vancomycin is the first-line drug used against *Bacillus spp.*

The genus *Pseudomonas* are Gram-negative, strictly aerobic organisms found in soil and water. They are part of the normal human flora but are predominantly isolated in cases of nosocomial infection [3]. *Pseudomonas aeruginosa* is the most common Gram-negative bacteria causing APIE, but other species have also been isolated [3, 16]. The pathogenesis of the infectious disease caused by *Pseudomonas* includes the production of extracellular enzymes and other toxic proteins and hemolysin, endotoxin, and exotoxin A, which explain the fulminant and severe nature of its clinical presentation [3]. *Pseudomonas spp.* are usually sensitive to aminoglycosides and ceftazidime [3].

Other bacteria members of the *Enterobacteriaceae* family may cause APIE. *Enterobacteriaceae* is a group of Gram-negative, facultative aerobes. They are distributed in the soil and plants, and colonize the human and animals' gastrointestinal tract [3].

Type of surgery	Most frequently isolated microorganisms
Cataract	Gram-positive bacteria (95% of culture-positive isolates). 70% of gram-positive bacteria are coagulase-negative Staphylococci
Trabeculectomy	Early-onset bleb related endophthalmitis: coagulase-negative staphylococcus. Late-onset: Streptococcus species
Glaucoma drainage implants	Streptococcus species, Staphlycoccus and *Haemophilus influenzae*
Vitrectomy	Gram-positive cocci account for more than 90% positive cultures
Penetrating keratoplasty	Coagulase-negative Staphylococci and Methicillin-resistant *Staphylococcus aureus*

Table 1.
Most frequently isolated microorganisms in different types of eye surgery [10, 12].

Fungal endophthalmitis is an infrequent cause of APIE; however, it should be considered as a possible pathogen [4]. *Candida, Aspergillus spp, Histoplasma*, and *Blastomyces dermatitidis* are some of the fungal microorganisms that may cause APIE.

Candida albicans is frequently found as part of the normal flora on the mucosal surfaces, and is the most common cause of fungal APIE, followed by *Aspergillus spp.* Patients that become immunocompromised by debilitating conditions such as AIDS, and other malignancies may also carry a higher risk for developing *Candida* APIE **Table 1** [4]. Summarizes the most frequently isolated microorganisms in different types of eye surgery.

5. Diagnosis

5.1 Signs and symptoms

The diagnosis of APIE is eminently clinical at onset. Intraocular surgery, mainly cataract surgery, is usually a painless procedure in the vast majority of cases [4, 12]. The sudden appearance of red eye, pain, and blurred vision as symptoms in the early postoperative period of patients that have undergone any intraocular surgery should always alert the surgeon to the possibility of APIE, although it is considered a rare but feared and devastating postoperative complication [3].

Common signs that may occur at onset are palpebral erythema and edema, ciliary injection, and conjunctival chemosis, corneal edema, hypopyon, anterior chamber cells, and vitreous haze due to vitritis (**Figures 1** and **2**). It is essential to mention that most endophthalmitis cases present between the third and tenth postoperative day, and 88% of the cases occur within six weeks after surgery (**Table 2**) [3, 4].

Fundus evaluation should be performed to determine the vitreous clarity, and to establish the status of the retina and the optic nerve. If fundus visualization is not feasible, linear B-ultrasound examination is mandatory to evaluate the posterior segment and rule out vitreous hemorrhage, retained lens material, retinal detachment, choroidal thickening, or the presence of membranes [4, 17].

5.2 Microbiology diagnosis

Samples obtained from anterior-chamber aspiration and vitreous needle biopsy or pars plana vitrectomy (PPV) should be process for smear and cultured

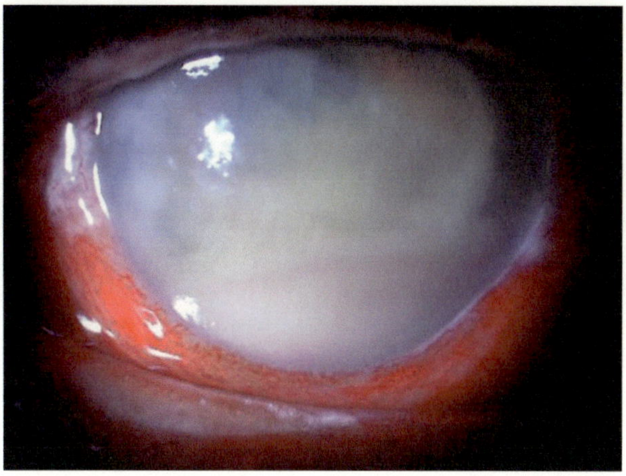

Figure 1.
Clinical image of a case of an acute postoperative infectious endophthalmitis caused by Pseudomonas aeruginosa, *showing prominent ciliary injection and conjunctival chemosis, a 3 mm hypopyon, and marked anterior chamber inflammatory infiltrate that obstructs visualizing the anterior segment details.*

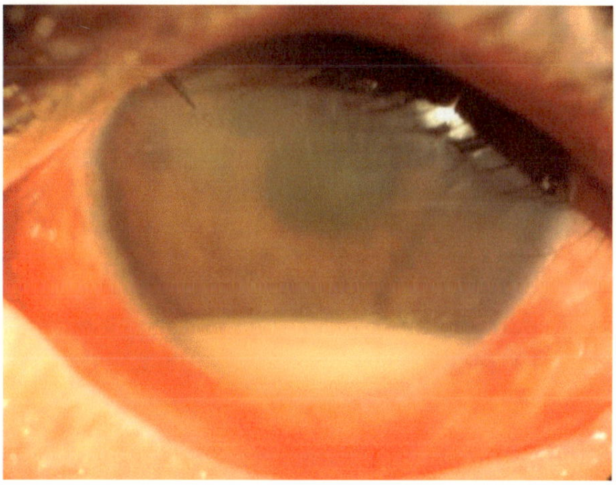

Figure 2.
Clinical image of a case of an infectious endophthalmitis 3 days after phacoemulsification surgery caused by Staphylococcus epidermidis. *The presence of hypopyon, corneal folds and edema, ciliary injection and cloudy media are observed.*

separately. The sample obtained from the vitreous should be undiluted and taken directly from the vitrectomy line. This has the potential advantage of having an adequate amount of bacterial load to grow in the culture plates, thus increasing the sensitivity of the culture to identify the possible APIE causative microorganism.

Alternatively, cassette washings from PPV should be concentrated by a centrifuge before culture and staining [3, 4]. Samples are placed on glass slides and stained using Gram and Giemsa stains. Obtained samples are plated on blood, thioglycolate, chocolate, and Saboraud agars and cultured under both, anaerobic and aerobic conditions. Whenever possible, it is advisable to place the obtained samples directly on agar plates in the operating room for better yield. They should be at room temperature by the time they are used, avoiding using them at refrigeration temperature because microbial growth might be reduced. Care should be taken to avoid contamination while placing the samples on the plates or transport media.

Symptoms	Percentage present in endophthalmitis patients
Blurred vision	94%
Red eye	82%
Pain	74%
Lid edema	36%
Signs	
Hypopyon	86%
Red eye	82%
Loss of fundus visualization	79%
Corneal infiltrate	5%

Table 2.
Percentage of presentation of common symptoms and signs in acute postoperative infectious endophthalmitis [4].

The endophthalmitis vitrectomy study (EVS) study reported positive cultures from 69.3% of biopsied cases using traditional agar plates and broth culture methods [13].

These conventional microbiology methods are commonly used for laboratory identification and antibiotic sensitivity tests of pathogens in APIE cases. Disadvantages of culture, include a low sensitivity and specificity for bacterial detection in the aqueous and vitreous humor, and are time-consuming [3, 4]. Nonetheless, whenever a minimal suspicion of infectious endophthalmitis exists, smear and culture are mandatory. Vitreous sample for culture gets a better yield than aqueous humour.

Disadvantages of lack of a microbiological confirmation in cases of APIE include non-response to IAI, increased morbidity from prolonged infection, repeated biopsies and IAI, and the potential to require performing more surgeries [4].

6. Polymerase chain reaction techniques and other novel methodologies for the diagnosis of acute postoperative endophthalmitis

Since the advent of PCR, molecular laboratory techniques have increased rapidly. Its use is part of many routine processing of clinical samples in microbiology laboratories, establishing a new era for diagnosing infectious diseases [17]. The use of PCR for APIE diagnosis increases significantly bacterial detection sensitivity and speed for etiologic diagnosis in vitreous and aqueous humors. The bacteria detection rate in aqueous and vitreous samples increased from approximately 48% to up to 95% using PCR techniques [17–21].

PCR and nested PCR protocols followed by post-PCR techniques such as RFLP (restriction fragment length polymorphism), DNA sequencing, and DNA-probe hybridization have all been utilized to improve the etiologic diagnosis of APIE [22, 23].

Reported sensitivities for bacterial identification in vitreous samples for several PCR techniques like nested PCR and real-time multiplex PCR are 84%, and 90–95%, respectively, although reported sensitivities vary among different publications [17].

Real-time PCR technology (RT-PCR) is a modification and enhancement of the PCR technique. It is a homogeneous technique in which DNA amplification and detection of the target sequence co-occur, decreasing PCR products' handling and risks of carryover contamination. Simultaneous DNA amplification and detection allow higher reliability as compared to other traditional multi-step techniques. One of the main advantages of real-time PCR technology is the rapid access to results, with microbial detection times of 30 to 50 minutes, compared to 1–14 days for previous PCR methods [18–21].

Green 16S rDNA–Based Universal PCR (SGRU-PCR) and a Multiplex Gram-Specific TaqMan–Based PCR (MGST-PCR) are useful for microorganism detection in many culture-negative samples. In one study, 90% were PCR positive among ten microbiologically negative samples, and five gave interpretable sequence data [17]. The pathogens identified included one coagulase-negative *Staphylococcus*, one *Moraxella spp*., and two *Streptococcus mitis* group, all APIE causative bacteria. Sequencing of PCR-positive/culture-negative samples also included the identification of a *Proteus spp*. causing APIE, which is a rare causative microorganism in postoperative endophthalmitis [17].

Albeit being useful in APIE diagnosis, molecular identification of pathogen microorganisms remains an expensive technique. It is not available in many small cities, underdeveloped countries, laboratory settings, and in many instances, it requires a high workload that makes it inadequate for routine use. Furthermore, clinical definitions of some species do not match those used for 16S rRNA identification [17, 18].

Among another novel microbial detection methods that could eventually be used in the expedite diagnosis of APIE cases are Matrix-Assisted Laser Desorption Ionization–Time of Flight Mass Spectrometry (MALDI-TOF MS) [24, 25] and the utilization of magneto-DNA nanoparticle Dovepress system [26]. The latter method was reported to simultaneously identify up to thirteen species of bacteria in under two hours [26].

Bacterial recognition directly from samples and colonies using MALDI-TOF MS has been described as a revolutionary method that better adapts to the clinical microbiology laboratory. MALDI-TOF MS is used to identify bacterial species and to detect microorganisms previously misidentified [24]. Moreover, detection of antimicrobial resistance using MALDI-TOF MS has been reported for many bacteria, including *Escherichia coli* and *Staphylococcus aureus*. Another advantage of MALDI-TOF MS is that the time required for pathogen identification declines by 55-fold and 169-fold and the cost by 5-fold and 96-fold compared with culture and molecular gene sequencing, respectively [24, 25].

The Magneto-DNA nanoparticle Dovepress system is an assay that utilizes magnetic nanoparticles and oligonucleotide probes to detect target nucleic acids from the pathogen. Rather than sequencing the whole RNA strand, a series of primers and probes were established to amplify and detect specific regions of interest within common bacterial types. They used a miniaturized micro-nuclear magnetic resonance system that requires only small volumes of sample for processing for signal readout [26].

It is hypothesized that ribosomal RNA sequence information from microorganisms such as bacteria could be used in a robust magneto-DNA assay. Because this magnetic detection strategy allows near background-free sensing, the assay steps are greatly simplified, and detection is much faster [26].

7. Treatment of acute postoperative infectious endophthalmitis

7.1 Intravitreal antibiotics and other pharmacologic therapies

Initial and one of the mainstays of treatment for APIE include intravitreal antibiotic therapy [3–5, 12]. Treatment with IAI should be started empirically before having any culture results. For many years, the EVS conclusions and recommended IAI had been a paradigm in APIE patients' care [4, 12]. Nonetheless, it is currently critical in most cases that clinical judgment should be used to determine treatment on a case-by-case basis. Moreover, first-line IAI recommendations have changed after EVS was published and, some authors have proposed vitrectomy as a concomitant treatment of IAI, for the treatment of APIE [27–29].

The EVS was a prospective, multicenter, randomized clinical trial evaluating the efficacy of immediate PPV and intravenous antibiotics to treat APIE. The EVS included endophthalmitis cases after cataract surgery. Patients were randomized to either vitrectomy or vitreous needle biopsy and intravenous antibiotics or no intravenous antibiotics [4, 13, 30]. The study endpoints were media clarity and best-corrected visual acuity. Patients received vancomycin and amikacin IAI. Furthermore, subconjunctival ceftazidime, vancomycin, dexamethasone, topical vancomycin, amikacin, cycloplegic, 1% topical prednisolone acetate and 30 mg bid of oral prednisone, for 5–10 days were prescribed as well [13, 30].

The EVS conclusions included no difference in final vision or media clarity whether or not intravenous antibiotics were used. In addition, patients with light perception visual acuity who received PPV had a three-fold increment in the probability of achieving 20/40, and a 50% reduction in the probability of severe visual loss than patients receiving only vitreous needle biopsy [13].

Patients with hand-motions or better vision showed no significant difference in final best-corrected visual acuity or media clarity whether or not an early vitrectomy was performed.

IAI recommendations have changed over the years. Initial treatment includes mainly intravitreal, as well as oral and topical antibiotics. Currently, two antibiotics are recommended by most retina specialists as first-line IAI treatment for APIE:

- Vancomycin (1 mg in 0.1 ml), and
- Ceftazidime (2.5 mg in 0.1 ml) [4, 11].

Vancomycin and/or amikacin are considered as intravitreal antibiotics alternatives in cases of cephalosporin allergy and/or the presence of ceftazidime resistant Gram-negative strains. Vancomycin has an excellent Gram-positive coverage despite isolated reports of resistance (**Table 3**) [4].

For fungal APE cases, voriconazole, 50–100 μg/0.1 ml, and amphotericine B, 5–10 μg/0.1 ml are described as first-line treatments.

Ceftazidime has emerged as first-line treatment for Gram-negative organisms due to its safer profile than amikacin. Another advantage of ceftazidime is that it may show synergy with vancomycin against gram-positive organisms [4, 12]. Oral, subconjunctival, and systemic antibiotics are used as adjuvant therapy in some hospital settings, although there is little or no evidence of their clinical effectiveness [3, 12]. Among all systemic antibiotics, ciprofloxacin is a first-generation fluoroquinolone that has been routinely used in APIE due to adequate ocular penetration and low side effect profile [4].

Third- and fourth-generation fluoroquinolones have shown a better Gram-positive coverage than ciprofloxacin while maintaining an adequate level of Gram-negative activity. Moxifloxacin has the most potent in vitro activity against Gram-negative and Gram-positive endophthalmitis pathogens [3–5]. It has been used as an intracameral antibiotic for cataract surgery prophylaxis, and there has been a three-fold decline in endophthalmitis rates with its use in phacoemulsification surgery. It is increasingly being used as an alternative intravitreal antibiotic for APIE cases [31]. Furthermore, moxifloxacin has also exhibited adequate ocular

Antimicrobial	Name	Class of drugs	Intravitreal dose
Antibiotics	Vancomycin*	Glycopeptide	1 mg/0.1 ml
	Ceftazidime*	Cephalosporin	2.25mgs/0.1 ml
	Amikacin	Aminoglycoside	0.4 mgs/0.1 ml
Antifungals	Voriconazole	Azol	50–100 μg/0.1 ml
	Amphotericine B	Polyene	5–10 μg/0.1 ml

**Vancomycin and ceftazidime are used as first-line treatment of acute postoperative endophthalmitis.*

Table 3.
Intravitreal antibiotics used for the management of acute postoperative infectious endophthalmitis [5]. Intravitreal injections of vancomycin and ceftazidime are currently recommended as first-line treatment in acute postoperative endophthalmitis.

penetration after systemic administration, with vitreous levels above minimum inhibitory concentration (MIC_{90}) for most bacteria [32].

Vitreous moxifloxacin pharmacokinetics have shown in several studies comparable bioavailability characteristics to ciprofloxacin, with reasonable safety [4, 5, 32]. Moreover, cases of vancomycin-resistant bacteria have been reported to respond adequately to intravitreal injection of moxifloxacin [4, 5, 32].

Linezolid is an oxazolidinone-class antibiotic that the FDA approved in 2000 [5, 33, 34]. It has excellent bioavailability when administered orally, and intraocular levels can reach therapeutic levels within one hour of being administered. Linezolid provides mainly gram-positive coverage [5, 33]. If Gram-positive organisms have shown resistance to vancomycin, it might be reasonable to supplement with oral linezolid, and likewise, oral ciprofloxacin or moxifloxacin may increase the antimicrobial properties of intravitreal ceftazidime [5, 33]. Other IAI used in animal models or humans for endophthalmitis include quinupristin-dalfopristin [5, 34–37], daptomycin [5, 38–40], tygecicline [5, 41], imipenem [5], among others [42, 43]. New antifungals for APIE, include miconazole, caspofungin, and micafungin [5]. In **Table 4**, some of the antibiotics that have been used in endophthalmitis are summarized.

Another debated topic in APIE treatment is the use of steroid therapy. Experimental endophthalmitis animal models have shown that the degree of retinal tissue damage is partly secondary to the elicited severe inflammatory response in the eye [4]. Hence, it is appropriate to address this issue besides the use of antimicrobial therapy, and aggressive steroid therapy should be prescribed in APIE patients, which include topical 1% prednisolone acetate as frequently as every hour as well as oral steroids [3, 4, 44]. Cycloplegic topical medication such as 1% atropine, BID should be prescribed as well, to help decrease pain.

Controversy, however, still prevails regarding the use of intravitreal steroids in APIE. Some authors reported an improvement in inflammation and final visual results with intravitreal injection of steroids and antibiotics, whereas other studies have described worse inflammation and worse visual outcomes [44]. Histopathology reports have also shown contradictory outcomes for intravitreal steroids. In addition, intravitreal triamcinolone has been shown a favorable effect for APIE when combined with IAI in some reports [44].

Dexamethasone implants have been approved for use in several forms of uveitis, which has led to evaluate their possible use in endophthalmitis patients. Moisseiev et al. [45] reported APIE patients treated with immediate intravitreal dexamethasone at the time of vitreous tap. Compared to a group without steroid use, a trend towards the reduced need for antibiotic re-injection was observed in the steroid group. Currently, intravitreal dexamethasone recommended dose is 400 μg in 0.1 ml.

Microorganism	Name of drug	Class of drug	Intravitreal dose
Gram positive	Linezolid	Oxazolindinone	300 μg/0.1 ml
	Quinupristine-dalfopristine	Streptogramin	0.4 mg/0.1 ml
	Daptomycin	Cyclic lipoglycopeptide	200 μg/0.1 ml
	Tigecycline	Glycylcycline	0.5–0.1 mg/0.1 ml
	Piperacillin/tazobactam	Ureidopenicillin/ß -lactamase inhibitor	250 μg/0.1 ml
Gram negative	Imipenem	Carbapenem	50 μg/0.1 ml
	Ciprofloxacin	Fluoroquinolone	0.1 mg/0.1 ml
	Levofloxacin	Fluoroquinolone	0.1 ml 0.5% solution
	Moxifloxacin*	Fluoroquinolone	0.2 mg/0.1 ml
Fungi	Miconazole	Azole	25 μg/0.1 ml
	Caspofungin	Echinocandin	50 μg/0.1 ml
	Micafungin	Echinocandin	0.025 mg/0.1 ml

**Moxifloxacin is increasingly being used as part of APIE prophylaxis and as alternative intravitreal antibiotic in acute postoperative endophthalmitis cases [5, 30].*

Table 4.
Main alternative antibiotics for potential use in the management of endophthalmitis caused by resistant microorganisms to standard IAI. Evidence of their use comes from case reports and case series in humans and animal models.

7.2 Vitrectomy for postoperative endophthalmitis

The EVS concluded that early vitrectomy in endophthalmitis was only beneficial in patients with visual acuity of light perception or worse [13]. Hence, delaying vitrectomy in APIE patients with a better presenting vision has been a common practice among retina specialists. Nonetheless, there is still debate on the adequate timing to perform vitrectomy in APIE patients.

The methods and results of EVS may not reflect modern surgery practice patterns. Furthermore, with the advent of more refined surgical techniques in recent years like minimally-invasive vitrectomy surgery (MIVS), which entail a lower complication rate compared to conventional vitrectomy, the EVS study's conclusions are possibly obsolete. Currently, performing both vitrectomy and IAI as first-line treatments might be more beneficial for many APIE cases [6, 7, 27–29, 46].

In many hospital settings, vitrectomy is usually performed in those APIE patients that do not respond to an initial dose of IAI. In these patients, repeating IAIs instead of performing PPV is likely to be of little benefit. Persisting levels of vitreous antibiotic above MIC_{90} for three days or more after IAI and repeating the same agents after 2–3 days may be deleterious to the eye due to an increased risk of retina toxicity. In addition, some authors [47] have hypothesized that bacterial sequestering or biofilm production might reduce the bacteria's sensitivity to IAI; furthermore, vitrectomy might help remove the bacterial load and increase antibiotic bioavailability in the vitreous cavity.

Peyman et al. were the first to report the use of early vitrectomy in endophthalmitis patients [48]. Cases underwent vitrectomy 24 hours after diagnosis, 65% achieving a final visual acuity of 20/400 or better.

The EVS evaluated the early vitrectomy role and contrasted immediate vitrectomy within six hours of diagnosis against inject-only as subgroups. Only core vitrectomy was performed on the included patients. While no advantage for performing PPV was found unless vision was light perception or worse, no disadvantage in the final visual outcome was found in performing vitrectomy [13].

Moreover, the induction of a posterior hyaloid separation and a complete vitrectomy were usually avoided in the EVS. Contrary to the EVS methods, some reports suggest that removing the posterior hyaloid and using silicone oil as a tamponade in APIE patients could improve anatomic and visual outcomes [13].

Kuhn et al. [46] described a series of patients who underwent early vitrectomy for endophthalmitis with a more thorough surgical vitrectomy and found no rhegmatogenous detachment cases. Ninety one percent of the cases had a final vision of 20/40 or better, contrary to 53% in the EVS study group. They postulated that removing the posterior vitreous cortex may remove the toxic load from proximity to the macula. Other case series have reached similar conclusions [6, 7, 27–29].

Current vitrectomy techniques include 23 Ga, 25 Ga, or 27 Ga MIVS rather than conventional 20 Ga techniques. In addition, some key points should be considered while performing vitrectomy in APIE patients:

First, because the media is frequently hazy for the surgeon to visualize a pars plana port, an infusion cannula sometimes cannot be used for the initial stages of the operation. It is advisable to place an inferotemporal port, reserving its use later in the procedure, once the tip's location in the vitreous cavity can be verified. Alternatively, an anterior chamber maintainer could be placed.

Second, opacities such as hypopyon and pupillary membranes should be aspirated from the anterior segment. Often, because of poor dilation of the pupil and visualization of the internal structures, the lens in phakic eyes must be removed. If the cornea remains too cloudy due to bacterial infiltration and inflammation, and it does not allow adequate visualization of the vitreous cavity, the use of keratoprosthesis should sometimes be considered.

Third, separation of the posterior hyaloid besides core vitrectomy should be attempted in some APIE cases. Some authors [46] have described performing complete vitrectomy to help decrease inflammatory cells and bacterial loads. It can be achieved with current vitrectomy systems, using high-cutting rates and low-flow to lessen the retina traction while removing vitreous strands, thus minimizing the risk of iatrogenic retinal breaks, as well. Nonetheless, caution should still prevail in performing peripheral vitrectomy, and posterior hyaloid separation in cases where the retina appears too necrotic since the risk of formation of retinal tears may increase in this scenario.

Video 1 (https://youtu.be/Q0lLB4Ozkoc) shows an APIE case where hypopyon aspiration, core and peripheral 23 Ga PPV, as well as posterior hyaloid separation were performed.

Fifth, the use of silicone oil as a tamponade has been shown to have a bactericidal effect in vitro and may be worth considering in the context of performing PPV in APIE patients, especially if retinal tamponade is also required in cases of retinal detachment. However, silicone oil's bactericidal effect has been challenging to prove in vivo [4, 6, 7, 27–29].

Another recently described surgical technique for endophthalmitis is endoscopic vitrectomy that uses an endoscopic probe inserted via pars plana to improve visualization in the vitreous cavity, identify intraocular structures, and avoid iatrogenic damage performing a PPV [49]. It has the advantage that it does not require clear anterior media, which is frequently compromised in endophthalmitis patients. It does not require waiting for media clearing, which carries an additional risk of tissue damage due to the infection and severe inflammation processes. Disadvantages of endoscopic vitrectomy include the steep curve for re-learning vitrectomy via an endoscope probe.

If an early vitrectomy is performed because of initial non-response to IAI or removing inflammatory debris, it is common to inject antibiotics concomitantly into the vitreous cavity. Antibiotics can be injected at the end of the vitrectomy or via the diluted solution infused into the vitreous cavity throughout the vitrectomy procedure.

The patient may be left with saline solution, air, gas, or silicone oil as tamponade. It is of the utmost relevance to consider that the volume of water-based fluid in the eye dictates the antibiotic's amount and concentration [4, 6, 7, 27–29, 46]. This is because high antibiotic levels present in the remaining meniscus of aqueous fluid may increase toxicity risk to the retinal tissue that may eventually induce further vision loss. Therefore, it is essential to consider injecting a third or fourth of the recommended intravitreal antibiotic dose in patients with gas or silicone oil-filled eyes to obtain an antibiotic's adequate concentration, as the concentration of the antibiotic changes in the small meniscus of aqueous fluid that will remain in the vitreous cavity.

Alternatively, antibiotic could be diluted at the proper concentration in the irrigation solution that enters the vitreous cavity, thus the remaining fluid will also have adequate antibiotic concentration. The antibiotic can be injected into the vitreous cavity before the tamponade [27–29, 46]. It may be necessary to position the patient face-down a few days after surgery to minimize macular exposure to antibiotics.

Some authors have described the successful use of infused vancomycin throughout vitrectomy at different concentrations. This approach might expose the retinal tissue to a more constant antibiotic level than an intravitreal injection. Nevertheless, it also may have the risk of using sub-therapeutic concentrations of the antibiotic [27].

7.3 Endophthalmitis prophylaxis

The single most effective prophylaxis of endophthalmitis includes preoperative application of 5% povidone-iodine (PI) conjunctival surface and cul-de-sac [50–53]. Bacteria have not developed resistance to PI, and PI is also effective against many microorganisms such as fungi and viruses. Several studies have proven the effectiveness of the aseptic technique and the use of PI in ophthalmological surgery. One report assessed the incidence of APIE over many years in the same hospital with the incorporation of PI, with no use of intraocular antibiotics. Over this time, the rate of APIE went from 0.38% to <0.03%. This rate is almost the same as the current studies looking into risk reduction using intracameral antibiotics [51].

Checking for lid infections like blepharitis, nasolacrimal duct obstruction, leaking wounds, and intracameral antibiotics like cefuroxime 1000 µg/0.1 ml or moxifloxacin at the end of the surgery, and the use topical postoperative antibiotics are some other measures that might decrease endophthalmitis incidence [3, 4].

A large study of eyes that underwent cataract surgery [54] showed that intracameral moxifloxacin declined postcataract surgery endophthalmitis incidence. Nonetheless, the routinary application of intracameral antibiotics has some risks, such as the development of resistant strains of pathogens, and retinal toxicity. For instance, hemorrhagic occlusive retinal vasculitis has been described after using intracameral vancomycin [53].

The most common causative bacteria in post intravitreal injections endophthalmitis are streptococci, common oral flora members. The use of masks and adhering to a strict no-talking policy has decreased post-injection endophthalmitis incidence.

Prompt surgical repair of open globe injuries and prophylactic IAI with or without systemic antibiotics have also been associated with reduced post-traumatic endophthalmitis incidence.

7.4 Other novel treatments and developments

Nakashizuka et al. [52] reported the safety and efficacy of 1.25% povidone-iodine (PI) intravitreal injection followed by vitrectomy using 0.025% irrigation to treat endophthalmitis. Most of the cases included in the study resolved rapidly, and good visual results were observed. No adverse events were reported. Moreover, the electrorretinogram (ERG) results showed increases in the oscillatory potentials amplitudes, flicker ERG and the a-wave's implicit time, suggesting the functional improvement in the retinal inner and outer layers after surgery. They concluded that intravitreal injection of PI followed by PPV was thought to be an effective and safe therapy for APIE. Other authors have reported similar findings [52, 53].

Other novel therapies under investigation for APIE include the development of microdevices such as biomimetic nanosponge to treat endophthalmitis caused by virulent pathogens such as *Enterococcus faecalis* isolates. *Enterococcus faecalis* produces the pore-forming bicomponent cytolysin that adds to retinal tissue damage in endophthalmitis. LaGrow et al. [55] hypothesized that a biomimetic nanosponge, which imitates erythrocytes, could adsorb subunits of the cytolysin and decrease damage to the retina, preserving vision in endophthalmitis patients.

They reported that biomimetic nanosponges nullified cytolysin activity and protected the retinal tissue from damage. These outcomes indicate that this therapeutic option could guard eyes against the deleterious effects of pore-forming toxins of various aggressive ocular bacteria [55].

8. Prognosis of acute postoperative endophthalmitis

One of the most important predictors of final visual outcome is presenting visual acuity. Patients with presenting vision of light perception or worse may have worse outcomes [3, 4]. Therefore, prompt treatment of endophthalmitis cases is associated with improved visual acuity outcomes. Prompt initiation of therapy is more important than any other factor, including PPV versus vitreous tap or the use of adjunctive systemic antibiotics.

Other predictors of worse visual outcomes include DM, older age, corneal infiltrate, high or low intraocular pressure, rubeosis iridis, an absent red reflex, and an open posterior capsule. Dense vitreous opacities, and vitreous membranes, retinal detachment, are also associated with a more unsatisfactory visual outcome [4].

9. Conclusions

Although many breathtaking advances have been described and applied for APIE treatment, further measures and prophylactic strategies are needed to decrease the incidence and improve the prognosis of this devastating complication of intraocular surgery.

Novel molecular biology techniques like RT-PCR have been developed to aid in the etiologic diagnosis of endophthalmitis, which has improved and expedited APIE patients' antibiotic treatment.

Advances in vitreoretinal surgery techniques such as the advent of MIVS and other improvements in vitrectomy systems have changed our way of thinking about early vitrectomy in the treatment of these patients.

However, controversy still prevails on many issues, such as the role of steroid use, vitrectomy timing, and the incorporation of other innovative diagnostic and therapeutic modalities for APIE.

Conflict of interest

The authors have no conflicts of interest to declare.

Nomenclature

Anti-VEGF	Anti-Vascular Endothelial Growth Factor
APIE	Acute Postoperative Infectious Endophthalmitis
DM	Diabetes Mellitus
EVS	Endophthalmitis Vitrectomy Study
ERG	Electroretinogram
IAI	Intravitreal Antibiotic Injection
MIVS	Minimally-invasive Vitrectomy Surgery
MGST-PCR	Multiplex Gram-Specific TaqMan–Based PCR
PCR	Polymerase Chain Reaction
RT-PCR	Real-Time Polymerase Chain Reaction
SGRU-PCR	Green 16S rDNA–Based Universal PCR
PPV	Pars Plana Vitrectomy
PI	Povidone-Iodine

Author details

Sergio E. Hernandez-Da Mota[1]*, Jose Luis Guerrero-Naranjo[2], Jose Dalma-Weiszhausz[2], Raul Velez-Montoya[2] and Jesus H. Gonzalez-Cortes[3]

1 Retina Department, David Clinic and Michoacan University School of Medicine "Dr. Ignacio Chavez", Morelia, Mexico

2 "Dr. Luis Sanchez Bulnes" Hospital, APEC, National Autonomous University of Mexico (UNAM), Mexico City, Mexico

3 Ophthalmology Department, Dr. Jose Eleuterio Gonzalez University Hospital, Autonomous University of Nuevo Leon, Monterrey, Mexico

*Address all correspondence to: tolodamota@yahoo.com.mx

References

[1] Schwartz SG, Flynn HW Jr, Das T, Mieler WF. Ocular Infection: Endophthalmitis. Dev Ophthalmol. 2016;55:176-88. DOI: 10.1159/000431195

[2] Packer M, Chang DF, Dewey SH, Little BC, Mamalis N, Oetting TA, Talley-Rostov A, Yoo SH; ASCRS Cataract Clinical Committee. Prevention, diagnosis, and management of acute postoperative bacterial endophthalmitis. J Cataract Refract Surg. 2011;37:1699-714. DOI: 10.1016/j. jcrs.2011.06.018

[3] Meredith TA, Ulrich JN. Infectious endophthalmitis. In: Wilkinson CP, Hinton DR, Sadda SR, Wiedemann P, editors. Ryan's Retina. 6th ed. Amsterdam:Elsevier; 2018. p. 2266-2281.

[4] Eichenbaum DA, Park RI, Topping TM. Postoperative endophthalmitis. In: Steinert RF, editor. Cataract surgery. 3rd ed. Saunders Elsevier; 2010. p. 671-680.

[5] Relhan N, Pathengay A, Schwartz SG, Flynn HW. Emerging Worldwide Antimicrobial Resistance, Antibiotic Stewardship and Alternative Intravitreal Agents for the Treatment of Endophthalmitis. Retina. . 2017;37:811-818. DOI: 10.1097/IAE.0000000 000001603

[6] Relhan N, Forster RK, Flynn HW Jr. Endophthalmitis: Then and Now. Am J Ophthalmol. 2018;187:20-27. DOI: 10.1016/j.ajo.2017.11.021

[7] Clarke B, Williamson TH, Gini G, Gupta B. Management of bacterial postoperative endophthalmitis and the role of vitrectomy. Surv Ophthalmol. 2018;63:677-693. DOI: 10.1016/j. survophthal.2018.02.003

[8] Gedde SJ, Herndon LW, Brandt JD, Budenz DL, Feuer WJ, Schiffman JC, Tube Versus Trabeculectomy Study Group. Postoperative complications in the tube versus trabeculectomy (TVT) study during five years of follow up. Am J Ophthalmol. 2012;153:804-814. DOI:10.1016/j. ajo.2011.10.024

[9] Olayanju JA, Hassan MB, Hodge DO, Khanna CL. Trabeculectomy related complications in Olmsted County, Minnesota, 1985-2010. JAMA Ophthalmol. 2015;133 (5):574-580. DOI:10.1001/jamaophthalmol. 2015.57

[10] Borkar DS, Wibbelsman TD, Buch PM, Rapuano SB, Obeid A, Ho AC, et al. Endophthalmitis Rates and Clinical Outcomes Following Penetrating and Endothelial Keratoplasty. Am J Ophthalmol. 2019;205:82-90. DOI: 10.1016/j. ajo.2019.05.004.

[11] Cao H, Zhang L, Li L, Lo S. Risk factors for acute endophthalmitis following cataract surgery: A systematic review and meta-analysis. PLoS One. 2013;8(8):e71731. DOI:10.1371/journal. pone.0071731

[12] Rahmani S, Eliott D. Postoperative Endophthalmitis: A Review of Risk Factors, Prophylaxis, Incidence, Microbiology, Treatment, and Outcomes. Review Semin Ophthalmol. 2018;33:95-101. DOI: 10.1080/ 08820538.2017.1353826

[13] Han DP, Wisniewski SR, Wilson, Barza M, Vine AK, Doft BH, Kelsey SF. Spectrum and susceptibilities of microbiologic isolates in the Endophthalmitis Vitrectomy Study, Am J Ophthalmol. 1996; 122:1-17. DOI: 10.1016/s0002-9394(14)71959-2

[14] O'Callaghan RJ. The Pathogenesis of Staphylococcus aureus Eye Infections. Pathogens. 2018;7:9. DOI: 10.3390/ pathogens7010009

[15] Astley R, Miller FC, Mursalin MH, Coburn PS, Callegan MC. An Eye on Staphylococcus aureus Toxins: Roles in Ocular Damage and Inflammation. Toxins (Basel). 2019;11:356. DOI: 10.3390/toxins11060356

[16] Choi JA, Chung SK. Postoperative Endophthalmitis following Cataract Surgery in Asia. ISRN Ophthalmol. 2011;2011:917265. DOI: 10.5402/2011/917265

[17] Cornut PL, Boisset S, Romanet JP, Maurin M, Carricajo A, Benito Y, Vandenesch F, Chiquet C. Principles and applications of molecular biology techniques for the microbiological diagnosis of acute postoperative endophthalmitis. Surv Ophthalmol. 2014;59:286-303. DOI: 10.1016/j.survophthal.2013.08.002

[18] Ogawa M, Sugita S, Shimizu N, Watanabe K, Nakagawa I, Mochizuki M. Broad-range real-time PCR assay for detection of bacterial DNA in ocular samples from infectious endophthalmitis. Jpn J Ophthalmol. 2012; 56:529-535. DOI: 10.1007/s10384-012-0174-z

[19] Bispo PJM, de Melo GB, Ho ing-Lima AL, Pignatari ACC. Detection and gram discrimination of bacterial pathogens from aqueous and vitreous humor using real-time PCR assays. Invest Ophthalmol Vis Sci. 2011;52:873-881. DOI: 10.1167/iovs.10-5712

[20] Ogawa M, Sugita S, Watanabe K, Shimizu N, Mochizuki M. Novel diagnosis of fungal endophthalmitis by broad-range real-time PCR detection of fungal 28S ribosomal DNA. Graefes Arch Clin Exp Ophthalmol. 2012;250:1877-1883. DOI: 10.1007/s00417-012-2015-7

[21] Sugita S, Kamoi K, Ogawa M, Watanabe K, Shimizu N, Mochizuki M. Detection of Candida and Aspergillus species DNA using broad-range real-time PCR for fungal endophthalmitis. Graefes Arch Clin Exp Ophthalmol. 2012;250:391-398. DOI: 10.1007/s00417-011-1819-1

[22] Nandi K, Ranjan P, Therese L, Biswas J. Polymerase chain reaction in intraocular inflammation. Open Ophthalmol J. 2008;2:141-5. DOI: 10.2174/1874364100802010141

[23] Biwas J, Bagyalakshmi R, Therese LK. Diagnosis of Aspergillus fumigatus endophthalmitis from formalin fixed paraffin-embedded tissue by polymerase chain reaction-based restriction fragment length polymorphism. Indian J Ophthalmol.2008;56:65-6. DOI: 10.4103/0301-4738.37600

[24] Lacroix C, Gicquel A, Sendid B, Meyer J, Accoceberry I, François N, Morio F, Desoubeaux G, Chandenier J, Kauffmann-Lacroix C, Hennequin C, Guitard J, Nassif X, Bougnoux ME. Evaluation of two matrix- assisted laser desorption ionization-time of ight mass spectrometry (MALDI-TOF MS) systems for the identi cation of Candida species. Clin Microbiol Infect. 2014;20:153-158. DOI: 10.1111/1469-0691.12210

[25] Seng P, Abat C, Rolain JM, Colson P, Lagier JC, Gouriet F, Fournier PE, Drancourt M, La Scola B, Raoult D. Identification of rare pathogenic bacteria in a clinical microbiology laboratory: impact of MALDI-TOF mass spectrometry. J Clin Microbiol. 2013;51:2182-2194. DOI: 10.1128/JCM.00492-13. DOI: 10.1128/JCM.00492-13

[26] Chung HJ, Castro CM, Im H, Lee H, Weissleder R. A magneto-DNA nanoparticle system for rapid detection and phenotyping of bacteria. Nat Nanotechnol. 2013;8:369-375. DOI: 10.1038/nnano.2013.70

[27] Clarke B, Williamson TH, Gini G, Gupta B. Management of bacterial postoperative endophthalmitis and the role of vitrectomy. Surv Ophthalmol. 2018;63:677-693. DOI: 10.1016/j.survophthal.2018.02.003

[28] Park JC, Ramasamy B, Shaw S, Ling RH, Prasad S. A prospective and nationwide study investigating endophthalmitis following pars plana vitrectomy: Clinical presentation, microbiology, management and outcome. Br J Ophthalmol. 2014;98:1080-1086. DOI:10.1136/bjophthalmol-2013-304486

[29] Grzybowski A, Turczynowska M, Kuhn F. The treatment of postoperative endophthalmitis: should we still follow the endophthalmitis vitrectomy study more than two decades after its publication? Acta Ophthalmol. 2018;96:e651-e654. DOI: 10.1111/aos.13623

[30] Doft BH, Barza M. Optimal management of postoperative endophthalmitis and results of the Endophthalmitis Vitrectomy Study. Curr Opin Ophthalmol. 1996;7:84-94. DOI: 10.1097/00055735-199606000-00015

[31] Haripriya A, Baam ZR, Chang DF. Endophthalmitis Prophylaxis for Cataract Surgery. Asia Pac J Ophthalmol (Phila). 2017;6:324-329. DOI: 10.22608/APO.2017200

[32] Sharma T, Kamath MM, Kamath MG, Nayak RR, Bairy KL, Musmade PB. Aqueous penetration of orally and topically administered moxifloxacin. Br J Ophthalmol. 2015;99:1182-5. DOI: 10.1136/bjophthalmol-2014-306502

[33] Duke SL, Kump LI, Yuan Y, et al. The safety of intraocular linezolid in rabbits. Invest Ophthalmol Vis Sci 2010;51:3115-3119. DOI: 10.1167/iovs.09-4244

[34] Babalola OE. Intravitreal linezolid in the management of vancomycin-resistant enterococcal endophthalmitis. Am J Ophthalmol Case Rep. 2020;20:100974. DOI: 10.1016/j.ajoc.2020.100974

[35] Hernandez-Da Mota SE. Quinupristin/dalfopristin in Staphylococcus aureus endophthalmitis: a case report. J Med Case Rep. 2011;5:130. DOI: 10.1186/1752-1947-5-130

[36] Stroh EM. Quinupristin/dalfopristin in vancomycin-resistant Staphylococcus aureus endophthalmitis. Arch Ophthalmol 2012;130:1323-1324. DOI: 10.1001/archophthalmol.2012.1504

[37] Giordano VE, Hernandez-Da Mota SE, Adabache-Guel TN, Castillejos-Chevez A, Corredor-Casas S, Salinas-Longoria SM, Romero-Vera R, Jimenez-Sierra JM, Guerrero-Naranjo JL, Morales-Canton V. Safety of intravitreal quinupristin/dalfopristin in an animal model. Int J Ophthalmol 2016;9:373-378. DOI: 10.18240/ijo.2016.03.08

[38] Buzzacco DM, Carroll CP. Intravitreal daptomycin in a case of bilateral endogenous endophthalmitis. Arch Ophthalmol 2012;130:940-941. DOI: 10.1001/archophthalmol.2011.2527

[39] Sim JM, Kapoor KG, Wagner AL. Intravitreal daptomycin for recalcitrant postoperative endophthalmitis. Case Rep Ophthalmol 2016;7:103-107. DOI: 10.1159/000444046

[40] Comer GM, Miller JB, Schneider EW, Khan NW, Reed DM, Elner VM, Zacks DN. Intravitreal daptomycin: a safety and efficacy study. Retina 2011;31:1199-1206. DOI: 10.1097/IAE.0b013e318207d1b9

[41] Horozoglu F, Metan G, Sever O, Percin D, Topal CS, Gonen T,

Keskinbora KH, Topcu B, Yanyali A. Intravitreal tigecycline treatment in experimental Acinetobacter baumannii endophthalmitis. J Chemother 2012;24:101-106. DOI: 10.1179/1120009X12Z.00000000018

[42] Aziza Y, Kodrat E, Saharman YR, Setiabudy R, Susiyanti M, Sjamsoe S. Efficacy of intravitreal Levofloxacin 0.5% ophthalmic solution in treating *Pseudomonas aeruginosa* endophthalmitis on a rabbit model. Asia Pac J Ophthalmol (Phila) 2013;2:199-205. DOI: 10.1097/APO.0b013e3182970cc9

[43] Ozkiriş A, Evereklioglu C, Eşel D, Akgün H, Erkiliç K. The efficacy of intravitreal piperacillin/tazobactam in rabbits with experimental *Staphylococcus epidermidis* endophthalmitis: a comparison with vancomycin. Ophthalmic Res. 2005;37:168-74. DOI: 10.1159/000086074.

[44] Ching Wen Ho D, Agarwal A, Lee CS, Chhablani J, Gupta V, Khatri M, Nirmal J, Pavesio C, Agrawal R. A Review of the Role of Intravitreal Corticosteroids as an Adjuvant to Antibiotics in Infectious Endophthalmitis. Ocul Immunol Inflamm. 2018;26:461-468. DOI: 10.1080/09273948.2016.1245758

[45] Moisseiev E, Abbassi S, Park SS. Intravitreal dexamethasone in the management of acute endophthalmitis: a comparative retrospective study. Eur J Ophthalmol. 2017;27:67-73. DOI: 10.5301/ejo.5000866.

[46] Kuhn F, Gini G. Vitrectomy for endophthalmitis. Ophthalmology. 2006;113:714. DOI: 10.1016/j.ophtha.2006.01.009

[47] Leung EH, Gibbons A. Environmental, Local, and Systemic Endophthalmitis Prophylaxis for Cataract Surgery. Int Ophthalmol Clin. 2020;60:113-126. DOI: 10.1097/IIO.0000000000000327

[48] Peyman GA, Rose M, Sanders D. Intravitreal antibiotic injection and vitrectomy in acute bacterial endophthalmitis. Can J Ophthalmol. 1976;11:188-90.

[49] Dave VP, Pappuru RR, Tyagi M, Pathengay A, Das T. Endoscopic vitrectomy in endophthalmitis: initial experience of 33 cases at a tertiary eye care center. Clin Ophthalmol. 2019;13:243-251. DOI: 10.2147/OPTH.S185716

[50] Otani K, Shimada H, Nakashizuka H, Okubo H Capsular bag irrigation using 0.025% povidone-iodine in balanced salt solution PLUS for the treatment of postoperative endophthalmitis. Int Ophthalmol. 2018;38:1787-1790. DOI: 10.1007/s10792-017-0645-9

[51] Shimada H, Hattori T, Mori R, Nakashizuka H, Fujita K, Yuzawa M. Minimizing the endophthalmitis rate following intravitreal injections using 0.25% povidone-iodine irrigation and surgical mask. Graefes Arch Clin Exp Ophthalmol. 2013;251:1885-90. DOI: 10.1007/s00417-013-2274

[52] Nakashizuka H, Shimada H, Hattori T, Noguchi T, Kokubo N, Yuzawa M. Vitrectomy using 0.025% povidone-iodine in balanced salt solution plus for the treatment of postoperative endophthalmitis. Retina. 2015;35:1087-94. DOI: 10.1097/IAE.0000000000000634

[53] Grzybowski A, Schwartz SG, Matsuura K, Ong Tone S, Arshinoff S, Ng JQ, et al. Endophthalmitis Prophylaxis in Cataract Surgery: Overview of Current Practice Patterns Around the World. Curr Pharm Des. 2017;23:565-573. DOI: 10.2174/1381612822666161216122230

[54] Melega MV, Alves M, Cavalcanti Lira RP, Cardoso da Silva I, Ferreira BG, Assis Filho HL, et al. Safety and efficacy

of intracameral moxifloxacin for prevention of post-cataract endophthalmitis: Randomized controlled clinical trial. J Cataract Refract Surg. 2019;45:343-350. DOI: 10.1016/j.jcrs.2018.10.044

[55] LaGrow AL, Coburn PS, Miller FC, Land C, Parkunan SM, Luk BT, Gao W, Zhang L, Callegan MC. A Novel Biomimetic Nanosponge Protects the Retina from the *Enterococcus faecalis* cytolysin. mSphere. 2017;2:e00335-17. DOI: 10.1128/mSphere.00335-17

Chapter 6

Endogenous Endophthalmitis: Etiology and Treatment

Sami Kabbara, Neil Kelkar, Mandi D. Conway and Gholam A. Peyman

Abstract

This chapter comprehensively covers all aspects of endogenous endophthalmitis from systemic infectious agents, with an emphasis on reported and newer etiologies to broaden the diagnostic and investigative acumen of treating ophthalmic providers. The discussion includes the etiology of metastatic endophthalmitis and diagnostic investigations, including polymerase chain reaction (PCR), for identification of bacterial and viral infections involving the eye in both immunosuppressed in non-immunosuppressed patients. Additionally, we present clinical and diagnostic findings of fungal infections, protozoal infections, and helminthic infections. Pediatric cases are also reported and etiologies described. We discuss both etiology and diagnostic challenges. Current therapeutic modalities and outcomes are reviewed. While no two cases of metastatic endophthalmitis are the same, some similarities may exist that allow us to generalize how to approach and treat this potentially sight- and life-threatening spectrum of diseases and find the underlying systemic cause.

Keywords: endophthalmitis, endogenous, bacterial, viral, fungal, protozoal, helminthic

1. Introduction to endogenous endophthalmitis: etiology and treatment

Endophthalmitis is defined any infectious inflammation of vitreous, retina, or choroid that may or may not involve the anterior chamber. A useful classification is to define the infectious agent as exogenous or endogenous depending the route of infection. Exogenous endophthalmitis occurs from direct entry of pathogen(s) after disruption of ocular tissues, whether from trauma (like an open globe injury) or from surgical interventions (such as cataract or glaucoma surgery, intravitreal injection, or retinal surgery). Alternatively, endogenous endophthalmitis occurs when pathogens spread from other parts of the body to the eye (mainly by hematogenous spread but can also be neuronal in case of some viruses) with a subsequent compromise to the blood-ocular barrier. Since the choroid and the retina are highly vascularized, these structures may be seeded early in the systemic infection. In this chapter, we discuss endogenous endophthalmitis including the incidence, causes, and management of bacterial, viral, fungal, and other less common infectious agents.

2. Endogenous bacterial endophthalmitis (EBE)

While endogenous bacterial endophthalmitis comprises the minority (2–8%) of endophthalmitis cases, it is a devastating intraocular infection that often results in poor visual outcomes, loss of the eye, and even mortality [1–4]. Nineteen percent of cases have a bilateral presentation [5]. Prompt recognition and treatment is vital for improved visual outcome. Unfortunately, many patients with EBE are either initially misdiagnosed (up to 25% of cases) or have a delay in diagnosis (a median of seven days) [2–4]. EBE is most commonly misdiagnosed as non-infectious uveitis but can also be mistaken for acute angle closure glaucoma, conjunctivitis, or orbital cellulitis [3, 4]. In children, EBE is most often misdiagnosed as retinoblastoma [3, 4].

Familiarity with common clinical features is crucial for proper diagnosis of EBE. Blurred vison (89%) and pain (48%) are common presentations, although they are not always present [3]. The most common systemic findings include fever (37%), often a low-grade fever and chills, and influenza-like features (20%) [3].

The absence of a clear view of the fundus is the most common ocular sign (40%), but other important exam findings include anterior chamber reaction (32%), hypopyon (35%), and vitritis (33%). Hypopyon color can be associated with different causative organisms. For example, *Staphylococcus aureus, Serratia marcescens*, and *Klebsiella* endophthalmitis can be associated with pink or blood-tinged hypopyon, whereas *Mycobacterium tuberculosis, Streptococcus bovis,* and *Listeria monocytogenes* endophthalmitis can present with tan or pigmented hypopyon [6]. Moreover, organisms such as *Listeria monocytogenes* and *Bacillus cereus* are commonly associated with elevated intraocular pressures [7].

Endogenous bacterial endophthalmitis is also known as metastatic endophthalmitis, since an extraocular (systemic) focus of infection is typically the source. Liver abscesses are the most common sources of infection followed by lung and cardiac infections [3]. Other foci include soft tissue infection, meningitis, urinary tract infection (UTI), brain, and renal abscesses. Moreover, patients diagnosed with EBE often have underlying medical conditions that lead to an immunosuppressed state such as Diabetes mellitus (DM), Human Immunodeficiency Virus (HIV) infection, autoimmune disease, and malignancy [3, 4]. Other predisposing factors for EBE include high-risk behaviors such as IV drug use (IVDU) and alcohol abuse [3].

These infections are often life-threatening, so investigations into underlying foci and risk factors are paramount. In fact, mortality rates as high as 5% have been reported in patients with EBE from an extraocular infection [4]. Blood cultures remain the most reliable way to establish a diagnosis. These cultures are routinely performed in a hospital setting, and although they are more likely to identify the underlying pathogen compared to intraocular cultures, results can be negative in up to half of cases [3–5, 8, 9]. Intraocular cultures become very important in cases of negative blood cultures. They can be obtained from the anterior chamber by paracentesis (AC tap) or from vitreous collection, either by needle aspiration or during pars plana vitrectomy (PPV). Experimental and clinical studies of exogenous bacterial endophthalmitis have found vitreous cultures to have a higher yield compared to aqueous cultures [10, 11]. It is less clear whether these results apply to EBE eyes. Nevertheless, a review of 342 cases of EBE found anterior chamber samples obtained alongside vitrectomy to be positive in 21% of the cases while a positive vitreous sample was obtained during vitrectomy in 41% of the cases [3]. Yet, AC tap has been advocated to be performed in eyes with more prominent anterior chamber inflammation and when the offending microorganism is still unknown [12]. Moreover, AC tap is a less invasive procedure than vitreous sampling. Due to its high sensitivity, PCR has emerged as an adjunct to cultures in diagnosing EBE. It is capable of amplifying DNA from a single bacterium in a few hours. Hence, it can establish a diagnosis days before culture results become finalized and identify organisms in a culture-negative specimen, even after antibiotic treatment has been initiated [13–16]. However, PCR has not replaced the utility of traditional cultures. It does not offer any insight into antibiotic sensitivity, which is important for antimicrobial stewardship, and its high sensitivity makes it vulnerable to false positive results from cross-contamination [17]. Nevertheless, due to increased affordability and reproducibility in addition to the aforementioned benefits, PCR is becoming increasingly utilized even in developing countries [18–20].

Regional variations exist regarding bacterial organisms that cause EBE. For example, Gram-positive bacteria comprise the majority of infections in North America and Europe, while Gram-negative organisms predominate in East Asia [1, 5]. This discrepancy can be attributed to *Klebsiella* being the most commonly reported organism behind EBE in East Asia [21]. In fact, up to 90% of EBE cases in East Asia were found to be result of *Klebsiella* spp., likely secondary to the high incidence of DM and hepatobiliary disease in that area [2, 6, 21]. Liver abscess is a common source for *Klebsiella*-induced EBE [2, 7, 22]. Other common Gram-negative species include *Pseudomonas aeruginosa, Neisseria meningitidis, Escherichia coli, Salmonella* spp., and *Serratia marcescens*. Patients with EBE from *P. aeruginosa* commonly have predisposing factors such as cystic fibrosis, immunosuppression, history of lung transplant, and endocarditis [23–25], although EBE by *P. aeruginosa* has been reported in an immunocompetent patient with an unknown source of infection [26]. *N. meningitidis* is also a common pathogen in children with EBE but has been on the decline with the advent of antibiotics [4]. It is important to suspect *N. meningitidis* in patients with sepsis, fever (which can be high and relapsing), rash involving the palms and soles, and meningismus; however, it is not always the culprit [27]. *N. meningitidis* has been isolated from eyes without the classic signs of meningococcemia [16, 28–32]. The majority of patients with *Escherichia coli* endogenous endophthalmitis have associated urinary tract infections and renal abscesses [4]. *Salmonella typhi* has been identified as a cause of endogenous endophthalmitis following typhoid fever [33, 34]. One study found that 7 out 14 patients were under one year of age [33]. Therefore, endogenous endophthalmitis should be suspected in all patients following typhoid fever, especially in infants. Other members of the *Salmonella* spp. have been implicated [35–37]. *Serratia marcescens* is commonly associated with nosocomial catheter-related infections in immunocompromised patients along with urogenital tract infections and IVDU [38–43].

The most common Gram-positive bacteria in EBE are *Staphylococcus aureus*, Group B streptococci, *Streptococcus pneumoniae, Listeria monocytogenes*, *Enterococcus faecalis*, *Bacillus cereus*, and *Nocardia* species [2, 44]. One study found that *S. aureus* was the single most common organism to cause EBE (25% of cases) [1]. *S. aureus* can be further divided into methicillin-sensitive *Staphylococcus aureus* (MSSA) and methicillin-resistant *Staphylococcus aureus* (MRSA). The latter group is typically more difficult to treat due to increased antibiotic resistance [45, 46]. MRSA infections are mainly found in hospitalized patients with predisposing risk factors such as DM, HIV, end-stage renal disease (ESRD), IVDU, skin/joint infections, and indwelling catheters; however, it has also been documented in immunocompetent patients without any known underlying risk factor [43, 47–52].

Group B *Streptococcus* endogenous endophthalmitis typically arises by hematogenous spread secondary to pneumonia, pharyngitis, UTIs, and skin infections [53, 54]. The endophthalmitis caused by this organism is commonly associated with endocarditis and septic arthritis [53, 54]. *Streptococcus pneumoniae* was found to be the most common isolated organism (20.8%) in a large Indian study that involved 173 eyes with EBE [55]. Interestingly, the majority of patients with EBE in this study were young (mean age 25 years) and without any predisposing illnesses ($\sim$68%). However, patients who are immunocompromised and asplenic, are susceptible to EBE by this microorganism [56–58]. Endogenous endophthalmitis has also been observed in patients with *S. pneumoniae* meningitis [59, 60].

Listeria monocytogenes is a Gram-positive rod that is typically transmitted via ingestion of contaminated food. Chronic uveitis has been documented as a sequela of this bacterial infection and requires long-term topical steroid therapy [7]. Blood cultures (23% positive yield) have significantly lower yield than intraocular tissue sampling such as aqueous (86%) and vitreous (78%) [7]. The source of infection is typically not found [7].

Enterococcus faecalis is a natural inhabitant of the GI tract and is a rare cause of EBE. A few documented cases identify some of the sources to be secondary to cholecystitis, indwelling catheter, and prosthetic valvular endocarditis [52, 61, 62]. One case has also been documented after gastrointestinal illness [63].

Nocardia spp. are ubiquitous filamentous bacteria found in water, soil, and decaying vegetation. These microorganisms are typically known to disseminate from a pulmonary focus in immunocompromised patients; however, EBE in immunocompetent patients has also been documented [64]. Up to half of patients are transplant patients, and a quarter have underlying autoimmune diseases [65]. Chorioretinal lesions are a common manifestation of *Nocardia* EBE and are believed to be the most frequent bacterial cause of subretinal abscesses [59, 65, 66]. They are found to occur in around 69% of patients, often requiring retinal biopsy and vitrectomy for diagnosis and treatment [65]. *Bacillus cereus* is very common in patients with history of IVDU [60, 67, 68]. Infection by this microorganism is known for its rapidly progressive and explosive course, which can often lead to panophthalmitis [60, 68–70].

3. Treatment of endogenous bacterial endophthalmitis

Treatment of EBE has evolved significantly in the last century, particularly after the introduction of antimicrobial agents. Initially, systemic administration was common practice and is still necessary to save the patient's life, but systemic therapy has lower efficacy of saving the eye. It has been established that antibiotic intraocular levels are insufficient to achieve any ocular clinical benefit [71, 72]. It is important to note that despite loss of vision, the infection in the eye should be treated to prevent meningitis and contiguous spread to the surrounding orbital tissues.

In the 1970s, Peyman et al. used animal models to better understand the blood-ocular barrier and to determine non-toxic doses of antimicrobials. They established the use of intravitreal antibiotic injections (IVI) as the standard of care for the treatment of endophthalmitis [73–76]. In the 1990s, the Endophthalmitis Vitrectomy Study (EVS), which studied only exogenous endophthalmitis, established IVI (IVI- of Pharmaceuticals) as standard of care and reported no additional benefit for using systemic ceftazidime and amikacin [77]. Nevertheless, the studied population was post-operative endophthalmitis patients, so the results may not be directly applicable to patients with EBE [77]. Also, they used systemic steroids rather than intravitreal steroids, the latter of which are known to be beneficial in saving visual function by decreasing intraocular inflammatory mediators and the former are questionably prudent in a systemic infection.

Although the treatment of EBE remains controversial due to a paucity of clinical trials, systemic antibiotics remain essential, as many patients have an underlying systemic infection or a distal infectious focus. In fact, in a study that looked at 342 cases of EBE, the two patients who did not receive systemic antibiotics died, while the 51 patients who did receive appropriate systemic treatment survived, although this was not statistically significant ($P = 0.10$) [4]. Currently, systemic antibiotics are seldom used as a monotherapy but are often used in combination with intravitreal antibiotics, and sometimes PPV [3].

Selection of appropriate antimicrobial agents for IVI depends on several factors, including the patient's allergies, the targeted organism, and antibiotic sensitivity and resistance. The most commonly used antimicrobials in IVI for empiric treatment are vancomycin for Gram-positive and ceftazidime for Gram-negative microorganisms [3]. Amikacin and gentamicin IVI can also be used for Gram-negative microorganisms [4]. A tap-and-inject technique is recommended: An intravitreal tap is initially performed through the pars plana to collect a sample of the vitreous for Gram staining and culture, followed by IVI.

Intravitreal corticosteroids have also been used to counter the inflammatory reaction associated with EBE. Dexamethasone is typically the agent of choice. It has been shown to be safe for all ocular structures up to 4 mg and may reduce the need for repeated antibiotic injections as well as improve visual outcomes [3, 25, 78].

The requirement for surgical intervention is not well established in the treatment of EBE. The EVS recommended PPV for patients with light perception vision, but as mentioned previously, the study involved patients with postoperative bacterial endophthalmitis only [77]. Nevertheless, there are several advantages of performing early vitrectomy on patients with EBE, including removing the infectious material from the vitreous and providing ample material for culture. A large series reported improved visual outcomes and lower rates of eviscerations and enucleation in a group of patients who received vitrectomy *versus* an IVI-only group [3]. For more on endophthalmitis treatment and management, please refer to the final section. [Addendum].

4. Endogenous spirochete endophthalmitis

Spirochetes are unique bacteria with distinct long helically coiled cells. Members of the phylum Spirochaetes include *Leptospira, Borrelia burgdorferi,* and *Treponema pallidum,* all of which are known to cause various systemic and intraocular inflammatory manifestations.

Treponema pallidum is the causative pathogen for the sexually transmitted infection syphilis. A recent report by the Centers for Disease Control and Prevention (CDC) has revealed that rates of syphilis are on the rise, particularly among HIV-positive patients and men who have sex with men [79, 80]. This rise in syphilis cases also correlates with an increase incidence of ocular syphilis, which is often the presenting feature of the disease [81–83]. The CDC considers a patient to have ocular syphilis if he/she has been diagnosed with syphilis, regardless of the stage, and any symptoms or ocular signs consistent with syphilis. Syphilis, also known as the "great imitator," can affect any ocular structure, including the cornea, sclera, uvea, retina, and optic nerve, and is often bilateral, and should be treated as a tertiary syphilis [84, 85].

The most common ocular manifestation of syphilis is generally agreed to be posterior uveitis followed by panuveitis, although some report granulomatous iridocyclitis as being most common [83, 86, 87]. Isolated intermediate and anterior uveitis can also occur [88]. Ocular syphilis can also present with necrotizing retinitis that can mimic acute retinal necrosis (ARN) or progressive outer retinal necrosis (PORN). However, these viral entities tend to progress quickly and are unresponsive to penicillin, whereas necrotizing retinitis secondary to syphilis tends to be slower and responsive to penicillin [89]. Moreover, retinal vasculitis can occur with occlusive manifestations [89, 90]. Patients with ocular syphilis may have several distinct retinal findings that could assist in diagnosis, such as creamy white preretinal precipitates that can migrate over time [91]. In addition, retinal lesions can heal with minimal retinal pigment epithelium involvement [23]. Acute syphilitic posterior placoid chorioretinitis is also a distinct and rare retinal manifestation of ocular syphilis characterized by discrete oval lesions of the outer retina and the inner choroid [83]. It is believed that these lesions occur secondary to inflammation from direct invasion of *Treponema pallidum* of the choriocapillaris, deposition of immune complexes, or a combination thereof [90]. Nevertheless, ocular syphilis is uncommon and constitutes a small percentage (1%–5%) of ocular inflammation cases in tertiary referral centers [80, 88, 92, 93].

One study examining 453 patients in an HIV clinic found incidence of syphilis to be 7.3%, of which 9% had ocular manifestations [94]. HIV-positive patients also showed higher rates of concurrent ocular syphilis at a younger age than immunocompetent patients [84, 88, 95]. Moreover, several studies have demonstrated that HIV-positive patients are more likely to have isolated anterior uveitis than HIV-negative patients [88, 96]. Therefore, the CDC recommends that all patients with HIV should be screened for syphilis, and all patients with syphilis should be screen for HIV. Screening for other common sexually transmitted diseases such as gonorrhea and chlamydia should also be performed. HIV-positive patients are more likely to present with acute, bilateral uveitis with more aggressive ocular involvement than HIV-negative patients [84, 85]. However, the CD4 count has not been shown to affect the frequency of ocular syphilis in HIV-positive patients [97].

Diagnosis of syphilis is achieved by nontreponemal and treponemal tests. Nontreponemal tests include Venereal Disease Research Lab (VDRL) and rapid plasma reagin (RPR) tests, which are commonly used for screening. These tests are sensitive but not specific; therefore, a positive result must be confirmed with a treponemal test such as fluorescent treponemal antibody absorption test (FTA-ABS), *T. pallidum* particle agglutination test (TPPA), or microhemagglutination-*T. pallidum* test (MHA-TP) due to their high specificity [98]. In very early or late stages of the infection, RPR can be negative, therefore, a more sensitive test such as enzyme immunoassay (EIA) or chemiluminescence immunoassays (CIA) can be used instead [99].

Ocular syphilis is categorized as a subtype of neurosyphilis and should receive prompt treatment, as delay in treatment may result in visual loss. Only 12% of patients diagnosed with neurosyphilis were found to have ocular involvement, and syphilitic meningitis does not always accompany ocular syphilis [97, 100]. Nevertheless, the CDC recommends a lumbar puncture to be performed on all patients with syphilis and ocular complaints, even in the absence of clinical neurological findings. Commonly, CSF-VDRL is the initial test followed by CSF-FTA-ABS if the former test is positive [101].

The recommended treatment by CDC for ocular syphilis includes intravenous aqueous crystalline penicillin G, 18 to 24 million units per day administered as 3 to 4 million units every four hours or continuous infusion over 10 to 14 days. An alternative regimen, if patient compliance is guaranteed, is 2.4 million units of intramuscular procaine penicillin G once daily in addition to 500 mg oral probenecid four times a day, both for 10 to 14 days.

Borrelia burgdorferi, the culprit behind Lyme disease, is another spirochete known to affect ocular structures. Like syphilis, Lyme disease progresses through different stages. Follicular conjunctivitis occurs in the early stage of the disease (7–11% of patients), while keratitis, episcleritis, uveitis, and neuroretinitis tend to occur in the second and third stages [93, 102, 103]. Anterior, intermediate, posterior, and panuveitis have all been reported to occur in Lyme disease, with the intermediate form being the most common one [104, 105]. Retinal vasculitis is also a common presentation in patients with uveitis [104, 106, 107]. Exudative retinal detachment and macular edema can also occur, along with involvement of the optic nerve such as papillitis and optic neuritis. However, Lyme-associated uveitis is rare. One study conducted in France found Lyme disease to be causative of uveitis in only 7 out of 1,006 cases [104]. Diagnosing Lyme-associated uveitis can be challenging, and it can be difficult to ascertain whether positive serologic testing was incidental in patients with uveitis. A study looking at 430 patients with uveitis found the incidence of positive Lyme serology to be similar to the general population [108]. Serology for Lyme disease without clinical suspicion (presentation of specific Lyme symptoms, tick bite, and/or presence in a *Borrelia burgdorferi*-endemic area) is discouraged due to high false positive rates [109]. The CDC currently recommends a two-step approach to establish the diagnosis [110]: ELISA, to be confirmed with western blot if positive or equivocal. Direct identification of intact spirochetes has also been reported in the vitreous post-vitrectomy [111]. Cultures and PCR of both vitreous samples and urine specimens have also been applied [112–114]. *Borrelia burgdorferi* is highly susceptible to systemic antimicrobial treatment. Oral doxycycline, amoxicillin, and ceftriaxone are routinely used in systemic treatment of Lyme disease [103, 104]. Intravenous ceftriaxone was observed to be more efficacious in treatment of uveitis compared to oral doxycycline, perhaps due to better penetration across the blood–brain barrier [104]. However, an optimal treatment regimen for uveitis remains elusive, and recurrences of uveitis after successful treatment are common. The etiology of such recurrences is unclear, but they are thought to be either a reinfection, relapse of the original infection (due to antibiotic resistance) or an autoimmune reaction. Steroids can be used as adjunct treatment and, in some cases, can be sufficient when used alone [104]. Intravitreal triamcinolone has been used to treat macular edema in Lyme disease [115].

Leptospirosis, caused by the spirochete *Leptospira,* is a common infection in tropical and subtropical areas such as the Caribbean, Central and South America, the Pacific Islands and Southeast Asia [116, 117]. The most common ocular manifestations include subconjunctival hemorrhage, chemosis, and conjunctival hyperemia. Uveitis, retinal vasculitis, retinal hemorrhages, and papillitis can also occur [118]. It is believed that 4–7 days after the onset of leptospirosis bacteremia, the immune system rapidly clears the pathogen from all host tissues except the eye and the brain, as they are somewhat immunologically privileged, resulting in uveitis 3–6 months post-systemic infection [119, 120]. The exact incidence of uveitis is unclear (3–92%) but can vary from anterior uveitis to panuveitis [119, 121]. Inflammation can be intense, leading to a formation of hypopyon. In fact, hypopyon secondary to leptospiral uveitis is the most common cause of hypopyon in tropical counties [119, 120]. Vitritis has been reported to occur in 76% of cases. Snow banking and vitreous precipitates can also occur in a linear pattern resembling the "string of pearls" that is characteristic of sarcoidosis [122]. The microscopic agglutination test is the gold standard for the diagnosis of leptospirosis; however, other tests such as PCR, ELISA, *Leptospira* dipstick test, and microscopic slide agglutination tests have been routinely used [123]. Intravenous penicillin G is typically reserved for severe infections, while oral doxycycline suffices for milder cases [124]. Topical, periocular and systemic steroids have also been used in the treatment of leptospiral uveitis [122].

5. Endogenous mycobacterial endophthalmitis

Mycobaterium tuberculosis, a rod shaped, aerobic bacterium, is known to infect around one third of the world's population [125]. Individuals are infected by inhalation of small airborne droplets containing the mycobacteria. The immune system is usually capable of containing the infection in immunocompetent patients; however, if that protective mechanism fails, mycobacteria are able to disseminate by hematogenous and lymphatic spread and seed in organs beyond the lungs, leading to extrapulmonary tuberculosis (TB) [126]. The eye is one of the organs that can be affected and represents 2–18% of extrapulmonary tuberculosis cases [127, 128]. *Mycobacterium tuberculosis* is an aerobic bacterium that has increased affinity to organs with high oxygen tension. The choroid is one of the tissues with the highest oxygen tension in the human body, making it especially vulnerable to seeding by mycobacteria.

The diagnosis of intraocular tuberculosis can be challenging, as it may have no pathognomonic eye findings. Instead, it has a protean presentation, which can appear similar to non-tubercular infections. Patients with HIV are more likely to develop intraocular TB than HIV-negative patients [3, 126]. However, severe intraocular TB can also occur in healthy individuals, which may cause a delay in diagnosis and treatment resulting in profound visual and organ loss [129, 130].

Uveitis is the most common ocular manifestation and can take the form of granulomatous anterior uveitis (12–36%), intermediate uveitis, posterior uveitis (11–20%) and most commonly, panuveitis (34–42%) [128]. Retinal manifestations can include multi-focal choroiditis, chorioretinitis, serpiginous-like choroiditis and choroidal tubercles [131–136]. Ocular tuberculosis can even be severe enough to cause panophthalmitis [137].

Identifying *M. tuberculosis* from body tissues and fluids is the gold standard for diagnosis. In the case of intraocular TB, this may require a major intervention such as enucleation, which may be clinically undesirable [138–140]. Moreover, most patients with intraocular TB present without signs of systemic manifestation, and tuberculin skin test (TST) can be negative in patients with disseminated TB [141, 142]. A recent review of endogenous TB endophthalmitis found that the majority of patients (63%) did not have a prior history of tuberculosis, and ocular manifestations were their presenting sign [141, 142]. Furthermore, half of the presenting patients denied any systemic symptoms such as fever, chills or hemoptysis prior to presentation at the eye clinic. The most common presenting symptom was decreased vision (90%), followed by pain (58%), eye redness (32%), and proptosis (6.5%), all of which are nonspecific signs [141, 142].

Together, these factors make accurate diagnosis of intraocular TB challenging. Nevertheless, certain ophthalmic findings can increase the likelihood of establishing the correct diagnosis. A study found that broad-based posterior synechiae, retinal vasculitis with or without choroiditis, and serpiginous-like choroiditis demonstrate a high likelihood of intraocular TB being present; however, the absence of these signs does not rule out the disease [143]. Moreover, retinal vasculitis in intraocular TB mainly involves the veins with perivascular cuffing and vitritis, and focal choroiditis lesions tend to be under the vessels [131, 144]. A presumed intraocular TB diagnosis can be made when these signs are present in addition to a positive tuberculosis test such as Tuberculin Skin Test (TST), QuantiFERON-TB Gold, chest radiograph, or computed tomography of the chest.

Being aware of the limitations of each diagnostic test is vital. As mentioned previously, TST can produce false negative results in some patients. These patients typically have anergy as result of immunosuppression or disseminated TB, hence TST should not be used to rule out TB when suspicion is high [145]. Moreover, spiral chest computed tomography is more sensitive in the detection of pulmonary TB and should be used in cases with normal radiography and high suspicion of the disease [146]. PPV can be an important diagnostic and therapeutic intervention, as it was found to have a higher yield than vitreous tap in returning positive for mycobacteria (87.5% vs. 14.3%, respectively) [142]. Moreover, PPV may have a similar role in improving visual outcomes and reducing the possibility of enucleation in intraocular TB as was demonstrated in EBE cases. PCR also has a high diagnostic value and can be more accurate than cultures in diagnosing intraocular TB [142].

In the absence of confirmatory tests such as direct visualization of the mycobacteria, positive response to antitubercular therapy (ATT) supports the diagnosis of presumed intraocular tuberculosis. In fact, any delay in treatment to establish a definitive diagnosis is discouraged. One study found that systemic antibiotics were started in 47.6% of endophthalmitis of unknown etiology cases prior to establishing a definitive diagnosis [142]. Antitubercular therapy comprises a four-drug regimen: isoniazid, rifampicin, ethambutol, and pyrazinamide. The role of steroids as part of ATT remains controversial. Some studies have found that steroids can be effective in reducing TB-associated mortality and recurrences of uveitis as well as treating macular edema [141, 147], while another multi-center study found the use of steroids was associated with higher treatment failure rates [148]. Failure rates were higher when steroid treatment was started prior to initiation of ATT compared to after [148]. Therefore, judicious use of steroids is recommended as part of ATT. In fact, there might be two different pathophysiological mechanisms behind the intraocular inflammation: an active mycobacterial infection of the eye and an immunological response to the pathogen located elsewhere in the body [3, 143]. Thus, steroids may be more beneficial in the latter case. Higher treatment failure rates were also observed in patients with choroidal involvement and associated vitreous haze [148]. Caution and close observation of patients on ATT is required as isoniazid and ethambutol can cause toxic optic neuropathy [149]. Nevertheless, TB-associated endophthalmitis has a very poor outcome. The majority of cases (83.7%) end in either evisceration, enucleation or exenteration of the eye [142]. Of note, this figure is significantly higher than for EBE which is reported to be 20% [3].

Nontuberculous mycobacteria (NTM) have also been shown to cause endogenous endophthalmitis [150]. They can be divided into slow and rapid growers [151]. The latter group comprises the most cases of overall ocular infections and carries worse visual outcomes [152, 153]. However, rapid growers are mainly associated with exogenous endophthalmitis and can occur in healthy individuals [150]. On the other hand, endogenous endophthalmitis is typically secondary to infection by slow growers and occurs almost exclusively in immunocompromised patients. The source of infection is often unknown but disseminated infections have been documented [150, 154]. Some of the NTM slow growers implicated in endogenous endophthalmitis include *Mycobacterium avium* (the most common), *Mycobacterium kansasii, Mycobacterium triplex and Mycobacterium haemophilum*. A case of a rapid grower NTM, *Mycobacterium chelonae,* has also been documented to cause endogenous endophthalmitis as has the slow-growing *Mycobacterium bovis* [155, 156]. NTM endophthalmitis is often misdiagnosed as fungal or bacterial infection as it can present as a chronic intraocular inflammation [152, 157]. Therefore, an infection by NTM should be suspected in any immunocompromised patient with chronic granulomatous intraocular inflammation and poor response to anti-inflammatory drugs. Guidelines for treatment of NTM infection have yet to be established; however, slow grower NTM can usually be treated by the standard ATT, while rapid grower NTM are more sensitive to macrolides, aminoglycosides and fluoroquinolones [158].

6. Endogenous viral endophthalmitis (EVE)

Viral infections represent a significant cause of posterior segment endogenous endophthalmitis due to their systemic spread, and viruses are more likely than other organisms to spread via a neuronal pathway. Viral infections can appear as isolated ocular manifestations or as part of a systemic infection. For example, Herpes Simplex virus 1 (HSV-1) and Varicella Zoster virus (VZV) spread via transaxonal route while Cytomegalovirus (CMV) and Epstein Barr virus (EBV) spread via hematogenous route within lymphocytes [159]. Infections causing posterior segment infections can lead to manifestations of the choroid, retina, and vitreous due to their highly vascularized nature [160, 161]. Prompt recognition and treatment can lead to improved visual outcomes in patients, but EVE is often misdiagnosed as non-infectious uveitis, anterior uveitis, or conjunctivitis, leading to poorer outcomes [160].

Patients with EVE often have an underlying immunosuppressed condition, so they should be evaluated for underlying immunosuppression if not already known [65]. DM, corticosteroid use, diminished lymphocyte response, HIV/AIDS, and malignancy can all encourage viruses to proliferate [162]. Patients with a history of travel to endemic areas or close contact with farm animals (particularly swine herders) should be evaluated for EVE [161]. Cases of EVE following systemic Ebola and COVID-19 infections have also been documented [163, 164]. There have been cases of viral endophthalmitis following intravitreal steroid injections that are exogenous in nature [160]. Identifying the common clinical features can aid in the prompt diagnosis of EVE. Common features include photophobia, decreased visual acuity, and eye pain [161]. Other presenting ocular features include conjunctival hemorrhages, peripapillary hemorrhage, narrowing of the inferior retinal vessels, anterior segment inflammation, focal lesion of the posterior pole, vitreous inflammation, occlusive vasculitis, keratic precipitates, chorioretinal scarring, ocular hypertension, and neovascularization [160, 163, 164]. EVE frequently presents as unilateral disease on presentation but can become bilateral as it progresses [160, 165–167].

Successful treatment of EVE requires prompt diagnosis using fluid from a vitreous tap [160]. PCR is the main laboratory test that has been effective in establishing diagnosis of viral infection such as HSV, VZV and CMV [160]. One study examined aqueous and vitreous fluid samples for HSV-1, HSV-2, VZV, EBV, CMV, and Human Herpesvirus 6 found PCR to have sensitivity and specificity of 91.3% and 98.8%, respectively in detection of herpes viruses as well as toxoplasma and fungal elements [168]. Viral serology of the vitreous is effective in confirming the pathogen involved in 80–90% of cases [160, 169, 170] and frequently changes the working diagnosis (23%) or confirms an uncertain diagnosis (39%) [170]. Moreover, PCR sensitivity can be further improved when combined with the calculation of Goldmann-Witmer coefficient (GWC) and immunoblotting for ocular fluid and serum antibodies. The GWC is a comparison of specific antibodies levels to total immunoglobulin in both aqueous humor and serum samples. Multiplex PCR allows testing of several organisms from a single ocular sample; however, this process, similar to monoplex PCR, does require the knowledge of a particular virion's sequence information prior to testing in order to design the primer necessary to generate a PCR product [171]. Fundus photography, retinal imaging, and optical coherence tomography (OCT) are all useful in diagnosing and monitoring EVE [160, 172].

Treatment of EVE requires systemic antivirals, intravitreal antivirals (or intraocular antiviral implants), and systemic corticosteroids for inflammation [160]. In the 1990s, Peyman and many others noted improvement of cytomegalovirus (CMV) retinitis after treatment with intravitreal ganciclovir and systemic antivirals [76, 173–179]. Studies also confirm the efficacy of systemic valaciclovir for appropriate management of EVE [179]. The role of systemic and intravitreal acyclovir for treatment of herpes virus retinitis has also been documented [174, 178]. Management of both ocular and systemic complications is essential for a favorable prognosis [160]. Long-term preventative antiviral therapy may be considered if patients present with recurrent inflammation. Patients may require anti-vascular endothelial growth factor agents for macular edema or neovascularization [160] and may also undergo vitrectomy for proper management. Vitrectomy should be considered when patients present with severe inflammation, retinal detachment, or traction that may create a detachment. Vitrectomy with silicone-oil tamponade and scleral buckle placement has been proven successful [179]. Caution should be taken in eyes of patients with a history of Ebola virus disease who present with evolving dark retinal regions, as these are characteristic of viable *Zaire ebolavirus* (EBOV) which poses a significant health risk during intraocular procedures [163]. Some eyes may experience neovascularization, for which they should undergo photocoagulation and/or retinal detachment surgery [160].

Several viruses have been implicated in the development of EVE. Most commonly, it is due to reactivation of the herpesvirus family, specifically varicella zoster virus (VZV), herpes simplex virus (HSV I and HSV II), CMV, and Epstein–Barr virus (EBV) [160, 180, 181]. The outcome of viral reactivation is influenced by multiple factors including strain virulence, human leukocyte antigen, and host immune response. HSV- EVE is generally well treated with systemic antiviral and corticosteroids with the resolution of symptoms [181]. However, as the virus remains latent in the trigeminal and dorsal root ganglion, recurrence is possible [181]. VZV-EVE may occur in adults with chickenpox but is rare in children [160]. It is more common in adults and may precede shingles in immunocompromised patients, but Acute Retinal Necrosis (ARN) can occur in patients with normal immune function; HSV I, HSV II, and VZV can cause ARN [182]. VZV generally has a poorer prognosis compared to HSV. EBV-EVE generally has a good prognosis and resolves rapidly with near-complete recovery [160]. Most people (90%) are CMV seropositive (it is thought to be latent in bone marrow) so it periodically actively replicates in both immunocompromised and normal patients. Therefore, culture of CMV shed in the patient's urine does not mean active systemic CMV infection to support the diagnosis of CMV retinitis. Patients can experience systemic symptoms, but ocular manifestations are more likely to be the initial finding [183]. CMV retinitis has historically had poor visual outcomes, although new antiretroviral therapies have decreased its incidence and improved outcomes [183]. Patients may experience reactivation of herpesvirus infections following other viral infections, such as COVID-19 [184].

Other causes implicated with EVE include pseudorabies, Zika virus, Dengue, Ebola, Chikungunya, and COVID-19 [163–165, 185]. Unlike herpesvirus infections, patients typically do not present with a history of immunosuppression. However, history is significant with respect to travel to endemic areas or known exposure to infected individuals [163–165, 185]. The posterior vitreous cavity may act as a reservoir for some viral infections. Zika and COVID-19 infections are notable for the presence of viral RNA in the tears [165]. In contrast, patients with Ebola Virus Disease (EBD) in the eye are negative for Ebola of the tears and conjunctiva [163]. However, virions have been recovered from the anterior chamber in eyes of recovered Ebola patients and poses a risk for cataract surgeons [163].

Patients with ocular viral infections are also at risk for reactivation of other bacterial or fungal agents in the eye. Cases of toxoplasmosis following Ebola infection have been documented in a small subset of patients [127]. Compared to more common causes, novel causes of EVE (Dengue and COVID) have no prospective, randomized therapeutic trials. As such, definitive therapies are not well established, and prognosis can range from full resolution to permanent vision loss [165, 185]. COVID-19 and Zika are more likely to cause poor visual outcomes compared to standard causes [164, 165]. Prompt diagnosis and early treatment are important for good visual outcomes of EVE.

7. Endogenous fungal endophthalmitis (EFE)

Fungi can lead to infection of the posterior chamber through hematogenous spread; in fact, this represents the most frequent cause of EFE [186, 187]. Most cases of fungal endogenous endophthalmitis have a predisposing systemic risk factor. Common risk factors for EFE include recent hospitalization, systemic surgery, indwelling catheter, broad-spectrum antibiotic use, steroids, parenteral nutrition, cytotoxic therapies, and gastrointestinal disease [186]. Lower abdominal procedures, including genitourinary procedures (e.g. uterine curettage, urinary tract dilation, lithiasis removal), and toe-nail extraction due advanced onychomycosis have been implicated with EFE [188]. Most cases of fungal endogenous endophthalmitis have a predisposing systemic risk factor [189]. Diagnosis of EFE is frequently missed, as these characteristic findings might mimic non-infectious uveitis and orbital cellulitis [190]. In the pediatric population, common misdiagnoses are orbital cellulitis, congenital glaucoma, conjunctivitis, and retinoblastoma [191]. Misdiagnosis rates range from 16% to 63% [4, 191].

Patients who experience misdiagnosis can experience a delay in diagnosis (mean of 13 days) [186, 192], but familiarity with the clinical features of EFE can aid in avoiding this. Patients frequently complain of blurry or decreased vision (77%), redness (49%), eye pain (34%), floaters (26%), and photophobia (12%) [192]. Systemic symptoms also include frequently mild and relapsing fever, scalp lesions, and other pain [193]. In a study that examined 65 eyes with EFE found most eyes to have diffuse anterior and posterior segment inflammation (71%), followed by focal posterior inflammation (28%) and focal anterior segment inflammation (2%) [186]. Eyes with EFE can have some characteristic exam findings that can help in establishing a proper diagnosis. For example, eyes with EFE from *Candida spp*. typically will have one or more creamy, white chorioretinal lesions most commonly found in the posterior pole [194]. These lesions tend to be less than 1 mm in diameter with an overlying vitritis. Moreover, fluffy white vitreous opacities connected by strands of inflammatory material ("string of pearls") can be noted [194]. Also, EFE from *Aspergillus* can have a characteristic macular chorioretinal lesion that can be associated with a gravitational layering of inflammatory exudates (pseudohypopyon) either in the preretinal or subretinal space [195].

Due to their systemic nature in immunocompromised patients, cases are more likely to be bilateral compared to other causes of endogenous endophthalmitis, but the majority are still unilateral [196]. Unlike bacterial causes, EFE is less associated with a known focal systemic lesion. About 44% of patients with EFE from *Candida* spp. had no known focal lesion [29]. However, patients frequently present with a history of IVDU, chemotherapy, DM, abdominopelvic procedures and renal failure. Mold infections, caused by organisms such as *Aspergillus*, commonly occur with a history of iatrogenic immunosuppression, corticosteroid use, neutropenic patients, or solid organ transplantation [188, 189, 196, 197]. It is rare for patients with AIDS or IVDU to have *Aspergillus* endophthalmitis [197], and those patients are more likely to have a history of pulmonary aspergillosis or disseminated aspergillosis [196].

An accurate diagnosis of the causative agent is essential to the treatment of EFE. Culture positivity for *Candida* spp. EFE rates range from 45% to 74% in the immunocompromised, perhaps leading to more frequent misdiagnosis in this population. PCR is increasingly becoming the gold standard diagnostic tool for the identification of EFE infections: Identification has been reported to be up to 100% compared to 37.5% in traditional culture techniques [198, 199]. However, PCR does experience the same pitfalls in the diagnosis of fungal infections as it does for EBE. Prompt diagnosis with PCR and intervention with early vitrectomy and/or chorioretinal biopsy have improved patient visual outcomes [200].

Candida spp. infections represent the most common cause of fungal endogenous endophthalmitis, with incidences ranging from 34–36% of cases of all EFE [29]. The *Candida* spp. are known to affect the eye and have a predilection toward the posterior segment [190, 196]. Reports show infection of *Candida* spp. after pacemaker implantation [196]. In immunocompromised patients, the most common cause of fungal endogenous endophthalmitis is *Candida* [199]. Infection with a new candida strain, *Candida dubliniensis*, has been noted in several countries. Although much less frequent than other *Candida* species, *C. dubliniensis* can present with fluconazole-resistance and no other systemic evidence for disseminated disease [201]. However, *C. dubliniensis* has better treatment outcomes compared to *C. albicans* [201]. Despite its low frequency in overall endophthalmitis cases, *Candida albicans* is the most common cause of endogenous endophthalmitis in pediatric populations worldwide. Risk of infection increases with a history of distant wound infection, meningitis, intravenous catheters, and UTIs [191, 202]. Common causes of pediatric fungal endophthalmitis include neonatal sepsis, poor hygiene, or an immunocompromised status [191]. Given the high rates of misdiagnosis in this population (63%), there is evidence that dilated ophthalmic examination of patients with invasive fungal disease and screening of at-risk children with evidence of fungal colonization has some therapeutic benefit [4, 191, 203].

The *Aspergillus* genus represents the second most common cause of fungal endophthalmitis (33%) [199]. Other common opportunistic fungi include *C. neoformans*, *Fusarium* spp., *Scedosporium*, *Rhodotorula* spp., *Mucor* spp., *Alternaria* spp., *Acremonium falciforme Pneumocystis jiroveci*, and many other less prevalent fungal species [167, 196, 198, 204]. Microsporidum has also been implicated with posterior segment etiology [205].

Pathogenic dimorphic fungi have also been implicated in EFE. Unlike opportunistic causes, pathogenic dimorphic fungi are usually regionally restricted. These infections can cause endophthalmitis in both immunocompetent and immunocom promised hosts. EFE is primarily a result of a disseminated pulmonary infection [196, 206]. Examination of the eye for dimorphic fungi shows fluffy yellow/white aggregates with retinal hemorrhages. *Coccidiodies immitis*, *Blastomyces dermatitidis, Histoplasma capsulatum,* and *S. schenckii* have all been implicated as regional causes of EFE [167, 196, 198, 204]. Patients who are suspected of having systemic *C. immitis* and *Blastomyces* should undergo serial eye examination given its insidious nature, especially for immunocompromised patients [196, 207, 208]. *C. immitis* does not always present with signs of systemic infection, so visual cues such as vitreous opacities are beneficial to a systemic diagnosis [207]. Despite early diagnosis and prompt treatment, it is reported that 50% of patients who do not succumb to the disseminated infection undergo enucleation of the infected eye [196, 207–209]. The initial treatment of suspected EFE should be intravitreal and systemic antifungal agents followed by early surgical intervention [193]. Depending on the specific cause and duration of EFE, medications used for treatment include amphotericin B, systemic fluconazole (oral or IV), voriconazole, and caspofungin, with preference depending on sensitivity of the infection and side effect profile. Like EBE, a tap-and-inject technique is recommended through the pars plana to collect a sample of the vitreous for culture followed by intravitreal injection of antifungals. Again, sometimes a chorioretinal biopsy may be required for identification of the fungus [171, 200, 210].

Treatment of endogenous fungal endophthalmitis in the eyes of pediatric population have shown favorable resolution with systemic and intravitreal antifungals, intravitreal steroids, and early surgical intervention. However, there is no specific guideline for dosing of pediatric patients with EFE with systemic and intravitreal antibiotics [192]. While patients with EFE have shown resolution of symptoms, as noted, with systemic and intravitreal antifungal medications, eyes that present with poor vision or are refractory to injected antifungals should undergo vitrectomy [198]. Surgical intervention via early PPV has been proven to have therapeutic efficacy [199].

Of all the fungal causes, infections with *Candida* spp. have shown the best visual acuity outcomes. Results for eyes with *Aspergillus* EFE are not as favorable because of increased rates of macular scarring secondary to infection [211].

8. Endogenous protozoal endophthalmitis

Protozoans, unicellular eukaryotic organisms, are a major cause of intraocular infections worldwide. Different protozoa have special animal hosts with varying routes of infection. Travel and dietary history as well as patient habits are important in establishing a diagnosis, since most transmission occurs through contaminated food and water sources in endemic areas. Protozoa such as *Giardia lamblia, Plasmodium falciparum, Acanthamoeba* spp., and *Toxoplasma gondii* can all present with intraocular manifestations; however, only toxoplasmosis is well established to cause endogenous endophthalmitis.

Acanthamoeba spp., typically associated with contact lens wear, trauma, and contaminated water exposure, can cause keratitis. Advanced stages can lead to corneal perforation and endophthalmitis; however, it is exogenous in nature secondary to direct corneal extension [212, 213]. Malaria, an infectious disease caused by *Plasmodium* and carried by *Anopheles* mosquitoes, leads to retinal ocular manifestation without any intraocular inflammation. Retinal findings, such as patchy retinal whitening and retinal hemorrhages, occur in severe cerebral malaria caused by *Palsmodium falciparum* but are secondary to microvascular obstruction and severe anemia [214, 215]. *Giardia lamblia*, the most common intestinal parasite worldwide, is acquired through ingestion of cysts from contaminated water [216]. Asymptomatic salt-and-pepper retinal degeneration is the most common ocular manifestation of giardiasis [217]. Only rare cases of retinal arteritis and anterior uveitis have been documented in the literature [218, 219]. Ocular sequalae of giardiasis is believed to occur as result of immune response to cross-reacting antigens or molecular mimicry rather than a direct invasion by the parasite [217, 220].

Toxoplasmosis gondii, a ubiquitous protozoan that infects roughly one third of the human population, is the most common cause of uveitis worldwide [221, 222]. Oocytes from cat (definitive host) feces infect humans (intermediate hosts) through consumption of contaminated water and undercooked meats (animals already infected) or from direct mishandling of domestic cat feces [223, 224]. In the past, all cases of ocular toxoplasmosis were believed to be reactivations of previous congenital infections; however, recent evidence has shown that most cases are in fact acquired postnatally [221, 225]. Congenital infection occurs when the mother is infected with the protozoa either just before conception or during gestation, which leads to vertical transmission through the placenta to the fetus. Fetal transmission only occurs if the mother is exposed to the parasite for the first time or to a novel strain [226]. Unless she is immunocompromised, a previously infected mother already possesses the immunity that protects her and the fetus from any new infection. Fetal infection during the first trimester will typically lead to a more severe form of congenital toxoplasmosis than later stages of pregnancy [227]. Retinochoroiditis is a common ocular manifestation, which may lead to blindness if left untreated [228]. Other extraocular clinical signs of congenital toxoplasmosis include seizures, sensorineural hearing loss, intracranial calcifications, microcephaly, and cognitive impairment. Prompt treatment of the newly infected mother with spiramycin has demonstrated a 60% reduction in congenital toxoplasmosis [229]. Moreover, prompt postnatal treatment of infants is also warranted. Infants who were treated after one year of life were more likely to develop new retinochoroidal lesions than patients who received earlier treatment (70% vs. 31%, respectively) [230]. It is important to note that clinical presentation of congenital toxoplasmosis can resemble congenital viral infections such as HSV, CMV, Zika virus, and rubella, which needs to be taken into consideration when making the diagnosis [228].

Other clinical classifications of toxoplasmosis include acquired cases in immunocompetent and immunocompromised patients. Toxoplasmosis is mainly asymptomatic in healthy patients. Painless cervical lymphadenopathy is the main clinical manifestation if symptoms do occur. Retinochoroiditis is also a common feature, since *Toxoplasma gondii* is the most common pathogen to infect the retina in immunocompetent patients [231]. Retinal lesions can present in acute or reactivation stages, and in the latter case, lesions are essentially similar whether the original infection was congenital or acquired [232, 233].

Retinochoroiditis is frequently subclinical but can result in retinal detachment and loss of vision [228, 234]. Other symptoms may include pain, photophobia and epiphora. Ophthalmic exam is vital in the diagnosis of retinochoroiditis, which typically presents as a focal white lesion with overlying vitritis. When vitritis is severe, a classic finding of "headlight in the fog" can be seen. Healed lesions become atrophic and develop a scar bordered with black pigment. Atypical lesions found in elderly and immunocompromised patients have distinctive characteristics including hemorrhages, multiple foci and features present in acute retinal necrosis (ARN) such as peripheral retinitis, vasculitis and vitritis [235, 236]. Early management of toxoplasmosis in immunodeficient patients is vital, as disseminated disease has 100% mortality if left untreated.

Recurrences of retinochoroiditis are common, roughly 80%, with a median interval of two years [237]. New lesions tend to occur at the border of an old, scarred lesion. Recurrences are more common after cataract extraction and in patients older than 40 years of age as well as in previously affected eyes [237–239]. Nevertheless, late sequelae and recurrences from congenital infection tend to be bilateral, more severe, and involve the macula, whereas acquired infections are usually unilateral, spare the macula, and are not associated with an old chorioretinal scar [228, 232, 240].

The diagnosis of toxoplasmosis is mainly clinical based on characteristic retinal lesions; however, serology can confirm the exposure to the protozoa. Various methods exist for detecting IgG and IgM immunoglobulins against *Toxoplasma gondii* such as immunocapture, immunoblot, immunosorbent agglutination, indirect immunofluorescence, enzyme-linked immunosorbent assays, and Chemiluminescence Immunoassay (CLIA) [241–243]. Each test has its own sensitivities and specificities which are beyond the scope of this chapter. Nevertheless, IgM antibodies indicate a primary infection and can be especially helpful in pregnant patients to determine whether infection occurred during or prior to pregnancy, while memory IgG antibodies demonstrate previous infection. IgM antibodies typically appears during the first week of infection and can remain detectable up to a year, while IgG appears approximately 2 weeks after the infection and typically remains detectable for life [244]. For example, patients with chronic and recurrent retinochoroiditis will typically only have IgG detected, whereas detection of both IgM and IgG typically indicates a primary and acute infection.

These serological tests only reveal previous exposure to *Toxoplasma gondii* and offer little insight into the mode of transmission. However, a new test using a protozoa-specific protein called *T. gondii* embryogenesis-related protein (TgERP) can be useful in determining the original source of infection [245]. PCR amplification has also been successfully utilized in the diagnosis of toxoplasmosis and can be especially useful in atypical patient presentations. PCR is also beneficial in testing for congenital infections, since it offers earlier diagnosis and avoids the invasiveness of serum testing on fetuses by sampling amniotic fluid [228, 246]. PCR can also utilize CSF, urine, fetal, and placental tissue [228, 247]. Moreover, a newer test that utilizes similar general principles of PCR, known as loop-mediated isothermal amplification method (LAMP), might offer a cheaper and simpler alternative in confirming *Toxoplasma gondii* exposure [248].

There is a lack of evidence supporting the utility of routine antibiotic and steroid regimens in the treatment of acute retinochoroiditis [249]. Not all cases necessarily warrant treatment; for example, small lesions in the periphery that are not vision-threatening tend to be self-limited and will heal spontaneously in immunocompetent patients [250–252]. Most clinicians will treat patients with disease persisting more than one month and associated with reduced visual acuity. Other indications for treatment include lesions that are vision-threatening such as those affecting the macula or the optic nerve, lesions larger than one disc diameter, lesions in monocular patients, presence of multiple lesions, lesions associated with moderate to severe vitritis, active lesions over a large vessel, or lesions in immunocompromised patients [253]. The classic triple therapy comprises oral pyrimethamine, sulfadiazine, and prednisolone. Pyrimethamine is prescribed with folinic acid to prevent bone marrow toxicity (anemia). Alternative treatments include oral trimethoprim-sulfamethoxazole (TMP-SMX), azithromycin, or clindamycin, all of which have shown favorable results [254–256]. Intravitreal treatment has also been studied for the treatment of ocular toxoplasmosis [257, 258]. Combined clindamycin and dexamethasone intravitreal injections were found to be comparable to a regimen of oral pyrimethamine and sulfadiazine [258–260]. Intravitreal TMP-SMX with dexamethasone also demonstrated benefit [261, 262]. Intravitreal injections can be favorable in pregnant patients due to their reduced systemic toxicity compared to oral medication [263, 264]. Photocoagulation around the foci of the scars and vitrectomy have also been performed; however, these studies are limited and did not show any preventive effect [265]. Fulminant ocular toxoplasmosis may occur with corticosteroid monotherapy, in which case vitrectomy may be warranted [266].

9. Endogenous helminthic endophthalmitis

Helminths at either the larval or adult stage can lead to the infection of ocular tissues through adjacent structures or may have a predilection for ocular tissue as they migrate through the vascular system [267]. Helminths generally only have a unilateral eye presentation, but there is no observed difference in eye predominance [192]. Although infrequent, helminth infections are more common in areas of consumption of contaminated water, raw meat, and freshwater fish [268, 269], so travel history to endemic areas is essential to ascertain the source of the infection. However, due to movement via rapid transport, such history might not be present [267]. Helminth endogenous endophthalmitis is much less frequent compared to bacterial, viral, and fungal causes. Pediatric populations are more likely to have zoonotic infections, such as *Toxocara canis*, due to ingestion of eggs or larvae in the feces of infected animals [270]. As such, rates for infections from parasitic sources are higher than the adult population [192] and more likely to be from less virulent organisms [192]. A common misdiagnosis in pediatric patients with an ocular helminth infection is retinoblastoma, requiring enucleation of the eye [192].

Due to the nature of these parasites, pathological lesions show a wider variety of clinical presentations compared to other causes of EE. Perhaps the most common cause of helminth infection is *Toxocara*, a notable cause of unilateral visual loss. Autopsy of affected individuals has shown infection of the brain, eye, lungs, and liver [268–270]. Human infection is noted in populations with a high prevalence of the consumption of freshwater raw fish [271]. Diagnosis of ocular toxocariasis is mainly a clinical one as the definitive diagnosis of histologic demonstration of larva is unfeasible and rarely done. Ophthalmic presentation of ocular toxocariasis include granuloma located in the posterior pole (25%) or the periphery with associated fibrous bands extending posteriorly (50%) [272]. Chronic endophthalmitis is also a common presentation (25%) [272]. Serum ELISA antibody test is commonly used to detect exposure to toxocariasis; however, intraocular fluid (aqueous humor and vitreous) ELISA antibody testing can be positive despite negative serum [270, 272]. Systemic or topical corticosteroid is commonly used to control the acute inflammatory reaction [270]. Albendazole is the current antihelminth drug of choice; however, it has yet to be proven that antihelminth drugs can kill intraocular larva [273, 274]. Pars plana vitrectomy or laser photocoagulation to remove the causal agent is also recommended in some patients [268, 270].

Two helminths with ocular manifestations are *Onchocerca volvulus* and *Loa loa*. Humans with an *Onchocerca volvulus* infection generally have an adult worm that produces microfilariae over a bony prominence. The microfilariae migrate throughout the connective tissue, skin, and ocular structures. Predominant ocular findings include punctate keratitis, iridocyclitis, chorioretinitis, and optic atrophy [268]. Diagnosis is accomplished via slit-lamp examination of microfilariae, with the aid of a punch biopsy [268, 275]. Treatment includes removal of the adult worm and administration of ivermectin. *Loa loa* is also diagnosed via circulating microfilariae; however, the adult worm is more commonly found in the conjunctiva [268]. Treatment of *Loa loa* includes removal of the worm and use of diethylcarbamazine [268]. Another helminth involved in EE is *Angiostrongylus cantonesis*. Patients generally present with blurred vision and poor visual acuity, and ocular symptoms generally occur two weeks to two months after ingestion of the *Pila* snail [268]. Patients are diagnosed via indirect ophthalmoscopy. Patients generally do not have favorable outcomes with an ocular infection of the nematode *Angiostrongylus*. Surgery, laser, and corticosteroid interventions do not improve visual acuity, as alteration of the RPE and retina are caused by the parasite directly. There is no specific therapy for *Angiostrongylus* EE [268]. Many other helminth infections have been implicated in endogenous helminth endophthalmitis, including dirofilarisis, taenia solium, fascioliasis, and schistosomiasis [268, 276, 277].

One helminth unique to the pediatric population is *Baylisascariasis procyonis*, a raccoon roundworm originating in North America. Seven cases document children with a history of pica and raccoon exposure who developed unilateral subacute neuroretinitis [278]. The worm can be identified via immunofluorescence assay of the serum or CSF, but the definitive diagnosis is visualization of the offending organism in the eye. Treatment options include albendazole and corticosteroids, but patients have a poor prognosis [279].

The most common helminths in the pediatric population are *Toxocara* and *Cysticercus*. Pediatric infections generally have fewer systemic symptoms, causing a delayed diagnosis of endogenous endophthalmitis [192]. Results in pediatric populations are not as favorable as in adult populations due to the delay in diagnosis and diffuse infection of the eye. Advantages of an early vitrectomy in pediatric populations include improved outcomes in patients, though visual rehabilitation is still a challenge for this population [192].

Helminths have also shown surprising manifestations in immunocompromised hosts. One patient with a history of systemic lupus erythematosus (SLE) presented with decreased bilateral vision in both eyes. Fundoscopy showed granulomas in the posterior poles bilaterally, with new granulomas developing in subsequent exams. Serology was positive for *Toxocara*. The patient was initially treated with intravitreal amphotericin B, vancomycin, and ceftazidime. After a full course of antibiotics and with albendazole, the patient had improved visual acuity of both eyes [280].

Another subset of immunocompromised patients who are at risk for helminth-induced endogenous endophthalmitis is the IVDU population. One patient with a history of IVDU reported two weeks of worsening right eye pain with decreased visual acuity. Endophthalmitis was suspected and a vitreous tap was performed. Gram stain showed no organisms, but rare white blood cells were present. Initial labs, bacterial and fungal cultures were negative. The patient was admitted for the endogenous spread of infection and placed on IV antibiotics. The patient's repeat serology was found to be positive for *Toxocara* titers [269].

Diagnosis of *Toxocara* or other helminths can be difficult in immunocompromised patients. Presentations can vary from granuloma formation to chronic retinal manifestations [269, 280]. Additionally, the parasitic load may not be high enough to give a positive serology result [269]. Serial optical coherence tomography (OCT) to observe for larval movement might aid diagnosis.

Immunocompromised patients with significant animal contact who present with suspicion of endogenous endophthalmitis should be considered for a helminth cause [4, 9]. Treatment of ocular toxocariasis should be tailored to the clinical presentation of the host, and patients with inflammation should be placed on steroids to reduce the risk of retinal detachment. Anti-helminthic agents and IV antibiotics have been successful, but surgical intervention may be necessary if complications occur [280].

10. Conclusion

Endogenous endophthalmitis can be a result of a systemic infection from a myriad of infectious agents including bacteria, viruses, fungi, protozoa, and helminthic organisms. Systemic infection should be suspected when there is no history of surgical intervention or trauma. Unlike exogenous endophthalmitis, the onset of clinical manifestations may be insidious and difficult to diagnose. This is particularly true in nonverbal patients.

Amikacin 200 *μg per* 0.1 *ml*	Step 1: Withdraw 0.4 ml from an amikacin vial (100 mg/2 ml)
	Step 2: Add the step 1 solution to a second 10 ml syringe containing 9.6 ml < 0.9% NaCl for injection USP (Preservative Free)
	Step 3: Withdraw 0.1 ml from step 2 solution (2 mg/ml), which will now contain 200 *μg*/0.1 ml of amikacin
Ceftazidime 2.2 mg/0.1 ml	Step 1: Reconstitue 1000 mg ceftazidime powder with 8 ml of 0.9% NaCl for injection USP (Preservative Free)
	Step 2: Withdraw all 8 mL of that the solution prepared in step 1 and add saline to create total volume of 10 ml. Then, withdraw 1 ml of that solution in a second syringe with 3.5 ml of 0.9% NaCl for injection USP (Preservative Free) (Total volume 4.5 mL)
	Step 3: Withdraw 0.1 from the step 2 solution (22.2 mg/ml), which will now contain 2.2 mg/0.1 ml of ceftazidime

Amikacin 200 μg per 0.1 ml	Step 1: Withdraw 0.4 ml from an amikacin vial (100 mg/2 ml)
	Step 2: Add the step 1 solution to a second 10 ml syringe containing 9.6 ml < 0.9% NaCl for injection USP (Preservative Free)
	Step 3: Withdraw 0.1 ml from step 2 solution (2 mg/ml), which will now contain 200 μg/0.1 ml of amikacin
Clindamycin 450 μg/0.1 ml	Step 1: Withdraw 0.3 ml from a vial of clindamycin (150 mg/ml)
	Step 2: Add the step 1 solution to a second 10 ml syringe containing 9.7 ml of 0.9% NaCl for injection USP (Preservative Free)
	Step 3: Withdraw 0.1 ml from step 2 solution (4.5 mg/ml), which will now contain 450 μg/0.1 of clindamycin
Gentamicin 100 μg/0.1 ml	Step 1: Withdraw 0.25 ml (10 mg) from a gentamicin vial (40 mg/ml)
	Step 2: Add the above 0.25 ml to a new 10 ml syringe containing 9.75 ml of 0.9% NaCl for injection USP (Preservative Free) (Final concentration 1mg/ml)
	Step 3: Withdraw 0.1 from step 2 solution (1 mg/ml), which will now contain 100 μg/0.1 ml of gentamicin
Vancomyci 1 mg/0.1 ml	Step 1: Dilute a vial of vancomycin powder (500 mg) with 10 ml 0.9% NaCI for injection USP (Preservative Free) Final concentration (50 mg/ml)
	Step 2: Withdraw 1 ml solution prepared in step 1 (50 mg/ml) into a new 5 ml syringe and add 4 ml of 0.9% NaCl for injection USP (Preservative Free) Final concentration (10 mg/ml)
	Step 3: Withdraw 0.1 from the step 2 solution (10 mg/ml), which will now contain 1 mg/0.1 ml of vancomycin
Dexamethasone 1000 μg (can inject to 1 mg)	Step 1: Withdraw 0.1 ml from a dexamethasone vial $_{u}$p containing 10 mg/ml vial
Amphotericin B 5 μg/0.1 ml	Step 1: one vial of 50 mg amphotericin B is diluted with 10 ml of sterile water (Preservative Free) Final concentration (5 mg/ml = 0.5 mg/0.1 ml)
	Step 2: Withdraw 0.1 ml of step 1 solution (0.5 mg/0.1 ml) and add it to 9.9 ml of sterile water (Preservative Free) Final concentration (0.05 mg/ml)
	Step 3: Withdraw 0.1 ml from step 2 solution, which will now contain 5 μg/0.1 ml of amphotericin B -final concentration 0.005mg/0.1 ml

Table 1.
Preparation of intravitreal pharmaceuticals.

1. Anesthetize the eyes with a topical anesthetic
2. Sterilize the eye with 5% povidone-iodine solution
3. Using a 25-gauge needle attached to a tuberculin syringe, position the needle perpendicular to the eye wall and enter 3.5 mm (in pseudophakic or aphakic eyes) or 4 mm (in phakic eyes)
4. Ensure the visualization of the needle from the pupil prior to aspirating the sample.
5. Gentle aspiration without excessive pressure then withdraw the needle.

Pearl 1: If 25-gauge needle is unsuccessful in obtaining a sample, then a 23-gauge needle can be used after making a small sclerotomy but a safer way is to use a 25 gauge vitrector through the sclerotomy site to obtain vitreous samples.
Pearl 2: Avoid attaching antibiotics to the original vitreous biopsy needle while in the eye due to increased risk of retinal injury. It is preferred to withdraw the biopsy needle and re-enter the eye with a new needle for antibiotic delivery.
Pearl 3: Injection of drugs should be limited to the smallest possible volume and the bevel of the needle

should be placed toward the lens, not toward the retina w.
Pearl 4: Do not combine dexamethasone and vancomycin in the syringe due to precipitation, but aminoglycosides and dexamethasone can be used in the same syringe. Of note, hemorrhagic occlusive retinal vasculitis has been reported with intravitreal gentamicin treatment

Table 2.
Vitreous tap technique [265].

- We recommend performing a PPV when endophthalmitis is suspected and when vitreous haze precludes the view of the disc or a large vessel.

- Goal of the PPV is to remove vitreous debris, obtain adequate sample for culture, reduce bacterial load, and prevent any further enzymatic degradation of the retina.

Table 3.
Pars Plana vitrectomy role Endophthalmitis [265].

1. In the absence of posterior view, we recommend insertion of a bent 23-gauge needle to infuse sterile air or balanced saline solution (BSS).

2. Resort to 23-gauge pneumovitrector or 25-gauge vitreous microinstrumentation to obtain diagnostic vitreous samples. These two instruments lead to minimal traction on the peripheral retina during vitreous collection.

3. In order to maintain IOP without sample dilution, the infusion fluid can be turn on as soon as the vitreous sample has been collected.

4. The vitrector aspiration port is attached to sterile syringe. Manual aspiration is applied as the surgeon performs the vitreous biopsy.

5. Lighted infusion cannula can be used as a source of light and infusion during both the vitreous biopsy collection and subsequent vitrectomy.

6. It is recommended that a separate posterior infusion cannula be placed early in the procedure.

7. Manipulation close to the retina should be avoided. A complete vitrectomy is not necessary at the first operation.

Pearl 1: Ensure avoidance of the retina in cases where the view is impaired, such as in eyes with a dense cataract.
Pearl 2: Vitrector can be safely placed behind the IOL in pseudophakic eyes.
Pearl 3: We recommend intravitreal and systemic therapy in endogenous endophthalmitis cases, especially in mycotic cases.
Pearl 4: Fluconazole 200 μ g/ml can be safely used in the infusion fluid during vitrectomy of eyes with endogenous fungal endophthalmitis.
Pearl 5: *(Silicone filled eyes)*
-Vitreous tap should be performed initially followed by intravitreal injection of one-quarter the recommended antibiotic dose for non-vitrectomized eye along with 1 mg dexamethasone.
-When purulent exudates are present in the vitreous cavity, we recommend the removal of silicone while using infusion fluid with recommended doses of antibiotics and steroids.
-The recommended infusion fluid composition for EBE: 20 μ g/ml vancomycin, 9 μ g/ml clindamycin, 8 μ g/ml gentamicin, 64 μ g/ml of dexamethasone.
-Silicone oil can be injected immediately after removal of infected eye's silicone oil or when inflammation is controlled.
Pearl 6: We recommend the reduced antibiotic dosage (25%) for retreatment in all vitrectomized eyes.

Table 4.
Pars Plana vitrectomy technique [265].

1. Perform a core pars plana vitrectomy
2. Perform endolaser around the desired biopsy site
3. Use 23-gauge vertical cutting intraocular scissors to incise the retinal specimen within the laser barrier to close the retinal vessels.
4. Hemostasis is achieved by raising the IOP by lifting the infusion fluid bottle, the vitrectomy instrument is used to slowly aspirate the retinal biopsy which is then removed from the aspiration tube slowly for culture and then proceed to close the sclerotomy.
5. Inject 20% or less sulfur hexafluoride gas/air into the eye.
6. Close the sclera and conjunctiva appropriately with suture if needed.

Pearl 1: Ensure that infusion bottle is raised during biopsy procedure to reduce the risk of intraocular hemorrhage. The infusion can then be turned off once hemostasis is achieved.
Pearl 2: Place the tissue specimen in the culture or fixation solution of choice and then promptly send it for microbiology and histology.
Pearl 3: Minimize any trauma to the biopsy during the procedure and transport.
Pearl 4: Often no further laser treatment or cryotherapy is required at the biopsy site.
Pearl 5: Instruct the patient to lay on the appropriate side to tamponade the site with gas during sleep.
Pearl 6: Closely follow up patients for any signs of retinal detachment.

Table 5.
Chorioretinal biopsy technique.

Infusion Fluid Upper limit of drug dosages without toxicity in non-vitrectomized eyes*	
Drug	**Nontoxic Dose (µg/ml)**
Single Drugs	
Amikacin	10
Amphotericin B methyl ester	75
Ceftazidime	40
Chloramphenicol	10
Clindamycin	9
Fluconazole	200
Gentamicin	8
Imipenem	16
Lincomycin	10
Methicillin	20
Netilmicin	4
Oxacillin	10
Penicillin	80
Teicoplanin	8
Tobramycin	10
Vancomycin	20
Dexamethasone	64
Combination Drugs	
Clindamycin/Gentamicin	9 / 8

Infusion Fluid Upper limit of drug dosages without toxicity in non-vitrectomized eyes*	
Drug	**Nontoxic Dose (μg/ml)**
Gentamicin/Oxacillin	8 / 10
Methicillin/Gentamicin	20 / 8
Penicillin/Gentamicin	80 / 8
**In vitrectomized eyes, one-quarter of the above doses should be used.*	

Table 6.
Antibiotics in the infusion fluid for pars Plana vitrectomy.

Causative agents of endogenous endophthalmitis discussed in this chapter
Gram-Positive Bacteria
Staphylococcus aureus
Streptococcus pneumoniae
Group B Streptococcus and other Streptococcus species
Listeria monocytogenes
Enterococcus faecalis
Nocardia species
Bacillus cereus
Gram-Negative Bacteria
Klebsiella pneumoniae
Pseudomonas aeruginosa
Neisseria meningitidis
Escherichia coli
Salmonella species
Serratia marcescens
Viruses
Cytomegalovirus
Ebola virus
Epstein–Barr virus
Herpes Simplex virus
SARS-CoV-2
Varicella-zoster virus
Zika virus
Protozoa
Toxoplasmosis gondii
Spirochetes
Borrelia burgdorferi
Leptospira
Treponema pallidum
Mycobacterium
Mycobacterium tuberculosis

Mycobacterium avium
Mycobacterium kansasii
Mycobacterium triplex
Mycobacterium haemophilum
Mycobacterium chelonae
Mycobacterium bovis

Table 7.
Causative agents of endogenous endophthalmitis discussed in this chapter.

Clinical presentations may be bilateral or unilateral. Vitreous and retinal involvement are potentially sight threatening and appropriate investigations should be performed to find the distal infection focus or systemic source(s) of the endogenous endophthalmitis and treatment usually involves systemic agents aimed at the offending organism as well as intravitreal pharmacotherapy and/or pars plana vitrectomy (PPV) to both obtain a microbiological sample both to identify the organism and to therapeutically debride the vitreous cavity of the organism, inflammatory cells, and destructive cytokines. Occasionally a chorioretinal biopsy may be required to identify the organism. Despite aggressive treatment, the eye (s) may lose vision, and some may require enucleation.

Addendum Treatment (**Tables 1–7**) [281].

Citation: Gholam A. Peyman, Stephen A. Meffert, Mandi D. Conway. Vitreoretinal Surgical Techniques, Second Edition, 2007.

Author details

Sami Kabbara[1], Neil Kelkar[2], Mandi D. Conway[1,2] and Gholam A. Peyman[1,2]*

1 Tulane University School of Medicine, Department of Ophthalmology, New Orleans, LA, USA

2 U of AZ College of Medicine-Phoenix Campus, Phoenix, AZ, USA

*Address all correspondence to: gpeyman1@yahoo.com

References

[1] Okada AA, Johnson RP, Liles WC Endogenous bacterial endophthalmitis: report of a ten-year retrospective study. Ophthalmology 101:832–8

[2] Silpa-Archa S, Ponwong A, Preble JM, Foster CS Culture-Positive Endogenous Endophthalmitis: An Eleven-Year Retrospective Study in the Central Region of Thailand. Ocul Immunol Inflamm 11:1–10

[3] Jackson TL, Paraskevopoulos T, Georgalas I Systematic review of 342 cases of endogenous bacterial endophthalmitis. Surv Ophthalmol. https://doi.org/10.1016/j.survophthal.2014.06.002.

[4] Jackson TL, Eykyn SJ, Graham EM, Stanford MR (2003) Endogenous bacterial endophthalmitis: A 17-year prospective series and review of 267 reported cases. Surv Ophthalmol 48: 403–423

[5] Wong JS, Chan TK, Lee HM Endogenous bacterial endophthalmitis: an East Asian experience and a reappraisal of a severe ocular affliction. Ophthalmology 107:1483–,

[6] Chersich MF, Takkinen J, Charlier C, et al Diagnosis and Treatment of Listeria monocytogenes Endophthalmitis: A Systematic Review. Ocul Immunol Inflamm 1:1–10

[7] Bajor A, Luhr A, Brockmann D Listeria monocytogenes endophthalmitis – case report and review of risk factors and treatment outcomes. BMC Infect Dis 16:332

[8] Chou FF, Kou HK Endogenous endophthalmitis associated with pyogenic hepatic abscess. J Am Col Surg 182:33–6

[9] Liao HR, Lee HW, Leu HS Endogenous Klebsiella pneumoniae endophthalmitis in diabetic patients. Can J Ophthalmol 27:143–7

[10] Koul S, Philipson A, Arvidson S Role of aqueous and vitreous cultures in diagnosing infectious endophthalmitis in rabbits. Acta Ophthalmol (Copenh. https://doi.org/10.1111/j.1755-3768.1990.tb01677.x.

[11] Liano C S-G, VF S-V, G S-V Sensitivity, specificity and predictive values of anterior chamber tap in cases of bacterial endophthalmitis. Eye Vis (l. https://doi.org/10.1186/s40662-017-0083-9

[12] Greenwald MJ, Wohl LG, Sell CH Metastatic bacterial endophthalmitis: a contemporary reappraisal. Surv Ophthalmol. https://doi.org/10.1016/0039-6257(86)90076-7.

[13] Okhravi N, Adamson P, Carroll N PCR-based evidence of bacterial involvement in eyes with suspected intraocular.

[14] Lohmann CP, Linde HJ, Reischl U Improved detection of microorganisms by polymerase chain reaction in delayed endophthalmitis after cataract surgery. Ophthalmology 107:1047–51

[15] RN VG Applications of the polymerase chain reac- tion to diagnosis of ophthalmic disease. Surv Ophthalmol 46:248–58

[16] Shah V, Garg A, Stanford M Endogenous Meningococcal Endophthalmitis with Isolated Joint Involvement in Immunocompetent Adults. Ocul Immunol Inflamm 27:1–4

[17] Lohmann CP, Gabel VP, Heep M Listeria monocyto- genes-induced endogenous endophthalmitis in an other- wise healthy individual: rapid PCR-diagnosis as the basis for effective treatment. Eur J Ophthalmol 9:53–7

[18] S.M. R, L J Polymerase Chain Reaction/Rapid Methods Are Gaining a Foothold in Developing Countries. PDA J Pharm Sci Technol 68:239–255

[19] A. A, W. F, W. P, W. L, L. Y, T B Identification of nine cryptic species of *Candida albicans*. BMC Infect Dis. https://doi.org/10.1186/s12879-018-3381-5.

[20] Franco-Duarte R, Černáková L, Kadam S Advances in Chemical and Biological Methods to Identify Microorganisms-From Past to Present. Microorganisms. https://doi.org/10.3390/microorganisms7050130

[21] Fung CP, Hu BS, Chang FY A 5-year study of the seroepidemiology of Klebsiella pneumoniae: high prevalence of capsular serotype K1 in Taiwan and implication for vaccine efficacy. J Infect Dis 181:2075–9

[22] Dodson D, Stewart R, Karcioglu Z, Conway MD, Mushatt D, Ayyala RS Klebsiella pneumoniae endophthalmitis secondary to liver abscess presenting as acute iridocyclitis. Ophthalmic Surg Lasers Imaging Sep-Oct;40:10 3928 15428877–20090901–17

[23] Reedy JS, Wood KE Endogenous Pseudomonas aeruginosa endophthalmitis: a case report and literature review. Intensive Care Med. https://doi.org/10.1007/s001340000623.

[24] Kresloff MS, Castellarin AA, Zarbin MA Endophthalmitis. Surv Ophthalmol 43:193–224

[25] Moisseiev E, Abbassi S, Park SS Intravitreal Dexamethasone in the Management of Acute Endophthalmitis: A Comparative Retrospective Study. Eur J Ophthalmol 27:67–73

[26] Menon J, Rennie IG Endogenous Pseudomonas endoph- thalmitis in an immunocompetent patient: a case for early diagnosis and treatment. Eye 14: 253–4

[27] CS R-GAF, MP G-D, LI L-A Pediatric endogenous endophthalmitis: Diagnostic challenge and review of the literature.

[28] Auerbach SB, Leach CT, B.J. Bateman, et al.Meningococcal endophthalmitis without concomitant septicemia or meningitis.

[29] Keynan Y, Finkelman Y, Lagacé-Wiens P (2012) The microbiology of endophthalmitis: Global trends and a local perspective. Eur J Clin Microbiol Infect Dis 31:2879–2886

[30] Brinser JH, J.B. HessMeningococcal endophthalmitis without meningitis.

[31] Kearns AM, M.S. Sprott-Endophthalmitis caused by Neisseria meningitides J Infect. 22:299–300

[32] Kerkhoff FT, Zee A, Bergmans AM Polymerase chain reaction detection of Neisseria meningitidis in the intraocular fluid of a patient with endogenous endophthalmitis but without associated meningitis. Ophthalmology 110:

[33] Dadia SD, Modi RR, Shirwadkar S, Potdar NA, Shinde CA, Nair AG Salmonella Typhi Associated Endogenous Endophthalmitis: A Case Report and a Review of Literature. Ocul Immunol Inflamm 28:1–6

[34] Sinha MK, Jalali S, Nalamada S Review of endogenous endophthalmitis caused by Salmonella species including delayed onset Salmonella typhi endophthalmitis. Semin Ophthalmol. https://doi.org/10.3109/08820538.2012.680642.

[35] Caravalho J, McMillan VM, Ellis Do RB, Betancourt A (1990) Endogenous endophthalmitis due to salmonella arizonae and hafnia alvei. South Med J 83:325–327

[36] Shohet I, Davidson S, Boichis H, Rubinstein E (1983) Endogenous

endophthalmitis due to Salmonella typhimurium - PubMed. Ann Ophthalmol 321–2

[37] YS Hwang SW LHJ-P Salmonella london endogenous endophthalmitis in a healthy infant.Yu. Dis J - June 1:578

[38] Memon M, Raman V Serratia marcescens endogenous endophthalmitis in an immunocompetent host. BMJ Case Rep. https://doi.org/10.1136/bcr-2015-209887.

[39] Gammon JA, Schwab I, Joseph P Gentamicin-Resistant Serratia marcescens Endophthalmitis. Arch Ophthalmol 98:1221–1223

[40] Breazzano MP, Jonna G, Nathan NR, Nickols HH, Agarwal A Endogenous Serratia marcescens panophthalmitis: A case series. Am J Ophthalmol Case Rep. https://doi.org/10.1016/j.ajoc.2019.100531.

[41] Shah SB, Bansal AS, Rabinowitz MP, Park C, EH Jr B, Eagle RC Endogenous Serratia marcescens endophthalmitis. Retin Cases Br Rep. https://doi.org/10.1097/ICB.0b013e318298bf6a.

[42] Marinella MA, Warwar R Endogenous endophthalmitis due to Serratia marcescens. South Med J. https://doi.org/10.1097/00007611-199804000-00016.

[43] Ma J, Carrell N, Baker CF Bilateral sequential choroidal abscess secondary to methicillin-resistant Staphylococcus aureus endogenous endophthalmitis. Can J Ophthalmol. https://doi.org/10.1016/j.jcjo.2020.01.008.

[44] RISHI EKTA, RISHI PUKHRAJ, NANDI KRISHNENDU, SHROFF DARAIUS, THERESE K ENDOPHTHALMITIS CAUSED BY ENTEROCOCCUS FAECALIS: A Case Series. Retina 29:214–217

[45] Bagga B, Reddy AK, Garg P Decreased susceptibility to quinolones in methicillin-resistant Staphylococcus aureus isolated from ocular infections at a tertiary eye care centre. Br J Ophthalmol 94:1407–1408

[46] Vola ME, Moriyama AS, Lisboa R Prevalence and antibiotic susceptibility of methicillin-resistant Staphylococcus aureus in ocular infections. Arq Bras Oftalmol 76:350–353

[47] Gorak EJ, Yamada SM, Brown JD Community-acquired methicillin-resistant Staphylococcus aureus in hospitalized adults and children without known risk factors. Clin Infect Dis 29: 797–800

[48] J. F, Y. M, A. B, al No Title. Ophthalmic Surg Lasers Imaging 48: 134–142

[49] B. P, J.W Y Mansoor A.M.: Subretinal abscess. BMJ Case Rep

[50] Shenoy SB, Thotakura M, Kamath Y, Bekur R Endogenous Endophthalmitis in Patients with MRSA Septicemia: A Case Series and Review of Literature. Ocul Immunol Inflamm. https://doi.org/10.3109/09273948.2015.1020173.

[51] Kansal V, Rahimy E, Garg S, Dollin M Endogenous methicillin-resistant Staphylococcus aureus endophthalmitis secondary to axillary phlegmon: a case report. Can J Ophthalmol. https://doi.org/10.1016/j.jcjo.2016.11.016.

[52] Sahin OZ, Kara E, Belice T, Ayaz T, Baydur Sahin S, Ozturk C, Yildirim S, Metin Y, Sahutoglu T Enterococcus faecalis endophthalmitis as a metastatic complication of hemodialysis vascular access-related sepsis: A case report and review of the literature. Hemodial Int. https://doi.org/10.1111/hdi.12356.

[53] Lee SY, Chee SP Group B Streptococcus endogenous

endophthalmitis : case reports and review of the literature. Ophthalmology 10:

[54] Yoshida M, Yokokura S, Nishida T, Mochizuki K, Suzuki T, Maruyama K, Otomo T, Nishiguchi KM, Kunikata H, Nakazawa T Endogenous endophthalmitis caused by group B streptococcus; case reports and review of 35 reported cases. BMC Ophthalmol. https://doi.org/10.1186/s12886-020-01378-0.

[55] Dave VP, Pathengay A, Panchal B, Jindal A, Datta A, Sharma S, Pappuru RR, Joseph J, Jalali S, Das T Clinical presentations, microbiology and management outcomes of culture-proven endogenous endophthalmitis in India. Indian J Ophthalmol 68:834–9

[56] Miller JJ, Scott IU, HW Jr F, Smiddy WE, Corey RP, Miller D Endophthalmitis caused by Streptococcus pneumoniae. Am J Ophthalmol. https://doi.org/10.1016/j.ajo.2004.03.008.

[57] M YY, R Y Pediatric endogenous endophthalmitis with presumed hyposplenism.Haruta. 10:

[58] V DG, N S, MJ T Endogenous pneumococcal endophthalmitis after splenectomy: report of two cases. Bull Soc Belge Ophtalmol 243:147–51

[59] Phillips WB, Shields CL, Shields JA, RC Jr E, Masciulli L, Yarian DL Nocardia choroidal abscess. Br J Ophthalmol. https://doi.org/10.1136/bjo.76.11.694.

[60] Kumar N, Garg N, Kumar N, Van Wagoner N Bacillus cereus panophthalmitis associated with injection drug use. Int J Infect Dis 26: 165–6

[61] Uchio E, Inamura M, Okada K, Hatano H, Saeki K, Ohno S A case of endogenous Enterococcus faecalis endophthalmitis. Jpn J Ophthalmol 36: 215–21

[62] Barge S, Rothwell R, Varandas R, Agrelos L Enterococcus faecalis Endogenous Endophthalmitis from Valvular Endocarditis. Case Rep Ophthalmol Med. https://doi.org/10.1155/2013/174869.

[63] Chaudhry IA, Shamsi FA, Al-Dhibi H, Khan AO Pediatric endogenous bacterial endophthalmitis: case report and review of the literature. J AAPOS. https://doi.org/10.1016/j.jaapos.2006.06.005.

[64] Milman T, Trubnik V, Shah M, McCormick SA, Finger PT Isolated Nocardia exalbida endogenous endophthalmitis. Ocul Immunol Inflamm. https://doi.org/10.3109/09273948.2011.563898.

[65] ME G-CY, TJ W Endogenous ocular nocardiosis: an interventional case report with a review of the literature. Surv Ophthalmol. https://doi.org/10.1016/j.survophthal.2011.03.003.

[66] Yap EY, Fam HB, Leong KP, Buettner H Nocardia choroidal abscess in a patient with systemic lupus erythematosus. Aust N Z J Ophthalmol. https://doi.org/10.1111/j.1442-9071.1998.tb01340.x.

[67] Masi RJ Endogenous endophthalmitis associated with bacillus cereus bacteremia in a cocaine addict. Ann Ophthalmol Oct;10(10):

[68] CL Jr C, WM M, GF H, JC M Endogenous Bacillus cereus panophthalmitis. Ann Ophthalmol Feb; 19(2):

[69] Hemady R, Zaltas M, Paton B, Foster CS, Baker AS Bacillus-induced endophthalmitis: new series of 10 cases and review of the literature. Br J Ophthalmol. https://doi.org/10.1136/bjo.74.1.26.

[70] Bouza E, Grant S, Jordan MC, Yook RH, Sulit HL Bacillus cereus Endogenous Panophthalmitis. Arch Ophthalmol 97:498–499

[71] D.F. M, L.A. F, H.E. A, S.K. G, L.A. W, T.A M Vitreous cefazolin levels after intravenous injection: effects of inflammation, repeated antibiotic doses, and surgery. Arch Ophthalmol 108:411–414

[72] J.L. A, R.M. K, R.L. B, M.Z S Human vitreous levels of selected antistaphylococcal antibiotics. Am J Ophthalmol 100:570–575

[73] Peyman GA, Spitznas M, Straatsma BR Chorioretinal diffusion of peroxidase before and after photocoagulation. Invest Ophthalmol 10:489–495

[74] Peyman GA, Spitznas M, Straatsma BR Peroxidase diffusion in the normal and photocoagulated retina. Invest Ophthalmol 10:181–189

[75] G.A P R.: Bacterial endophthalmitis. Treatment with intraocular injection of gentamicin and dexamethasone. Arch Ophthalmol 91:416–418

[76] G.A. P, E.M. L, D.M M Intravitreal injection of therapeutic agents. Retina 29:875–912

[77] The Endophthalmitis Vitrectomy Study Group: Results of the endophthalmitis vitrectomy study. Arch Ophthalmol 113:1479–1496

[78] Graham RO, Peyman GA Intravitreal injection of dexamethasone. Treatment of experimentally induced endophthalmitis. Arch Ophthalmol 92: 149–154

[79] Centers for Disease Control and Prevention. Sexually transmitted disease surveillance.

[80] Shalaby IA, Dunn JP, Semba RD, Jabs DA Syphilitic uveitis in human immunodeficiency virus-infected patients. Arch Ophthalmol 115:469–473

[81] Oliver SE, Cope AB, Rinsky JL, Williams C, Liu G, Hawks S, Peterman TA, Markowitz L, Fleischauer AT Erika Samoff, for the Ocular Syphilis Disease Investigation Specialists Workgroup, Increases in Ocular Syphilis—North Carolina, 2014–2015. Clin Infect Dis 65:15

[82] Doris JP, Saha K, Jones NP, al Ocular syphilis: the new epidemic. Eye (l 20: 703–705

[83] Eandi CM, Neri P, Adelman RA, Yannuzzi LA, ET Jr C International Syphilis Study Group. Acute syphilitic posterior placoid chorioretinitis: report of a case series and comprehensive review of the literature. Retina 32:1915–1941

[84] Becerra LI, Ksiazek SM, Savino PJ, al Syphilis uveitis in human immunodeficiency virus-infected and noninfected patients. Ophthalmology 96:1727–1730

[85] TH CN, B B, C F, E C, P L Syphilitic uveitis in patients infected with human immuno- deficiency virus. Graefes Arch Clin Exp Ophthalmol 243:863–869

[86] Barile GR, Flynn TE Syphilis exposure in patients with uveitis. Ophthalmology 104:1605–9

[87] LiJZ,TuckerJD,LoboAM,etal. OcularsyphilisamongHIV- infected individuals. Clin Infect Dis 51:468–471

[88] Moradi A, Salek S, Daniel E, Gangaputra S, Ostheimer TA, Burkholder BM, Leung TG, Butler NJ, Dunn JP, Thorne JE Clinical features and incidence rates of ocular complications in patients with ocular syphilis. Am J Ophthalmol. https://doi.org/10.1016/j.ajo.2014.10.030.

[89] Kiss S, Damico FM, Young LH Ocular manifestations and treatment of syphilis. Semin Ophthalmol 20:161–7

[90] P DM, EJ C, J S, D CWH, J B, L SY, V G, C P, R A Ocular Syphilis: An Update. Ocul Immunol Inflamm 27:117–125

[91] Fu EX, Geraets RL, Dodds EM Superficial retinal precipitates in patients with syphilitic retinitis. Retina 30:1135–1143

[92] Tamesis RR, Foster CS Ocular syphilis. Ophthalmology 97:1281–1287

[93] Puech C, Gennai S, Pavese P Ocular manifestations of syphilis: Recent cases over a 2.5-year period. Graefes Arch Clin Exp Ophthalmol 248:1623–1629

[94] Balba GP, Kumar PN, James AN Ocular syphilis in HIV- positive patients receiving highly active antiretroviral therapy. Am J Med 119:

[95] Levy JH, Liss RA, Maguire AM Neurosyphilis and ocular syphilis in patients with concurrent human immunodeficiency virus infection. Retina 9:175–180

[96] Amaratunge BC, Camuglia JE, Hall AJ Syphilitic uveitis: a review of clinical manifestations and treatment outcomes of syphilitic uveitis in human immunodeficiency virus-positive and negative patients. Clin Exp Ophthalmol 38:68–74

[97] Marra C, Sahi S, Tantalo L Enhanced molecular typing of Treponema pallidum: geographical distribution of strain types and association with neurosyphilis. J Infect Dis 202:1380–8

[98] Singh AE, Romanowski B Syphilis: review with emphasis on clinical, epidemiologic, and some biologic features. Clin Microbiol Rev 12:187–209

[99] Davis J Ocular syphilis. Curr Opin Ophthalmol 25:513–518

[100] Marra CM, Maxwell CL, Smith SL Cerebrospinal fluid ab- normalities in patients with syphilis: association with clinical and laboratory features. J Infect Dis 189:369–76

[101] Aldave AJ, King JA, Cunningham Jr ET Ocular syphilis. Curr Opin Ophthalmol 12:433–41

[102] Weinberg R Ocular involvement in Lyme disease. Am. Acad. Ophtalmol.

[103] Stanek G, Wormser GP, Gray J Lyme borreliosis. Lancet 379:461–473

[104] Bernard A, Seve P, Abukhashabh A, Roure-Sobas C, Boibieux A, Denis P, Broussolle C, Mathis T, Kodjikian L Lyme-associated uveitis: Clinical spectrum and review of literature. Eur J Ophthalmol. https://doi.org/10.1177/1120672119856943.

[105] Huppertz H, D M, Lieb W Ocular manifesta- tions in children and adolescents with Lyme arthritis. Br J Ophthalmol 83:1149–1152

[106] HO SIJ, MR V The expanding clinical spectrum of ocular Lyme borreliosis. Ophthalmology 107:581–587

[107] AM SU, GE L Retinal vasculitis in Lyme borreliosis. Bull Soc Belge Ophtalmol 259:205–214

[108] Bernard A, Kodjikian L, Abukhashabh A Diagnosis of Lyme-associated uveitis: value of serological testing in a tertiary centre. Br J Ophthalmol 102:369–372

[109] Tugwell P, Dennis DT, Weinstein A, Wells G, Shea B, Nichol G, Hayward R, Lightfoot R, Baker P, Steere AC Laboratory evaluation in the diagnosis of Lyme disease. Ann Intern Med 15;127(12):10 7326 0003–4819–127–12–199712150–00011

[110] Case definitions for infectious conditions under public health surveillance. Centers for Disease

Control and Prevention. MMWR Recomm Rep 1997:

[111] DJ K, GP W Ocular Lyme disease: case report and review of the literature. Br J Ophthalmol 74:325–327

[112] Steere AC, Duray PH, Kauffmann DJ Unilateral blindness caused by infection with the Lyme disease spi- rochete, Borrelia burgdorferi. Ann Intern Med 103:382–384

[113] Secondary reti- nitis pigmentosa and cerebral demyelination in Lyme bor- reliosis. Br J Ophthalmol 77:120–122

[114] Pleyer U, Priem S, Bergmann L Detection of Borrelia burgdorferi DNA in urine of patients with ocular Lyme bor- reliosis. Br J Ophthalmol 85:552–555

[115] Reibaldi M, Faro S, Motta L, al Intravitreal triamcinolone for macular edema in Lyme disease. Graefes Arch Clin Exp Ophthalmol 246:457–458

[116] Bharti AR, Nally JE, Ricaldi JN, et al Peru-United States Leptospirosis Consortium. Leptospirosis: a zoonotic disease of global importance. Lancet Infect Dis. https://doi.org/10.1016/s1473-3099(03)00830-2.

[117] Shah I Leptospirosis. Pediatr Infect Dis 4:4–8

[118] Martins MG, Matos KT, Silva M V, Abreu MT Ocular manifestations in the acute phase of Leptospirosis. Ocul Immunol Inflam 6:75–9

[119] Rathinam SR Ocular manifestations of leptospirosis. J Postgr. Med Jul-Sep; 51:

[120] Sturman RM, Laval J, Weil VJ Leptospiral Uveitis. Arch Ophthalmol 61:633–9

[121] Feigin RD, Anderson DC Human Leptospirosis. CRC Crit Rev Clin Lab Sci 5:413–67

[122] Rathinam SR R, S S, S D, D N, RA N, P. Uveitis associated with an epidemic outbreak of Leptospirosis. Am J Ophthalmol 124:71–9

[123] Picardeau M, Bertherat E, Jancloes M, al Rapid tests for diagnosis of leptospirosis: current tools and emerging technologies. Diagn Microbiol Infect Dis 78:1–8

[124] Brett-Major DM, Coldren R Antibiotics for leptospirosis. Cochrane Database Syst Rev

[125] World Health Organization.

[126] Sanches I, Carvalho A, Duarte R Who are the patients with extra-pulmonary tuberculosis? Rev Port Pneumol 21:90–93

[127] Steptoe PJ, Momorie F, Fornah AD, et al (2020) Evolving Longitudinal Retinal Observations in a Cohort of Survivors of Ebola Virus Disease. JAMA Ophthalmol 138:395–403

[128] Dalvin LA, Smith WM Intraocular manifestations of mycobacterium tuberculosis: a review of the literature. J Clin Tuberc Other Mycobact Dis 7:13–21

[129] Patel SS, Saraiya N V, Tessler HH, Goldstein DA Mycobacterial ocular inflammation: delay in diagnosis and other factors impacting morbidity. JAMA Ophthalmol. https://doi.org/10.1001/jamaophthalmol.2013.71.

[130] Vaziri K, Schwartz SG, Kishor K, Flynn HW Endophthalmitis: state of the art. Clin Ophthalmol 9:95–108

[131] Gupta V, Gupta A, Rao NA Intraocular tuberculosis – an update. Surv Ophthalmol 52:561–587

[132] Gupta V, Gupta A, Arora S, Bambery P, Dogra MR, Agarwal A Presumed tubercular serpiginouslike choroiditis: clinical presenta- tions and

management. Ophthalmology 110:1744–1749

[133] Khochtali S, Gargouri S, Abroug N The spectrum of presumed tubercular uveitis in Tunisia, North Africa. Int Ophthalmol 35:663–671

[134] Sharma A, Thapa B, Lavaju P Ocular tuberculosis: an update. Nepal J Ophthalmol 3:52–67

[135] Gan WL, Jones NP Serpiginous-like choroiditis as a marker for tuberculosis in a non-endemic area. Br J Ophthalmol 97:644–647

[136] Tejada P, Mendez MJ, Negreira S Choroidal tubercles with tubercu- lous meningitis. Int Ophthalmol 18:115–118

[137] Srichatrapimuk S, Wattanatranon D Somnuek Sungkanuparph,"Tuberculous Panophthalmitis with Lymphadenitis and Central Nervous System Tuberculoma". Case Rep Infect Dis. https://doi.org/10.1155/2016/6785382

[138] Helm CJ, Holland GN Ocular tuberculosis. Surv Ophthal

[139] Barondes MJ, Sponsel WE, Stevens TS, Plotnik RD Tuber- culous choroiditis diagnosed by chorioretinal endobiopsy. Am J Ophthalmol 112:460–461

[140] Sen S, Kashyap S, Singh UB Intraocular tuberculosis mimicking retinoblastoma: a case report. Diagn Cytopathol 28:107–109

[141] Bansal R, Gupta A, Gupta V Role of anti-tubercular therapy in uveitis with latent/manifest tuberculosis. Am J Ophthalmol 146;772–77:

[142] Antaki F, Javidi S, Touma S, Aubin MJ Endogenous Tuberculous Endophthalmitis and Panophthalmitis: A Systematic Review of Case Reports and Case Series. Clin Ophthalmol 14: 3075–3096

[143] Gupta A, Bansal R, Gupta V, Sharma A, Bambery P Ocular signs predictive of tubercular uveitis. Am J Ophthalmol. https://doi.org/10.1016/j.ajo.2009.11.020.

[144] Gupta A, Gupta V, Arora S PCR-positive tubercular retinal vasculitis: clinical characteristics and management. Retina 21:444

[145] Nayak S, Acharjya B Mantoux test and its interpretation. Indian Dermatol Online J 3:2–6

[146] Alkabab YM, Enani MA, Indarkiri NY, Heysell SK Performance of computed tomography versus chest radiography in patients with pulmonary tuberculosis with and without diabetes at a tertiary hospi- tal in Riyadh, Saudi Arabia. Infect Drug Resist 11:37–43

[147] Critchley JA, Young F, Orton L, Garner P Corticosteroids for prevention of mortality in people with tuberculosis: a systematic review and meta-analysis. Lancet Infect Dis 13:223–237

[148] Agrawal R, Gunasekeran D V, Grant R, Agarwal A, Kon OM, Nguyen QD, Pavesio C, Gupta V Collaborative Ocular Tuberculosis Study (COTS)–1 Study Group. Clinical Features and Outcomes of Patients With Tubercular Uveitis Treated With Antitubercular Therapy in the Collaborative Ocular Tuberculosis Study (COTS)-1. JAMA Ophthalmol. https://doi.org/10.1001/jamaophthalmol.2017.4485.

[149] Jimenez-Lucho VE, Del Busto R, Odel J Isoniazid and ethambutol as a cause of optic neuropathy. Eur J Respir Dis 71:42–45

[150] Pinitpuwadol W, Tesavibul N, Boonsopon S, Sakiyalak D, Sarunket S, Choopong P Nontuberculous

mycobacterial endophthalmitis: case series and review of literature. BMC Infect Dis. https://doi.org/10.1186/s12879-020-05606-2.

[151] Runyon EH Anonymous mycobacteria in pulmonary disease. Med Clin North Am 43:273–90

[152] Matieli LC V, De Freitas D, Sampaio J, al Mycobacterium abscessus endophthalmitis: treatment dilemma and review of the literature. Retina 26: 826–829

[153] Girgis DO, Karp CL, Miller D Ocular infections caused by non-tuberculous mycobacteria: update on epidemiology and management. Clin Exp Ophthalmol 40:467–75

[154] Sinawat S, Yospaiboon Y, Sinawat S Bilateral endogenous endophthalmitis in disseminated NTM infection: a case report. J Med Assoc Thai May;94(5):

[155] Ambler JS, Meisler DM, Zakov ZN, Hall GS, Spech TJ Endogenous Mycobacterium chelonae endophthalmitis. Am J Ophthalmol 108: 338–9

[156] Antaki F, Marchand-Senécal X, Aubin MJ Endogenous endophthalmitis and bilateral optic neuropathy secondary to Mycobacterium bovis. Can J Ophthalmol. https://doi.org/10.1016/j.jcjo.2019.10.008.

[157] Garg P Fungal, mycobacterial, and Nocardia infections and the eye: an update. Eye (l 26:245–51

[158] Moorthy RS, Valluri S, Rao NA Nontuberculous mycobacterial ocular and adnexal infections. Surv Ophthalmol 57:202–35

[159] Ludlow M, Kortekaas J, Herden C Neurotropic virus infections as the cause of immediate and delayed neuropathology. Acta Neuropathol 131: 159–184

[160] Lee JH, Agarwal A, Mahendradas P, Lee CS, Gupta V, Pavesio CE, Agrawal R (2017) Viral posterior uveitis. Surv Ophthalmol 62: 404–445

[161] Ai JW, Weng SS, Cheng Q, Cui P, Li YJ, Wu HL, Zhu YM, Xu B, Zhang WH (2018) Human endophthalmitis caused by pseudorabies virus infection, China, 2017. Emerg Infect Dis 24:1087–1090

[162] Rochat C, Polla BS, Herbort CP (1996) Immunological profiles in patients with acute retinal necrosis. Graefe's Arch Clin Exp Ophthalmol 234: 547–552

[163] Varkey JB, Shantha JG, Crozier I, et al (2015) Persistence of Ebola Virus in Ocular Fluid during Convalescence. N Engl J Med 372:2423–2427

[164] François J, Collery AS, Hayek G, Sot M, Zaidi M, Lhuillier L, Perone JM (2020) Coronavirus Disease 2019-Associated Ocular Neuropathy with Panuveitis: A Case Report. JAMA Ophthalmol. https://doi.org/10.1001/jamaophthalmol.2020.5695

[165] Kodati S, Palmore TN, Spellman FA, Cunningham D, Weistrop B, Sen HN (2017) Bilateral posterior uveitis associated with Zika virus infection. Lancet 389: 125–126

[166] Heinemann MH (1992) Characteristics of cytomegalovirus retinitis in patients with acquired immunodeficiency syndrome. Am J Med. https://doi.org/10.1016/0002-9343(92)90331-5

[167] Glasgow BJ, Engstrom RE, Holland GN, Kreiger AE, Wool MG (1996) Bilateral endogenous Fusarium endophthalmitis associated with acquired immunodeficiency syndrome. Arch Ophthalmol 114:873–877

[168] S. S, M. O, N. S, al Use of a comprehensive polymerase chain reaction system for diagnosis of ocular infectious diseases. Ophthalmology 120: 1761–1768

[169] Harper TW, Miller D, Schiffman JC, Davis JL (2009) Polymerase Chain Reaction Analysis of Aqueous and Vitreous Specimens in the Diagnosis of Posterior Segment Infectious Uveitis. Am J Ophthalmol. https://doi.org/10.1016/j.ajo.2008.07.043

[170] Scheepers MA, Lecuona KA, Rogers G, Bunce C, Corcoran C, Michaelides M (2013) The value of routine polymerase chain reaction analysis of intraocular fluid specimens in the diagnosis of infectious posterior Uveitis. Sci World J. https://doi.org/10.1155/2013/545149

[171] Riddell J, Comer GM, Kauffman CA (2011) Treatment of Endogenous Fungal Endophthalmitis: Focus on New Antifungal Agents. Clin Infect Dis 52: 648–653

[172] Gupta V, Al-Dhibi HA, Arevalo JF (2014) Retinal imaging in uveitis. Saudi J Ophthalmol 28:95–103

[173] Akula SK, Ma PE, Peyman GA, Rahimy MH, Hyslop NE, Janney A, Ashton P (1994) Treatment of cytomegalovirus retinitis with intravitreal injection of liposome encapsulated ganciclovir in a patient with AIDS. Br J Ophthalmol 78:677–680

[174] Schulman JA, Peyman GA, Fiscella RG, Pulido J, Sugar J (1984) Parenterally Administered Acyclovir for Viral Retinitis Associated with Aids. Arch Ophthalmol 102:1750

[175] Peyman GA (2018) Intravitreal injections: A historic background. J Ophthalmic Vis Res 13:91–92

[176] Yoshizumi MO, Lee D, Vinci V, Fajardo S (1990) Ocular toxicity of multiple intravitreal DHPG injections. Graefe's Arch Clin Exp Ophthalmol 228: 350–355

[177] Peyman G, Goldberg M, Uninsky E, Tessler H, Hendricks R (1984) Vitrectomy and intravitreal antiviral drug therapy in acute retinal necrosis syndrome Report of two cases. Arch Ophthalmol 102:1618–1621

[178] Schulman J, Peyman GA, Pulido J (1985) Viral retinitis and its management. Afro-Asian J Ophthalmol 4:76–80

[179] Almeida DRP, Chin EK, Tarantola RM, et al (2015) Long-term outcomes in patients undergoing vitrectomy for retinal detachment due to viral retinitis. Clin Ophthalmol 9: 1307–1314

[180] Kim SJ, Barañano DE, Grossniklaus HE, Martin DF (2011) Epstein-Barr infection of the retina: Case report and review of the literature. Retin Cases Br Reports 5:1 5

[181] Grutzmacher RD, Henderson D, McDonald PJ, Coster DJ (1983) Herpes simplex chorioretinitis in a healthy adult. Am J Ophthalmol 96:788–796

[182] Ganatra JB, Chandler D, Santos C, Kuppermann B, Margolis TP (2000) Viral causes of the acute retinal necrosis syndrome. Am J Ophthalmol 129:166–172

[183] Jabs DA, Van Natta ML, Thorne JE, Weinberg D V., Meredith TA, Kuppermann BD, Sepkowitz K, Li HK (2004) Course of cytomegalovirus retinitis in the era of highly active antiretroviral therapy: 1. Retinitis progression. Ophthalmology 111:2224–2231.e3

[184] Gupta A, Dixit B, Stamoulas K, Akshikar R (2020) Atypical bilateral acute retinal necrosis in a coronavirus disease 2019 positive

immunosuppressed patient. Eur J Ophthalmol. https://doi.org/10.1177/1120672120974941

[185] Ng AW, Teoh SC (2015) Dengue eye disease. Surv Ophthalmol 60:106–114

[186] Lingappan A, Wykoff CC, Albini TA, Miller D, Pathengay A, Davis JL, Flynn HW (2012) Endogenous fungal endophthalmitis: Causative organisms, management strategies, and visual acuity outcomes. Am J Ophthalmol 153:162–166.e1

[187] Essman TF, Flynn HW, Smiddy WE, Brod RD, Murray TG, Davis JL, Rubsamen PE (1997) Treatment outcomes in a 10-year study of endogenous fungal endophthalmitis. Ophthalmic Surg Lasers 28:185–194

[188] Tamez-Peña A, González-González LA, López-Jaime GR, Rodríguez-García A (2010) Endoftalmitis endógena por Fusarium spp en un paciente con onicomicosis: reporte de un caso.

[189] Sridhar J, Flynn HW, Kuriyan AE, Miller D, Albini T (2013) Endogenous fungal endophthalmitis: Risk factors, clinical features, and treatment outcomes in mold and yeast infections. J Ophthalmic Inflamm Infect 3:1–6

[190] Smith SR, Kroll AJ, Lou PL, Ryan EA (2007) Endogenous Bacterial and Fungal Endophthalmitis. Int Ophthalmol Clin 47:173–183

[191] Murugan G, Shah PK, Narendran V (2016) Clinical profile and outcomes of pediatric endogenous endophthalmitis: A report of 11 cases from South India. World J Clin Pediatr 5:370

[192] Maitray A, Rishi E, Rishi P, Gopal L, Bhende P, Ray R, Therese K (2019) Endogenous endophthalmitis in children and adolescents: Case series and literature review. Indian J Ophthalmol 67:795–800

[193] Martínez-Vázquez C, Fernández-Ulloa J, Bordón J, Sopeña B, De La Fuente J, Ocampo A, Rubianes M (1998) *Candida albicans* endophthalmitis in brown heroin addicts: Response to early vitrectomy preceded and followed by antifungal therapy. Clin Infect Dis 27: 1130–1136

[194] Nagao M, Saito T, Doi S, al Clinical characteristics and risk factors of ocular candidiasis. Diagn Microbiol Infect Dis 73:149–152

[195] Weishaar PD, Flynn HW, Murray TG, al Endogenous Aspergillus endophthalmitis: clinical features and treatment outcomes. Ophthalmology 105:57–65

[196] Vilela RRC, Vilela L, Vilela P, Vilela RRC, Motta R, Pôssa AP, De Almeida C, Mendoza L (2014) Etiological agents of fungal endophthalmitis: Diagnosis and management. Int Ophthalmol 34:707–721

[197] Smith JR, Chee SP (2000) Endogenous Aspergillus endophthalmitis occurring in a child with normal immune function [11]. Eye 14:670–671

[198] Connell PP, O'neill EC, Amirul Islam FM, et al (2010) ENDOGENOUS ENDOPHTHALMITIS ASSOCIATED WITH INTRAVENOUS DRUG ABUSE. Retina 30:1721–1725

[199] Smith WM, Fahle G, Nussenblatt RB, Sen HN (2013) A rare case of endogenous Aspergillus conicus endophthalmitis in an immunocompromised patient. J Ophthalmic Inflamm Infect 3:1–4

[200] Birnbaum FA, Gupta G (2016) The Role of Early Vitrectomy in the Treatment of Fungal Endogenous

Endophthalmitis. Retin Cases Br Reports 10:232–235

[201] Moloney TP, Park J (2013) *Candida dubliniensis* endophthalmitis: Five cases over 15 years. J Ophthalmic Inflamm Infect 3:1–6

[202] Khan S, Athwal L, Zarbin M, Bhagat N (2014) Pediatric infectious endophthalmitis: A review. J Pediatr Ophthalmol Strabismus 51:140–153

[203] Enzenauer RW, Levin A V., Elder JE, Morin JD, Calderwood S (1992) Screening for Fungal Endophthalmitis in Children at Risk. Pediatrics 90:

[204] Vagefi MR, Kim ET, Alvarado RG, Duncan JL, Howes EL, Crawford JB (2005) Bilateral endogenous Scedosporium prolificans endophthalmitis after lung transplantation. Am J Ophthalmol 139: 370–373

[205] Mietz H, Franzen C, Hoppe T, Bartz-Schmidt KU (2002) Microsporidia-induced sclerouveitis with retinal detachment. Arch Ophthalmol 120:864–865

[206] Klotz SA, Penn CC, Negvesky GJ, Butrus SI (2000) Fungal and parasitic infections of the eye. Clin Microbiol Rev 13:662–685

[207] Vasconcelos-Santos D V., Lim JI, Rao NA (2010) Chronic coccidioidomycosis endophthalmitis without concomitant systemic involvement: A clinicopathological case report. Ophthalmology 117:1839–1842

[208] Cutler JE, Binder PS, Paul TO, Beamis JF (1978) Metastatic Coccidioidal Endophthalmitis. Arch Ophthalmol 96:689–691

[209] Rodenbiker HT, Ganley JP (1980) Ocular coccidioidomycosis. Surv Ophthalmol 24:263–290

[210] Modjtahedi BS, Finn AP, Barb SM, MacLachlan MJ, van Zyl T, Papakostas TD, Eliott D (2019) Characteristics and Outcomes of Endogenous Endophthalmitis: Eight-Year Experience at a Tertiary Care Center. Ophthalmol Retin 3:61–72

[211] Sadiq MA, Hassan M, Agarwal A, Sarwar S, Toufeeq S, Soliman MK, Hanout M, Sepah YJ, Do D V., Nguyen QD (2015) Endogenous endophthalmitis: diagnosis, management, and prognosis. J Ophthalmic Inflamm Infect 5:1–11

[212] Mammo Z, Almeida D, MD MBA ACANTHAMOEBA ENDOPHTHALMITIS AFTER RECURRENT KERATITIS AND NODULAR SCLERITIS. Retin cases Br rep 11:180–182

[213] Moshari A, McLean IW, Dodds MT Chorioretinitis after keratitis caused by Acanthamoeba: case report and review of the literature. Ophthalmology 108: 2232–2236

[214] Maude RJ, Dondorp AM, Abu Sayeed A, Day NP, White NJ, Beare NA The eye in cerebral malaria: what can it teach us? Trans R Soc Trop Med Hyg. https://doi.org/10.1016/j.trstmh.2008.11.003.

[215] Kochar DK, Shubhakaran BLK, Thanvi I, Joshi A, Vyas SP Ophthalmoscopic abnormalities in adults with falciparum malaria., QJM. An Int. J. Med. 91:

[216] Ali SA, Hill DR Giardia intestinalis. Curr Opin Infect Dis 16:

[217] Corsi A, Nucci C, Knafelz D Ocular changes associated with *Giardia lamblia*infection in children. Br J Ophthalmol 82:59–62

[218] Knox DL, J Jr K Retinal arteritis, iridocyclitis, and giardiasis. Ophthalmology 10:6891764

[219] Turnbull A, Lin Z, Matthews B Severe bilateral anterior uveitis secondary to giardiasis, initially misdiagnosed as a side effect of metronidazole. Eye 27:1225–1226

[220] Khalifa E, El-Nouby K, Ali A, El-Mashad A, Negm O Ocular changes in giardiasis: Human and experimental studies. Tanta Med Sci J 2:119–31

[221] Pleyer U Schlu¨ ter D M nz M Ocular toxoplasmosis: recent aspects of pathophysiology and clinical implications. Ophthalmic Res 52:

[222] McCannel CA, Holland GN, Helm CJ Causes of uveitis in the general practice of ophthalmology. Am J Ophthalmol 121:35–46,

[223] Derouin F, Pelloux H Prevention of toxoplasmosis in transplant patients. Clin Microbiol Infect 14:

[224] Dubey JP, Miller NL, Frenkel JK The Toxoplasma gondii oocyst from cat feces. J Exp Med 132:

[225] Furtado JM, Ashander LM, Mohs K Toxoplasma gondii migration within and infection of human retina. PLoS One 8:

[226] Elbez-Rubinstein A, Ajzenberg D, Darde ML, al Congenital toxoplasmosis and reinfection during pregnancy: case report, strain characterization, experimental model of reinfection, and review. J Infect Dis 199:280–285

[227] Desmonts G, Couvreur J Congenital toxoplasmosis. A prospective study of the offspring of 542 women who acquired toxoplasmosis during pregnancy.Thalhammer OPollak ABaumgarten KPathophysiology of Congenital Disease.

[228] Peyron F, Wallon M, Kieffer F, al Toxoplasmosis.Wilson CBNizet VMaldonado Y et. al.Remington and Klein's Infectious Diseases of the Fetus and Newborn Infant.2015.Saunders/ ElsevierPhiladelphia:pp.

[229] Thiebaut R, Leproust S, Chene G, al Effectiveness of prenatal treatment for congenital toxoplasmosis: a meta-analysis of individual patients' data. Lancet 369:115–122

[230] Phan L, Kasza K, Jalbrzikowski J, al Longitudinal study of new eye lesions in children with toxoplasmosis who were not treated during the first year of life. Am J Ophthalmol 146:375–384

[231] Holland GN Reconsidering the pathogenesis of ocular toxoplasmosis. Am J Ophthalmol 128:502–505

[232] Montoya JG, Remington JS Toxoplasmic chorioretinitis in the setting of acute acquired toxoplasmosis. Clin Infect Dis 23:277–282

[233] Delair E, Monnet D, Grabar S, al Respective roles of acquired and congenital infections in presumed ocular toxoplasmosis. Am J Ophthalmol 146:851–855

[234] Faridi A, Yeh S, Suhler EB, Smith JR F, C.J. Retinal detachment associated with ocular toxoplasmosis. Retina. https://doi.org/10.1097/IAE.0000000000000279.

[235] Danise A, Cinque P, Vergani S, al Use of the polymerase chain reaction assays of aqueous humor in the differential diagnosis of retinitis in patients infected with human immunodeficiency virus. Clin Infect Dis 24:1100–1106

[236] Johnson MW, Greven CM, Jaffe GJ, al Atypical, severe toxoplasmic retinochoroiditis in elderly patients. Ophthalmology 104:48–57

[237] Bosch-Driessen LH, Plaisier MB, Stilma JS, al Reactivations of ocular toxoplasmosis after cataract extraction. Ophthalmology 109:41–45

[238] Bosch-Driessen LE, Berendschot TT, Ongkosuwito J V, Rothova A Ocular toxoplasmosis: clinical features and prognosis of 154 patients. Ophthalmology 10:11986090

[239] Holland GN, Crespi CM, Dam-van Loon N, al Analysis of recurrence patterns associated with toxoplasmic retinochoroiditis. Am J Ophthalmol 145: 1007–1013

[240] Burnett AJ, Shortt SG, Isaac-Renton J, al Multiple cases of acquired toxoplasmosis retinitis presenting in an outbreak. Ophthalmology 105:1032–1037

[241] O'Connor G Manifestations and management of ocular toxoplasmosis. Bull N Y Acad Med 50:192–210

[242] Levigne P, Peyron F, Wallon M Assessment of the diagnostic performance of the IDS-iSYS tests for toxo IgG, toxo IgM and avidity. Diagn Microbiol Infect Dis. Epub. https://doi.org/10.1016/j.diagmicrobio.2016.07.006.

[243] Mathis T, Beccat S, Sève P, al Comparison of immunoblotting (IgA and IgG) and the Goldmann-Witmer coefficient for diagnosis of ocular toxoplasmosis in immunocompetent patients. Br J Ophthalmol 102:1454–1458

[244] Dard C, Fricker-Hidalgo H, Brenier-Pinchart MP, Pelloux H Relevance of and New Developments in Serology for Toxoplasmosis. Trends Parasitol. https://doi.org/10.1016/j.pt.2016.04.001.

[245] Hill D, Coss C, Dubey JP, et al Identification of a sporozoite-specific antigen from Toxoplasma gondii. J Parasitol. https://doi.org/10.1645/GE-2782.1.

[246] Grover CM, Thulliez P, Remington JS, al No Title. J Clin Microbiol 28:2297–2301

[247] Sterkers Y, Varlet-Marie E, Marty P, Bastien P, Group ANOFELT-PCRQC Diversity and evolution of methods and practices for the molecular diagnosis of congenital toxoplasmosis in France: a 4-year survey. Clin Microbiol Infect. https://doi.org/10.1111/j.1469-0691.2009.03101.x.

[248] Lau YL, Meganathan P, Sonaimuthu P, al Specific, sensitive, and rapid diagnosis of active toxoplasmosis by loop-mediated isothermal amplification method using blood samples from patients. J Clin Microbiol 48:3698–3702

[249] Kim SJ, Scott IU, Brown GC, Brown MM, Ho AC, Ip MS, Recchia FM Interventions for toxoplasma retinochoroiditis: a report by the American Academy of Ophthalmology. Ophthalmology. https://doi.org/10.1016/j.ophtha.2012.07.061.

[250] Holland GN Ocular toxoplasmosis: a global reassessment, Part I. Epidemiology and course of disease. Am J Ophthalmol 136:973–988

[251] Holland GN Ocular toxoplasmosis: a global reassessment, Part II. Disease manifestations and management. Am J Ophthalmol 137:1–17

[252] Holland GN Ocular toxoplasmosis: new directions for clinical investigation. Ocul Immunol Inflamm Mar;8(1):1:

[253] Wakefield D, Cunningham ET, Pavesio C, al Controversies in ocular toxoplasmosis. Ocul Immunol Inflamm 19:2–9

[254] Holland GN, Lewis KG An update on current practices in the management of ocular toxoplasmosis. Am J Ophthalmol 134:102–114

[255] Soheilian M, Sadoughi MM, Ghajarnia M, al Prospective randomized trial of trimethoprim/sulfamethoxazole versus pyrimethamine and sulfadiazine

in the treatment of ocular toxoplasmosis. Ophthalmology 112: 1876–1882

[256] Lashay A, Mirshahi A, Parandin N, al A prospective randomized trial of azithromycin versus trimethoprim/ sulfamethoxazole in treatment of toxoplasmic retinochoroiditis. J Curr Ophthalmol 29:120–125

[257] Peyman GA, Charles HC, Liu KR, Khoobehi B, Niesman M Intravitreal liposome-encapsulated drugs: a preliminary human report. Int Ophthalmol 12:175–82

[258] Soheilian M, Ramezani A, Azimzadeh A, Sadoughi MM, Dehghan MH, Shahghadami R, Yaseri M, Peyman GA Randomized trial of intravitreal clindamycin and dexamethasone versus pyrimethamine, sulfadiazine, and prednisolone in treatment of ocular toxoplasmosis. Ophthalmology. https://doi.org/ 10.1016/j.ophtha.2010.04.020.

[259] Kishore K, Conway MD, Peyman GA Intravitreal clindamycin and dexamethasone for toxoplasmic retinochoroiditis. Ophthalmic Surg Lasers May-Jun;32:11371084

[260] Cazenave J, Forestier F, Bessieres M, al Contribution of a new PCR assay to the prenatal diagnosis of congenital toxoplasmosis. Prenat Diagn 12:119–127

[261] Souza CE, Nascimento H, Lima A, al Intravitreal injection of sulfamethoxazole and trimethoprim associated with dexamethasone as an alternative therapy for ocular toxoplasmosis. Ocul Immunol Inflamm 1–4

[262] Choudhury H, Jindal A, Pathengay A, al No Title. Ophthalmic Surg Lasers Imaging Retin 46:137–140

[263] Nath R, Guy E, Morrison A, Kelly SP Toxoplasma retinochoroiditis in pregnancy: Using current evidence to inform management. Clin Ophthalmol 3:657–661

[264] Martinez CE, Zhang D, Conway MD, Peyman GA Successful management of ocular toxoplasmosis during pregnancy using combined intraocular clindamycin and dexamethasone with systemic sulfadiazine. Int Ophthalmol 1998–1999.:85–88

[265] T. D, P. L, B. F, al Laser photocoagulation around the foci of toxoplasma retinochoroiditis: a descriptive statistical analysis of 35 patients with long-term follow-up. Ophthalmologica 210:90–94

[266] Oray M, Ozdal PC, Cebeci Z, Kir N, Tugal-Tutkun I Fulminant Ocular Toxoplasmosis: The Hazards of Corticosteroid Monotherapy. Ocul Immunol Inflamm. https://doi.org/ 10.3109/09273948.2015.1057599.

[267] Laver N V., Specht CS (2016) Pathogenic Properties of Infectious Organisms and Tissue Reactions. In: Infected Eye. Springer International Publishing, pp 13–35

[268] Nimir AR, Saliem A, Ibrahim IAA (2012) Ophthalmic parasitosis: A review article. Interdiscip Perspect Infect Dis. https://doi.org/10.1155/2012/587402

[269] Singh PP, Robbins CB, Feng HL, Borkar DS, Fekrat S (2020) Ocular Toxocariasis Presenting as Endophthalmitis in a Young Adult Intravenous Drug User. J Vitreoretin Dis 247412642094658

[270] Woodhall D, Starr MC, Montgomery SP, Jones JL, Lum F, Read RW, Moorthy RS (2012) Ocular toxocariasis: Epidemiologic, anatomic, and therapeutic variations based on a survey of ophthalmic subspecialists. Ophthalmology 119:1211–1217

[271] Baquera-Heredia J, Cruz-Reyes A, Flores-Gaxiola A, López-Pulido G, Díaz-Simental E, Alderrama-Valenzuela L (2002) Case report: Ocular gnathostomiasis in Northwestern Mexico. Am J Trop Med Hyg 66:572–574

[272] JR MD PhD. PREVALENCE CF, Retina. COFVLAPWOT 2005;25(8): 1005–1013. Cited Journals@Ovid Full Text

[273] Toxocariasis Clinical Aspects, Epidemiology, Medical Ecology, and Molecular Aspects. Dickson Despommier. Clin Microbiol Rev Apr 16:265–272

[274] Shields JA Ocular toxocariasis: a review. Surv Ophthalmol 28:361–381

[275] Richards FO, Boatin B, Sauerbrey M, Sékétéli A (2001) Control of onchocerciasis today: Status and challenges. Trends Parasitol 17:558–563

[276] Gorezis S, Psilla M, Asproudis I, Peschos D, Papadopoulou C, Stefaniotou M (2006) Intravitreal dirofilariasis: A rare ocular infection. Orbit 25:57–59

[277] Dalimi A, Jabarvand M (2005) *Fasciola hepatica* in the human eye. Trans R Soc Trop Med Hyg 99:798–800

[278] Mets MB, Noble AG, Basti S, Gavin P, Davis AT, Shulman ST, Kazacos KR (2003) Eye findings of diffuse unilateral subacute neuroretinitis and multiple choroidal infiltrates associated with neural larva migrans due to Baylisascaris procyonis. Am J Ophthalmol 135:888–890

[279] Pradhan ZS, Jacob P (2013) Infectious scleritis: Clinical spectrum and management outcomes in India. Indian J Ophthalmol 61:590–593

[280] Gan YK, Ahmad SS, Alexander SM (2016) Two case reports of toxocariasis mimicking endophthalmitis in immunosuppresed adults. J Coast Life Med 4:248–250

[281] Conway MD, Peyman GA (2019) Management of endophthalmitis. In: Vitreoretin. Surg. Tech. Routledge, pp 534–558

Section 4

COVID-19-related Eye Infections

Chapter 7

Potency of SARS-CoV-2 on Ocular Tissues

Saliha Durak, Hande Eda Sutova, Abuzer Alp Yetisgin, Ozlem Kutlu and Sibel Cetinel

Abstract

The current COVID-19 pandemic has affected more than 100 million people and resulted in morbidity and mortality around the world. Even though the disease caused by SARS-CoV-2 is characterized by respiratory tract involvement, previous and recent data also indicates ocular manifestation. Not surprisingly, cell entry point of the virus, ACE2 receptor, is widely expressed in ocular tissues ranging from conjunctiva to retina. Despite the sensibility of ocular tissues, the sophisticated defense mechanism of the eye might eliminate viral transmission. Nevertheless, the potential of systemic transmission through the nasolacrimal duct may not be eliminated. In the case of ocular involvement, the disease outcomes might be as treatable as conjunctivitis or as serious as retinal degeneration and the treatment regimen vary accordingly. Within these contingencies, our aim with this chapter is to shed light on molecular bases of SARS-CoV-2 infection, systemic invasiveness following ocular transmission, manifestation and permanent effects on ocular tissues.

Keywords: COVID-19, SARS-CoV-2, conjunctivitis, conjunctiva, retina, ACE2, TMPRSS2

1. Introduction

Coronaviruses are enveloped, positive-sense RNA viruses belonging to the subfamily Coronavirinae in the family Coronaviridae and cause serious respiratory ailments in humans [1]. In the last 20 years, three different types of coronavirus, including Middle-East respiratory syndrome coronavirus (MERS-CoV), severe acute respiratory syndrome coronavirus (SARS-CoV) and SARS-CoV-2, respectively, have caused severe respiratory tract infections and fatal outbreaks. SARS-CoV-2 emerged in Wuhan, China in December 2019 and has rapidly become an international health emergency [2]. In March 2020, the World Health Organization (WHO) has declared novel coronavirus disease 2019 (COVID-19) pandemic.

SARS-CoV-2 uses the angiotensin-converting enzyme 2 (ACE2) receptor for viral entry, as in SARS-CoV [3]. One of the major structural proteins, the glycoprotein Spike (S) of the SARS-CoV-2 binds to surface receptor (ACE2) of the host cell and mediates viral entry. S protein is composed of two domains; S1 domain contains receptor-binding region, while S2 domain manages viral fusion with the membrane of the host cell. Host transmembrane protease serine type 2 (TMPRSS2) cleaves the S protein into S1 and S2 domains upon virus binding to ACE2 [3–5]. SARS-CoV-2 receptor binding and fusion of viral membrane and cell membrane initiate viral infection.

ACE2 protein is expressed in a variety of human organs and tissues, including ocular tissues ranging from conjunctiva to retina [6, 7]. Understanding the transmission paths of SARS-CoV-2 is crucial to prevent the viral spread. Current studies show that SARS-CoV-2 could be transmitted via direct contact or aerosol droplets. Ocular surfaces are possible viral entry and infection sites, or gateway for spread of the virus to the respiratory system [8, 9]. Although ocular symptoms are rare in COVID-19 patients, manifestations affecting the ocular surfaces such as conjunctivitis, epiphora, chemosis [10, 11], retinal hemorrhages, central retinal vein occlusion (CRVO), ischemia [12–15] as well as blurred vision and vision loss [16, 17] have been reported.

This chapter focuses on the presence and the effects of cellular receptors of SARS-CoV-2 on ocular tissues, evaluates the potential ocular transmission through the eyes, and discusses the short and long-term effects and manifestations of the virus on ocular surfaces at the molecular level.

2. ACE2 and TMPRSS2 expression profiles in ocular tissues

In 2020, various cases of positive conjunctival swabs and conjunctivitis were reported as COVID-19 symptoms. Therefore, several researchers have investigated the ocular surfaces as a potential infection route for SARS-CoV-2 [18, 19]. To this end, intensive research focused on the presence of ACE2 and TMPRSS2 receptors in various ocular tissues since both receptors play important roles in the entry of SARS-CoV-2 to the host cells [20, 21].

ACE2 is an important component of Renin-Angiotensin System (RAS). The circulatory RAS is composed of certain enzymes and active-inactive peptides and plays crucial roles in human body including the regulation of blood pressure, fluid volumes and electrolyte homeostasis [22–27]. These regulations are controlled through the digestion of Angiotensinogen by Renin to generate Angiotensin I and transformation of Angiotensin I to the active form Angiotensin II by angiotensin-converting enzyme (ACE). Recently, Renin and ACE independent generation of Angiotensin II has also been reported [27]. In addition to the circulatory system, RAS is also found locally in some tissues and two separate research groups, Fischer-Ferraro *et al.* and Ganten *et al.* discovered the first clues on local RAS and its tissue-specific roles in 1971 [28, 29]. To date, local RAS has been reported in various organs such as brain, heart, intestine, kidney, and the eye [30, 31]. The presence of RAS in the eye suggested its involvement in various ocular diseases such as age-related macular degeneration (AMD), diabetic retinopathy, and glaucoma [22].

ACE2 is a carboxypeptidase found in circulatory system and in some tissues and regulates RAS negatively by cleaving angiotensin II [21]. This carboxypeptidase is structurally similar to angiotensin converting enzyme (ACE) with a 42% sequence similarity [32]. ACE2 was first discovered and cloned in 2000 as a counter-regulator of ACE, which generates Angiotensin (1–7) by cleaving a single residue from Angiotensin II or Angiotensin (1–9) by removing single residue from Angiotensin I [32–35]. In the eye, ACE2 expression has been demonstrated in a wide variety of ocular tissues, including aqueous humor, retina, corneal epithelium, conjunctival epithelium, and limbal epithelium [6, 7, 22]. ACE2 is found to decrease intraocular pressure (IOP) upon activation with chemical inducers [36].

In addition to ACE2, recent studies showed that TMPRSS2 receptor was also contributing to the cell entry of SARS-CoV-2 by cleaving the spike protein after its' binding to ACE2 receptor [6, 37, 38]. TMPRSS2 is one of the serine proteases, involved in various physiological and pathological processes, including protein catabolism, blood coagulation and tissue rearrangement [39, 40]. As a homologous to enterokinase, the function of TMPRSS2 is suggested to be similar to enterokinase that cleaves acidic pro-peptide from trypsinogen to generate active enzyme. However, exact physiological functions of TMPRSS2 are still not clear [40, 41]. Many ocular surfaces express TMPRSS2 receptor such as conjunctiva and corneal stroma [42].

Due to the important roles of ACE2 and TMPRSS2 in SARS-CoV-2 infection, their individual and co-expression in ocular tissues is investigated [43]. In an early study, local ACE2 expression in rodent retina was evaluated by using immunoblotting, immunohistochemistry analyses and mRNA levels. Expression of ACE2 was broadly localized in the inner nuclear layer and photoreceptors of rodent retinas [44]. Similarly, TMPRSS2 expression was also shown in the retina [45]. One of the most comprehensive studies on this subject was the investigation of coronavirus-2 (CoV-2) tropism in ocular tissues [6]. Here, co-expression of ACE2 receptor and TMPRSS2 protease was shown in human adult conjunctival, limbal and corneal epithelium but not in embryonic and fetal ocular tissues [6]. On the other hand, comparative RNA expression levels of ACE2 and TMPRSS2 in various tissues suggested ACE2 being the limiting factor for infection because TMPRSS2 expression showed a broader tissue distribution [46]. Similarly, expression of ACE2 and TMPRSS2 in post-mortem eyes of non-diabetic and diabetic retinopathy specimens revealed significantly strong expression of ACE2 in corneal and conjunctival epithelium while broad expression of TMPRSS2 in all ocular surfaces [42]. A comparable expression pattern with post-mortem eyes was found in five surgical conjunctival specimens as well, only with higher ACE2 staining intensity in the surgical specimen [42].

Co-expression profile of ACE2 and TMPRSS2 genes shows some contradicting expression profiles between human primary conjunctival and pterygium cells and different cell lines including ARPE-19, HUVEC, HaCaT, HepG2, and A549 [37]. For instance, persistent expression of ACE2 and TMPRSS were observed in conjunctival and pterygium cells of some patients, which was concluded not to be enough for SARS-CoV-2 cell entry [37]. In contrast, a significantly higher gene expression of TMPRSS2 and a lower but notable ACE2 gene expression in studied ocular (ARPE-19, HUVEC) and lung cell (A549) lines were observed [37]. Investigation of healthy and diseased conjunctival samples for mRNA expression levels of ACE2 and TMPRRS2, and ACE2 protein expression by immunostaining revealed ACE2 expression in conjunctival samples [47]. However, protein

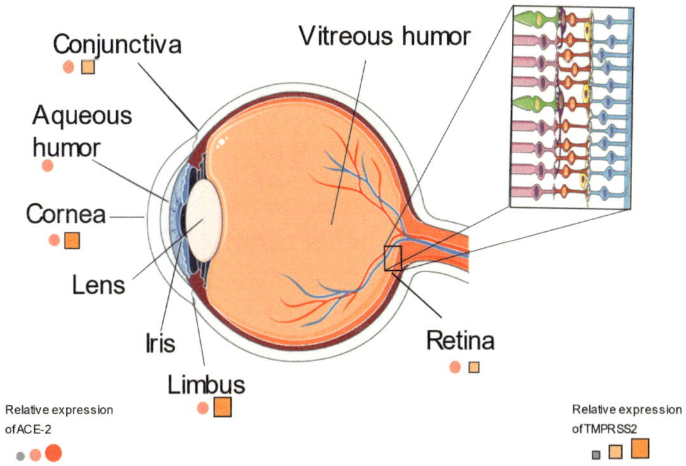

Figure 1.
Representative schematic of the relative expression profile of ACE2 and TMPRSS2 in ocular surfaces. (This schematic was created using Servier Medical Art templates, which are licensed under a Creative Commons Attribution 3.0 Unported License; https://smart.servier.com).

expression of ACE2 and other SARS-CoV-2 mediators of cell entry found not significant enough for the infection [47]. On the other hand, the expression of ACE2 and TMPRSS2 in ocular epithelium such as corneal epithelial cells, conjunctival epithelial cells and corneal endothelial cells is also reported. Herein, co-expression of ACE2 and TMPRSS2 in corneal epithelium and endothelium suggested the susceptibility of cornea for a potential SARS-CoV-2 infection site (**Figure 1**) [48].

3. Potential systemic invasiveness of SARS-CoV-2 following ocular transmission

The three human coronaviruses, SARS-CoV, MERS-CoV, and SARS-CoV-2 are highly infectious compared to HCoV-229-E, HCoV-NL63, HCoV-OV43, and HCoV-HKU1, which infect upper respiratory tract with mild symptoms. On the other hand, SARS-CoV, MERS-CoV, and SARS-CoV-2 cause severe lower respiratory tract infection, which then leads to pneumonia [49]. The transmission mechanism of SARS-CoV and SARS-CoV-2 are similar in many aspects. These viruses could be transmitted with direct contact, droplet, or aerosolized particle contact with the eye surface, nose, and mouth [9]. SARS-CoV and SARS-CoV-2 are genetically similar as well. However, the number of patients infected with SARS-CoV-2 is hundreds of times higher, indicating a significantly higher transmission rate compared to SARS-CoV and MERS-CoV [50]. It's also recently shown that the rate of SARS-CoV-2 replication in conjunctiva is higher than SARS-CoV and MERS-CoV [51].

Potency of viral infections are mainly affected by the virus invasiveness, receptor repertoire of the host cell membrane, and the immune system response. The first step for the viral invasion is the binding of the virus to the host cell by its receptors [52]. Glycoproteins and spike proteins are well-known proteins for all coronaviruses that bind to the receptor of the host cell and trigger the viral entry. The spike proteins are encoded in β-coronaviruses and today, it has been known that SARS-CoV-2 spike protein has the receptor-binding domain, mediating the interaction with the host cell membrane receptor, ACE2 [53].

The eye is an organ representing a large surface area and could be easily exposed to external pathogenic factors. The large surface area of the eye is a potential landing zone for viral particles [54]. Importantly, the expression of TMPRSS2, CD147, ACE2, and CTSL proteins in ocular tissues indicate their potential as SARS-CoV-2 entry route [55–57]. Confirmed expression of ACE2 and TMPRSS2 in conjunctival and corneal tissues [46] suggest conjunctiva and cornea as ocular regions for SARS-CoV-2 entry [8, 49].

Ocular exposure may lead to systemic transmission of the SARS-CoV-2 virus via two pathways. In first pathway, cornea, conjunctiva, lacrimal gland, meibomian glands could be directly exposed to the infection. Particularly, the conjunctival tissue could be easily infected via droplets or a close contact with infected individuals and contaminated hands. Due to its potency as an entry site of viruses, conjunctiva is accepted as an important pathway for infection of the respiratory viruses [52]. In second pathway, virus in tear can migrate through the nasolacrimal duct and infect the nasal or gastrointestinal epithelium [9].

SARS-CoV-2 may indirectly enhance the possibility of ocular complications as well. For instance, the cytokine storm, vascular endothelial dysfunction, and hypercoagulability may lead to not only retinal microangiopathic changes but also congestion of the central retinal vessels, or micro-vascularization of the optic nerve head [14, 58, 59]. It has been also reported that SARS-CoV-2 led to paracentral acute middle maculopathy and acute macular neuro-retinopathy [60, 61]. In May 2020, retinal changes in 12 adult COVID-19 patients were analyzed by using optical coherence tomography (OCT). Hyper-reflective lesions were observed at the ganglion cell level and interestingly, inner plexiform layers were found more prominently at the papillomacular bundle in both eyes [14]. A 40-year-old man diagnosed with SARS-CoV-2 infection reported that he had right calf pain and blurred vision in both eyes. His ophthalmic exam revealed retinal vein occlusion (RVO) on both eyes, indicating COVID-19 as a potential cause for RVO [12].

On the other hand, the viral infection can occur at the upper respiratory tract and viruses can migrate to the nasolacrimal duct and to the conjunctiva, resulting in viral conjunctivitis [62]. Furthermore, SARS-CoV-2 infection via the conjunctival tissues may also occur in non-human primates that the SARS-CoV-2 inoculation has been shown to cause mild COVID-19 in rhesus macaques [63].

3.1 Natural ocular defense mechanisms

The eye has natural anatomical and physiological protection mechanisms that prevent the entry of large amounts of virus-loaded particles to the ocular surface [64]. The eye has three defense mechanisms against different types of microorganisms and toxic substances. These are; mechanical, immunological, and anatomical defense mechanisms which are critical to recognize and eliminate the pathogens from the ocular surface for eye protection [65].

Mechanical defense system is composed of eyelids, eyelashes, corneal epithelium containing tight intercellular junctions, and conjunctival mucosa. Corneal epithelial cells also protects the ocular surface by secreting cytokines and causing immune defense activation against the viral invasion [65]. Eyelid protects the eye surface against any mechanical injury. When the eyelids and lashes are closed, the eye is also protected from any exposure of pathogens and other foreign molecules such as dust, dirt, and any other debris [66].

Anatomical defense system is based on the barriers of anterior and posterior segments of the eye. The drugs administered to the eye is extensively drained by the precorneal barriers present in the anterior segment (around 90%) and tears migrate through the nasolacrimal duct [67]. Aqueous humor is secreted by the ciliary body and the flow direction of the aqueous humor is towards the cornea, which is an opposite direction of topically administrated drug. The aqueous humor can be a limiting factor for the drugs to show therapeutic effects. Sclera presents at the posterior segment of the eye and protects the eye from the exogenous substances. Surface charge, physicochemical properties, and molecular radius are the parameters affecting the drug permeability across sclera. The drug with greater molecular radius and lipophilicity can lead to inhibition of permeation across sclera [67]. On the other hand, the pathogens are also cleaned from the ocular surface with the lacrimal drainage system. However, this physical self-cleaning system may cause SARS-CoV-2 infection via the migration of infected tears throughout the nasolacrimal drainage system and this passage can function as an alternative entry route of the virus from ocular surface to the respiratory tract [68].

Immune defense at the ocular surface is important for preservation of the eye. Particularly, cornea have a variety of defense mechanisms; classified as native, nonspecific, and acquired immunological defenses.

Innate immunity is the first line of defense mechanism in corneal infection; presents at birth and provides a nonspecific defense system [65]. This system can function in case of viral load and pathogenesis. Innate immune response is given at first encounter with the pathogen and can vary between different pathogens. For instance, among SARS-CoV viruses, the replication of the SARS-CoV-2 has been more extensive in the bronchus than SARS-CoV and the higher plasma concentrations of proinflammatory cytokines have been observed in the SARS-CoV-2-infected patients [9].

Tears, corneal nerves, epithelium, keratocytes, polymorphonuclear cells and some cytokines are other cellular and molecular elements for protection of cornea against microorganisms. The first function of tears is to keep the cornea not to be dried. Tears clean the foreign particles from the ocular surface and transports antimicrobial proteins lactoferrin, lysozyme, lipocalin, and beta-lysine to prevent the infections. In addition to these proteins, immunoglobulins protect the cornea from infections [65]. Lactoferrin is able to inhibit the binding of SARS-CoV-2 to ACE2, and IgA shows an effective immune response against different types of microorganisms [65, 69]. For instance, secreted IgA protects the corneal epithelium by binding to bacteria and prevents it from attaching to epithelium. Besides, IgG has the ability to bind bacteria and neutralize some viruses.

Corneal epithelial cells activate immune response by secreting cytokines to preserve the eye against microbial invasion. They store IL-1α to release it passively, when the trauma or any foreign agent stimulates the membrane. Keratocytes synthesize IL-6 and defensins as a defense mechanism. IL-6 and IL-1 show a synergetic effect against microbial activity. Defesin has antimicrobial activity in ocular infections and induce epithelial healing. It is also found in neutrophils located in conjunctiva. Corneal nerves send sensory information and therefore control the reflexive movements for protection of the eye. Furthermore, several other eye complements, composed of a variety of effectors and regulatory proteins activating each other to produce biologically active molecules, such as opsonins, enzymes and chemotaxins [65].

There are early and late defense stages of relevant innate and acquired immune responses. The immediate immune response takes minutes to several hours against microbial infection. When the innate immunity is unable to fight against the microorganisms or their antigens, acquired immunity can control microbial replication. Langerhans cells, antigen-presenting cells of the cornea, recognize the foreign antigen and can respond within 24–48 hours [65]. They recognize, process and present the antigens with MHC class II molecules, which are present on their surface. When they recognize an antigenic foreign molecule, they process the antigen and transport it to the surface by MHC molecules both class I and class II. The presentation of peptides by MHC molecules activates T cells and T-cell receptors, which then lead to the binding of MHC molecules to each other. If the MHC II molecule presents the antigen, then CD4 helper T cells kill the pathogen by secretion of cytokines that activates the other effector cells such as macrophages [65].

3.2 Nasolacrimal duct can play a role in SARS-CoV-2 systemic transmission

The human tear ducts consist of the upper and lower lacrimal canaliculus, lacrimal sac, and nasolacrimal duct (**Figure 2**) [70]. The nasolacrimal system functions as a bridge between the ocular surface mucosa and upper respiratory tract for migration of the viruses with the help of tears to the inferior meatus of the nose. It allows the virus to move from the ocular surface to the respiratory tract throughout the nasolacrimal duct [52, 71]. The fluid may be taken up by the conjunctiva, sclera, or cornea but the highest percent of the liquid is drained into the nasopharyngeal space. Additionally, the epithelial lining of the lacrimal duct can absorb the tear fluid, which allows immunizing agents to be drained to nasal tissue [72].

In addition to the above-mentioned functions of nasolacrimal duct, it has a role in nonspecific immune defense. Nasolacrimal duct protects against dacryocystitis; thus, the epithelial cells produce a variety of antimicrobial substances, such as

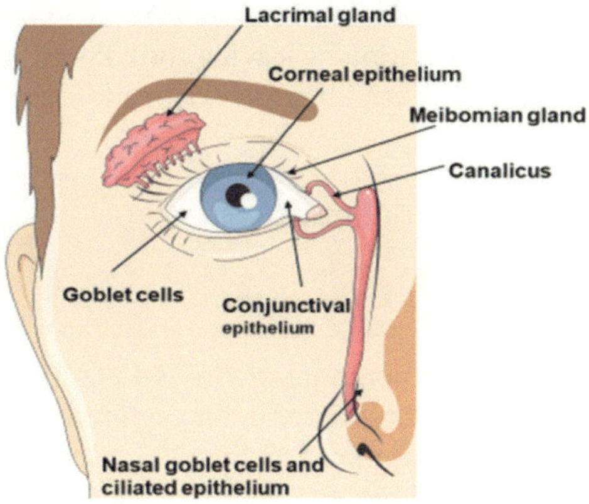

Figure 2.
Representative schematic of ocular surface and tear ducts (This schematic was created using Servier Medical Art templates, which are licensed under a Creative Commons Attribution 3.0 Unported License; https://smart.servier.com).

lysozyme and lactoferrin. In case of an infection or an inflammatory dacryocystitis, antimicrobial peptides human inducible beta defensins 2 and 3 are produced. Moreover, the secretory products of the mucus component mucins (MUC1, MUC2, MUC4, MUC5AC, MUC5B, and MUC7) are produced by goblet and epithelial cells. Mucins preserve mucosal surfaces against pathogenic substances. It has been observed that MUC5B protects the patient against the SARS-CoV-2. There is a lower allelic frequency of the MUC5B genetic variant in the COVID-19 patient's body compared the healthy people, which is related to a higher level of MUC5B expression [73]. On the other hand, the expression of MUC1 and the soluble mucin MUC5AC were observed in cells that also express ACE2, indicating that the mucins may function in entry and transmission of the SARS-CoV-2 [46, 74]. However, it was revealed that the increased levels of secreted MUC1 and MUC5AC in the sputum cleaned from the trachea of COVID-19 patients [75]. The epithelium present in the nasolacrimal duct produces TFF peptides TFF1 and TFF3. The efferent tear ducts also contain lymphocytes and other defense cells that function in adaptive immune mechanisms [70].

Nasolacrimal duct has common entry receptors for some respiratory viruses. For instance, the glycoproteins of host epithelial cell, carrying terminal sialic acid (SA), are distributed through the ocular tissue and the respiratory tract through the lacrimal passage. Thus, the patient becomes infected with pneumonia [71]. α2–6-linked SA is significantly abundant in trachea and nasal mucosa, while α2–3- linked SA are more prominent in ocular tissues and the lower respiratory tract tissues [72]. There are several reports hypothesized that the exposure of the ocular surface to SARS-CoV-2 may lead to infection, because of the drainage of the virus particles via the nasolacrimal duct [76]. Siedlecki *et al.* has shown that SARS-CoV-2 can infect the ocular surface by migrating into the respiratory tract with the help of tears through the nasolacrimal duct [77]. Supporting to this, the highest expression level of SARS-CoV-2 entry factors was shown in nasal epithelial cells (clusters of goblet cells and ciliated cells), among all cells present in the respiratory tree [46]. Unlike all these infection routes, SARS-CoV-2 infection may also possible with the hematogenous spread from the lacrimal gland [8].

Consequently, the human eye has three roles in coronavirus infection. Firstly, it is one of the target organs for coronavirus infection. Secondly, the conjunctiva can function as a transporter for human coronavirus to enter the respiratory tract.

SARS-CoV-2 can reach to nasal mucosa with nasolacrimal epithelium, gastrointestinal tract, and systemic circulation by leaving the conjunctivitis [19]. Thirdly, conjunctival secretions and tears can function to spread human coronavirus [52].

4. SARS-CoV-2 related ocular manifestations

4.1 Ocular surface manifestations

Since ocular surfaces hold the potential for SARS-CoV-2 transmission, clinical research focusing the COVID-19-associated ocular symptoms have attracted great attention. Even though, the incidence of SARS-CoV-2 infection through ocular surfaces is low, ocular manifestations are various. Dry eyes, epiphora, hyperemia were the most prevalent symptoms in COVID-19 patients, while chemosis, photophobia and conjunctivitis are barely seen. Other reported ocular surface symptoms were conjunctival congestion, conjunctival secretions, foreign body sensations, blurred vision, itching/irritation, ocular pain, and eye redness. The prevalence of SARS-CoV-2 and profiling ocular symptoms related to COVID-19 are summarized in **Table 1** by including 2660 patients from 43 independent studies [10–14, 16, 17, 59–61, 69, 78–108].

In a large study, including 535 patients, 5.0% of the patients (27 patients) displayed conjunctival congestion. Conjunctival congestion was in fact, the first symptom in four patients, which explains that ocular manifestations may be observed in early times of SARS-CoV-2 infection. However, SARS-CoV-2 nucleic acid could not be identified in ocular swabs. Other ocular manifestations were dry eye, blurred vision, foreign body sensation, tearing, itching, ocular pain and photophobia. Conjunctival congestion has lasted for 5.9 ± 4.5 days among the patients and ofloxacin, tobramycin and ganciclovir eye drops were supplied for

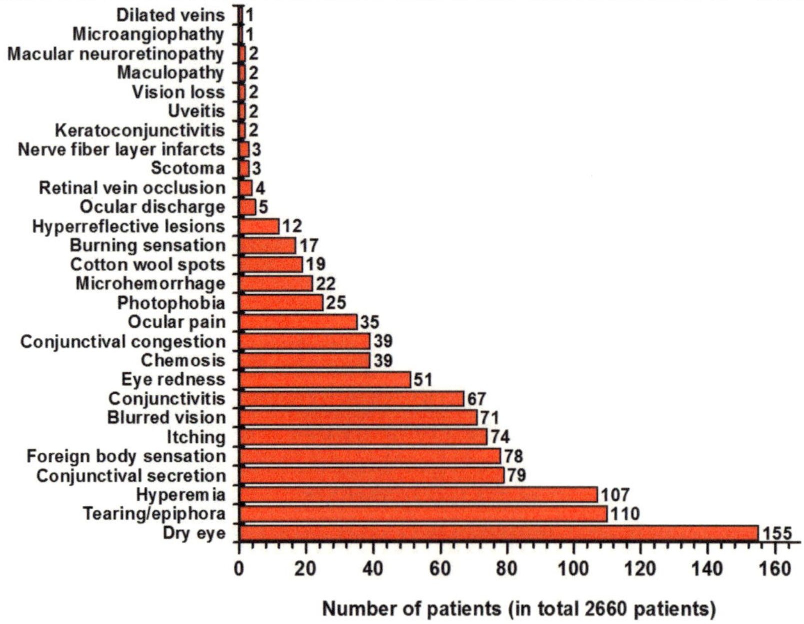

Table 1.
The number of ocular findings observed in a total of 2660 patients with COVID-19 [10–14, 16, 17, 59–61, 69, 78–108].

treatment. Conjunctival congestion was a more widespread symptom in patients with frequent hand-eye contact [10].

In some studies, the presence of SARS-CoV-2 viral RNA on the ocular surfaces was confirmed. In February 2020, a study including 30 COVID-19 patients has declared SARS-CoV-2 nucleic acid in tear, conjunctival secretion as well as in sputum samples in one patient with conjunctivitis at the third day of the disease. The presence of the virus in the eye allowed speculation that transmission with the aerosols could be possible. However, this was one of the early studies and at that time there was not enough information about the transmission routes of virus [104]. In another study, involving 72 COVID-19 patients, conjunctivitis was detected in two patients (2.8%) and SARS-CoV-2 nucleic acid was identified in ocular discharges of one patient [106]. Detection of virus RNA in the eye suggests that the ocular pathway may be a gateway for viral transmission. In a case study, SARS-CoV-2 RNA was detected on the ocular swab of a woman with conjunctivitis at the third day of the COVID-19 diagnosis. Conjunctival samples were continuously taken on a daily basis and viral RNA was detected, despite in a decreasing curve for 21 days. However, the viral RNA became observable again 5 days after it became unobservable in the ocular swabs. To understand the presence of viral replication in the conjunctiva, researchers have inoculated the first positive viral RNA samples in Vero E6 cells and 5 days later, they have observed cytopathic effect and confirmed viral replication by RT-PCR with RNA purified from Vero E6 cell growth media [83].

On the other hand, SARS-CoV-2 viral RNA was also present in some patients without conjunctivitis. Viral RNA was detected in ocular swabs in two patients among 33 COVID-19 patients (6.1%) without any ocular manifestation [19]. In another study, including 121 patients diagnosed with COVID-19, ocular manifestations such as itching, tearing, redness, foreign body sensation and discharge were obtained in only eight patients (6.6%). Ocular swab was positive for SARS-CoV-2 RNA in one of them and in two patients without ocular manifestations [107]. The presence of SARS-CoV-2 on normal ocular surfaces may indicate that both symptomatic and asymptomatic ocular surface contact also has a risk of virus transmission.

There are several cases, where ocular manifestations were reported as the first presenting manifestation of COVID-19. A 65-year-old patient applied to ophthalmology department with a complaint of burning sensation and discharge for the last two days was diagnosed with conjunctivitis. After 2 days, the patient was admitted to the hospital with symptoms associated with COVID-19 and SARS-CoV-2 infection was confirmed with positive RT-PCR results of the nasopharyngeal and conjunctival swabs as well as computed tomography (CT) scanning of the lungs [88]. In a study, 12 out of 38 COVID-19 patients (31.6%) presented ocular symptoms, including conjunctivitis, hyperemia, epiphora, chemosis and increased secretions. SARS-CoV-2 nucleic acid was detected in conjunctival swabs of two patients. In these patients, conjunctivitis was the first symptom in one patient [11]. The occurrence of ocular symptoms primarily suggests that ocular surface is the potential transmission site of the virus in these patients.

Conjunctivitis could be seen in both early and late stages in the course of COVID-19. In February 2020, bilateral conjunctivitis, including redness, tearing and foreign body sensation was observed 13 days after the onset of the disease in a COVID-19 patient. Although the presence of SARS-CoV-2 nucleic acid was less in the nasopharyngeal and sputum swabs, it was confirmed in conjunctival swabs by RT-PCR at days 13, 14 and 17 in a gradually decreasing manner. Ribavirin eye drops helped the treatment of the symptoms and the RT-PCR test from ocular swabs turned negative on day 19 [82]. In a COVID-19 patient at intensive care unit, ocular symptoms started on the 17th day of the disease with conjunctival hyperemia and clear secretions and pseudomembranous. On the 19th day, hemorrhagic conjunctivitis was defined, however, SARS-CoV-2 RNA was not detectable in the patient's conjunctival and tear samples. Azithromycin eyedrop and dexamethasone were used for treatment and ocular manifestations were started to decrease from day 21 [95]. Conjunctivitis, seen in the middle and late phases of the COVID-19, may have developed due to systemic viral infection or auto-inflammatory and autoimmune responses. Considering the nasolacrimal duct forms a connection between the eye and the respiratory tract; it is likely that the virus in the respiratory tract may subsequently infect the eye. The fact that ACE2 receptor is expressed predominantly in the respiratory tract than epithelial cells in the eye surface confirms this theory.

In the first study where keratoconjunctivitis was reported as the main symptom of COVID-19, virus was detected in ocular swabs with much lower titers than respiratory swabs. The corneal findings in this case involved pseudodendrite, subepithelial infiltrate and multiple epithelial defects spreading through the cornea [81]. The first case of COVID-19 related acute anterior uveitis associated with acute follicular conjunctivitis and conjunctival hyperemia was reported in Italy. Acute anterior uveitis was characterized by bilateral eye redness lasting two weeks, unilateral photophobia, lacrimation, miosis, aqueous humour flare and anterior lens opacity causing blurred vision [16].

The low rate of ocular symptoms seen in patients with COVID-19 may be due to the under diagnosis. Particularly, for the diagnosis of conjunctivitis, an ophthalmologist is required. Otherwise, disease can be unnoticed and treated silently during systemic COVID-19 treatment regimen. Besides, since the ocular inoculation of SARS-CoV-2 cannot be fully elucidated, sampling time in the course of disease may also be a factor affecting detection of the presence of the virus on ocular surfaces. Since the virus may have been eliminated by ocular defense mechanisms or may have already entered the respiratory tract, the duration time of the virus on ocular surfaces may be very short. The sensitivity threshold of RT-PCR, which is the conventional method used to confirm the presence of the virus, may also cause false negative results. However, in order to declare that conjunctivitis occurs due to SARS-CoV-2 infection, virus detection through ocular swabs is mandatory since conjunctivitis may be of different viral, bacterial and allergic origin in patients with COVID-19. It should also be taken into account that ocular manifestations may be the only symptoms of the COVID-19.

4.2 Retinal findings in patients with COVID-19

In viral infections, the cytopathic effect of the viral agent on retinal cells or damage to the retinal vasculature are common pathological findings of the retina. Systemic damage caused by SARS-CoV-2 made it necessary to enlighten additional viral involvement sites in addition to the respiratory system. Presence of ACE2 in aqueous humor [7] and retina [15] has allowed researchers to raise query on the possible injury caused by COVID-19 in the posterior part of the eye.

The first report published in May 2020 declaring COVID-19 related retinal alterations has paved the way for further studies. Retinal cotton wool spots and microhemorrhages in four patients as well as hyperreflective lesions at ganglion cell layer and inner plexiform layer in 12 patients was reported. Of the 12 patients, three had high blood pressure, one had diabetes and one had dyslipidemia. Examination was performed on 11–33 days after the onset of COVID-19 symptoms using optical coherence tomography (OCT). Intraocular inflammation was not noticed in any of the patients, however the presence of SARS-CoV-2 in the intraocular fluids was not tested in this study [14]. Similarly, in another study, 10 out of 18 intensive care unit patients had retinal abnormalities characterized by cotton wool spots, flame-shaped hemorrhages, peripheral retinal hemorrhages, macular hemorrhages, retinal pigment epithelium hyperplasia and choroidal naevus. Nine of them had a history of diabetes and 12 of them had high blood pressure [96]. In another study of 25 patients, 3 patients (12%) displayed retinal changes including microhemorrhages, flame-shaped hemorrhage and nerve fiber layer infarcts (**Figure 3**). Retinal examinations were performed at 12–59 days after the onset of symptoms and only one patient had a medical history of hypertension. Another patient had hypotension, severe anemia, kidney and peripheral nervous system damage, which may explain microhemorrhages and nerve fiber layer infarcts [89]. These findings suggest that retinal alterations may occur depending on the patients' medical histories, yet it may also be due to the cytokine storm, which is developed as a result of immune response induced by COVID-19 and reaches to the retina by passing through the blood retina barrier.

In the fundus examination of a COVID-19 patient who was admitted to the hospital with the complaint of scotoma and decreased vision in one eye, fern-like retinal whitening, hyperreflective inner layers, increased venular tortuosity and retinal hemorrhages were found in the right eye and the patient was diagnosed with impending central retinal vein occlusion (iCRVO). After 10 days of treatment with steroids, patient's retinal changes and blood flow in central retinal vein almost returned to normal [87]. The iCRVO in this patient is thought to be due to the systemic response of COVID-19, as it can be treated with steroid therapy and the patient has no risk-bearing medical history. In the examination of a patient with lower leg pain and blurred vision in addition to common COVID-19 symptoms, deep venous thrombosis in the leg, bilateral CRVO, intraretinal hemorrhages, optic disk swelling, and cotton wool spots were detected. After 2 weeks of anticoagulant treatment, the patient's complaints returned to normal [12]. Similar to this, vascular occlusions may occur in the cases of hypertension, obesity and high cholesterol. In another study, bilateral cotton wool spots were detected on fundus examination during the late stage of COVID-19 in one patient, suffering an arcuate visual field defect in one eye. It was the first study to report COVID-19 induced vision loss. Retinal microvascular ischemia in the superficial plexus, which corresponded to the arcuate scotoma was detected by optical coherence tomography (OCT) angiography

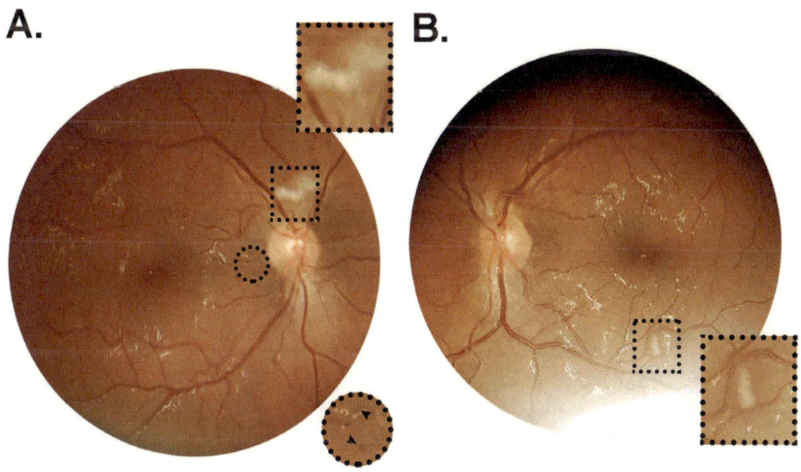

Figure 3.
Retinal photograph of a patient with COVID-19. (A) Nerve fiber layer infarct above the optic nerve head, and microhemorrhages in the papillomacular bundle close to the optic disc was present in the right eye. (B) Nerve fiber layer infarcts at the inferior temporal vascular arcade, approximately 1.5-disc diameters inferior to the macula was present in the left eye. Reproduced from Reference [89] (CC BY 4.0).

[17]. These retinal changes can be related to microangiopathy and ischemia that are characterized in different anatomic parts in COVID-19 pathogenesis [109, 110].

In a study involving 54 COVID-19 patients, 15 patients had dilated veins, tortuous vessels was observed in seven patients, retinal hemorrhages in five patients, cotton wools spots in four patients and drusen in six patients were reported during fundus examination. Both mean artery diameters for severe cases and mean vein diameters for severe or non-severe cases were significantly higher in 54 COVID-19 patients, compared to 133 unexposed subjects [13]. Retinal vessel diameters and retinal circulation are parallel to the systemic circulation. Alterations in the retinal vessels can provide an insight into alterations in other organs. Enlargement of the vessels can be explained by the increased blood supply and effect of inflammatory mediators together with the inflammatory response to COVID-19 or a direct effect of the SARS-CoV-2 to endothelium. Moreover, two patients with COVID-19 had paracentral acute middle maculopathy and acute macular neuroretinopathy accompanied by scotoma [60]. In another study, scotoma, acute vision loss and several retinal hemorrhages related with acute macular neuroretinopathy and paracentral acute middle maculopathy were reported in one patient [61]. It has been reported that paracentral acute middle maculopathy is associated with the reduced blood supply to intermediate, deep, superficial capillary plexuses and acute macular neuroretinopathy is associated with the reduced blood supply to deep capillary plexus [111].

Venous thromboembolism is also a reported condition in COVID-19 patients; however, it is not known whether this is caused by the direct effect of the virus or the inflammatory response of the COVID-19. Cotton wool spots are characterized by disruption of axoplasmic flow in nerve tissue layer due to microvascular occlusion, and retina is extremely sensitive to ischemic events in the body. Considering the thrombotic conditions caused in COVID-19 patients, it can be thought that cotton wool spots in the retina are a result of the occlusion of terminal retinal arterioles.

The fact that the SARS-CoV-2 affects the central nervous system [112, 113] and the presence of its nucleic acid in retina [114] suggests that as a part of central nervous system, retina may be directly affected by the virus. Considering that the effect of SARS-CoV-2 on the central nervous system also effects the vital organ brain, non-invasive retinal examinations could be a prediction of the scope of COVID-19 in other organs like brain and heart, which has been implemented before for different diseases such as stroke, Alzheimer disease, multiple sclerosis and Parkinson disease [115].

In some studies, there was no link between retinal findings and ocular surface changes suggesting that retinal findings may be a marker of systemic alterations, and thus the importance of fundus examination should not be underestimated even in patients without any ocular complaints during the COVID-19 pandemic.

4.3 COVID-19 related expected long-term effects on eye

Ocular manifestations of COVID-19 range from redness to acute anterior uveitis on the anterior segment of the eye and from microhemorrhages to retinal microvascular ischemia on the retina. Some of these manifestations may cause vision loss and blurred vision.

Retinal changes such as damage of retinal cells or retinal vasculature may be the precursor of a long-term retinal disease. When the peripapillary vascular impairment is compared between the control group and patients recovered from COVID-19, lower radial peripapillary capillary plexus perfusion density and reduced blood supply to peripapillary retinal nerve fiber layer were present in post COVID-19 patients [98]. Older and systemic hypertensive patients were more prone to this microvascular damage. The radial peripapillary capillary plexus is very important for function of the retinal ganglion cells and axons and it is related to nerve fiber layer thickness and visual field loss in glaucoma [116]. Decrease in radial peripapillary capillary plexus density and nerve fiber layer thinning have been characterized in patients with early stage of glaucoma [117, 118]. Besides, it is more prominent in patients with glaucoma for more than ten years than in patients with glaucoma less than ten years [119]. However, whether the peripapillary capillary changes in patients with COVID-19 are reversible will be seen in further studies. Although these patients are at risk of developing glaucoma in the future, it should be kept in mind that there are several effective physiological parameters for disease development.

Looking at MERS and SARS outbreaks, it is difficult to predict the long-term ocular effect of COVID-19, due to the insufficient ocular findings and limited number of patients. Although different mechanisms cause the ocular effects of coronaviruses in animals, studies in animal models and understanding these mechanisms could give an idea about the long-term ocular effects of coronavirus in humans. Investigation of the effect of the coronavirus-related immune responses in retinal disease using experimental coronavirus retinopathy (ECOR) model indicated that levels of some cytokine molecules (TNF-α, TNF receptors) and signaling molecules (nitric oxide) increased in mice infected with murine coronavirus (mouse hepatitis virus) [120]. It was stated that TNF-α induction of nitric oxide may cause retina degeneration and loss of photoreceptor cells. In addition to that, following the primary immune response to virus, increased TNF receptor molecules and T cell reactivity may trigger autoimmunity.

The RAS system and its component ACE2 have important regulatory functions in the eye. ACE2 activation is known to reduce intraocular pressure [36]. Decreased expression of ACE2 to prevent viral spread can lead to misbalance of ACE-Angiotensin II/ACE-Angiotensin (1–7) balance, increase in intraocular pressure, vasoconstriction [61] and subsequently cause glaucoma. Hypothetically, in the light of this information, it is difficult to say that COVID-19 can cause a medium- or long-term serious ocular diseases such as glaucoma. However, ocular follow-up of COVID-19 patients with retinal symptoms may present whether these assumptions are justified as well as may benefit understanding virus tropism and immune responses to the virus.

5. Conclusion

With the emergence of SARS-CoV-2 in December 2019, the reporting of ocular symptoms observed in COVID-19 patients attracted many researchers and numerous publications were published in a short time to clarify the interaction between SARS-CoV-2 and the eye. Despite the fact that ocular symptoms present a low prevalence relative to respiratory and systemic symptoms, there is strong evidence for the ocular transmission of the SARS-CoV-2. The eye surfaces are one of the primary infection sites for SARS-CoV-2 and conjunctival secretions and tears can cause systemic spread of the virus. Additionally, the virus can use the ocular surfaces as a gateway to the respiratory tract.

Revealing the relationship between coronaviruses and the eye is of great importance in the diagnosis, treatment and infection control in both present and potential viral infections. Although many studies are investigating the ocular tropism of respiratory viruses, ocular transmission routes should be better understood in order to develop novel treatment methods such as antiviral agents that can be used in ocular treatments against RNA viruses. Besides, non-invasive retinal examinations can be evaluated as a reflection of the patients' current systemic thrombotic condition and can be used in long-term patient follow-up related to COVID-19.

Considering that the first or only symptom of the COVID-19 may be conjunctivitis and virus can spread via tears even from asymptomatic patients, ophthalmologists and healthcare professionals should be aware of the risk and take necessary precautionary measures.

Conflict of interest

The authors declare no conflict of interest.

Author details

Saliha Durak[1,2], Hande Eda Sutova[1,2], Abuzer Alp Yetisgin[1,3], Ozlem Kutlu[1] and Sibel Cetinel[1*]

1 Nanotechnology Research and Application Center (SUNUM), Sabanci University, Istanbul, Turkey

2 Faculty of Engineering and Natural Sciences, Molecular Biology, Genetics and Bioengineering Program, Sabanci University, Istanbul, Turkey

3 Faculty of Engineering and Natural Sciences, Materials Science and Nano-Engineering Program, Sabanci University, Istanbul, Turkey

*Address all correspondence to: cetinel@sabanciuniv.edu

References

[1] Masters PS. The molecular biology of coronaviruses. Adv Virus Res. 2006;66:193-292.

[2] Zhu N, Zhang D, Wang W, Li X, Yang B, Song J, et al. A Novel Coronavirus from Patients with Pneumonia in China, 2019. New England Journal of Medicine. 2020;382(8):727-33.

[3] Hoffmann M, Kleine-Weber H, Schroeder S, Krüger N, Herrler T, Erichsen S, et al. SARS-CoV-2 Cell Entry Depends on ACE2 and TMPRSS2 and Is Blocked by a Clinically Proven Protease Inhibitor. Cell. 2020.

[4] Tang T, Bidon M, Jaimes JA, Whittaker GR, Daniel S. *Corona*virus membrane fusion mechanism offers a potential target for antiviral development. Antiviral Research. 2020;178:104792.

[5] Walls AC, Park Y-J, Tortorici MA, Wall A, McGuire AT, Veesler D. Structure, Function, and Antigenicity of the SARS-CoV-2 Spike Glycoprotein. Cell. 2020;181(2):281-92.e6.

[6] Collin J, Queen R, Zerti D, Dorgau B, Georgiou M, Djidrovski I, et al. Co-expression of SARS-CoV-2 entry genes in the superficial adult human conjunctival, limbal and corneal epithelium suggests an additional route of entry via the ocular surface. The Ocular Surface. 2020.

[7] Holappa M, Valjakka J, Vaajanen A. Angiotensin(1-7) and ACE2, "The Hot Spots" of Renin-Angiotensin System, Detected in the Human Aqueous Humor. Open Ophthalmol J. 2015;9:28-32.

[8] Ho D, Low R, Tong L, Gupta V, Veeraraghavan A, Agrawal R. COVID-19 and the Ocular Surface: A Review of Transmission and Manifestations. Ocular Immunology and Inflammation. 2020;28(5):726-34.

[9] Barnett BP, Wahlin K, Krawczyk M, Spencer D, Welsbie D, Afshari N, et al. Potential of Ocular Transmission of SARS-CoV-2: A Review. Vision. 2020;4(3):40.

[10] Chen L, Deng C, Chen X, Zhang X, Chen B, Yu H, et al. Ocular manifestations and clinical characteristics of 535 cases of COVID-19 in Wuhan, China: a cross-sectional study. Acta Ophthalmologica. 2020;98(8):e951-e9.

[11] Wu P, Duan F, Luo C, Liu Q, Qu X, Liang L, et al. Characteristics of Ocular Findings of Patients With Coronavirus Disease 2019 (COVID-19) in Hubei Province, China. JAMA Ophthalmol. 2020;138(5):575-8.

[12] Gaba WH, Ahmed D, Al Nuaimi RK, Dhanhani AA, Eatamadi H. Bilateral Central Retinal Vein Occlusion in a 40-Year-Old Man with Severe Coronavirus Disease 2019 (COVID-19) Pneumonia. Am J Case Rep. 2020;21:e927691-e.

[13] Invernizzi A, Torre A, Parrulli S, Zicarelli F, Schiuma M, Colombo V, et al. Retinal findings in patients with COVID-19: Results from the SERPICO-19 study. EClinicalMedicine. 2020;27:100550.

[14] Marinho PM, Marcos AAA, Romano AC, Nascimento H, Belfort R. Retinal findings in patients with COVID-19. The Lancet. 2020;395(10237):1610.

[15] Senanayake Pd, Drazba J, Shadrach K, Milsted A, Rungger-Brandle E, Nishiyama K, et al. Angiotensin II and Its Receptor Subtypes in the Human Retina. Investigative Ophthalmology & Visual Science. 2007;48(7):3301-11.

[16] Mazzotta C, Giancipoli E. Anterior Acute Uveitis Report in a SARS-CoV-2 Patient Managed with Adjunctive Topical Antiseptic Prophylaxis Preventing 2019-nCoV Spread Through the Ocular Surface Route. Int Med Case Rep J. 2020;13:513-20.

[17] Gonzalez-Lopez JJ, Felix Espinar B, Ye-Zhu C. Symptomatic Retinal Microangiophaty in a Patient with Coronavirus Disease 2019 (COVID-19): Single Case Report. Ocular Immunology and Inflammation. 2020:1-3.

[18] Leonardi A, Rosani U, Brun P. Ocular Surface Expression of SARS-CoV-2 Receptors. Ocul Immunol Inflamm. 2020;28(5):735-8.

[19] Xie H-T, Jiang S-Y, Xu K-K, Liu X, Xu B, Wang L, et al. SARS-CoV-2 in the ocular surface of COVID-19 patients. Eye and Vision. 2020;7(1):23.

[20] Aiello F, Gallo Afflitto G, Mancino R, Li JO, Cesareo M, Giannini C, et al. Coronavirus disease 2019 (SARS-CoV-2) and colonization of ocular tissues and secretions: a systematic review. Eye (Lond). 2020;34(7):1206-11.

[21] Hikmet F, Mear L, Edvinsson A, Micke P, Uhlen M, Lindskog C. The protein expression profile of ACE2 in human tissues. Mol Syst Biol. 2020;16(7):e9610.

[22] Choudhary R, Kapoor MS, Singh A, Bodakhe SH. Therapeutic targets of renin-angiotensin system in ocular disorders. J Curr Ophthalmol. 2017;29(1):7-16.

[23] Holappa M, Vapaatalo H, Vaajanen A. Many Faces of Renin-angiotensin System - Focus on Eye. Open Ophthalmol J. 2017;11:122-42.

[24] Medina-Enriquez MM, Lopez-Leon S, Carlos-Escalante JA, Aponte-Torres Z, Cuapio A, Wegman-Ostrosky T. ACE2: the molecular doorway to SARS-CoV-2. Cell Biosci. 2020;10(1):148.

[25] Mirabito Colafella KM, Bovee DM, Danser AHJ. The renin-angiotensin-aldosterone system and its therapeutic targets. Exp Eye Res. 2019;186:107680.

[26] Paz Ocaranza M, Riquelme JA, Garcia L, Jalil JE, Chiong M, Santos RAS, et al. Counter-regulatory renin-angiotensin system in cardiovascular disease. Nat Rev Cardiol. 2020;17(2):116-29.

[27] Oakes JM, Fuchs RM, Gardner JD, Lazartigues E, Yue X. Nicotine and the renin-angiotensin system. American Journal of Physiology-Regulatory, Integrative and Comparative Physiology. 2018;315(5):R895-R906.

[28] Fischer-Ferraro C, Nahmod VE, Goldstein DJ, Finkielman S. Angiotensin and renin in rat and dog brain. J Exp Med. 1971;133(2):353-61.

[29] Ganten D, Marquez-Julio A, Granger P, Hayduk K, Karsunky KP, Boucher R, et al. Renin in dog brain. Am J Physiol. 1971;221(6):1733-7.

[30] Wagner J, Jan Danser AH, Derkx FH, de Jong TV, Paul M, Mullins JJ, et al. Demonstration of renin mRNA, angiotensinogen mRNA, and angiotensin converting enzyme mRNA expression in the human eye: evidence for an intraocular renin-angiotensin system. Br J Ophthalmol. 1996;80(2):159-63.

[31] Holappa M, Vapaatalo H, Vaajanen A. Local ocular renin-angiotensin-aldosterone system: any connection with intraocular pressure? A comprehensive review. Ann Med. 2020;52(5):191-206.

[32] Luhtala S, Vaajanen A, Oksala O, Valjakka J, Vapaatalo H. Activities of angiotensin-converting enzymes ACE1

and ACE2 and inhibition by bioactive peptides in porcine ocular tissues. J Ocul Pharmacol Ther. 2009;25(1):23-8.

[33] Tipnis SR, Hooper NM, Hyde R, Karran E, Christie G, Turner AJ. A human homolog of angiotensin-converting enzyme. Cloning and functional expression as a captopril-insensitive carboxypeptidase. J Biol Chem. 2000;275(43):33238-43.

[34] Imai Y, Kuba K, Penninger JM. The discovery of angiotensin-converting enzyme 2 and its role in acute lung injury in mice. Exp Physiol. 2008;93(5):543-8.

[35] Chhabra KH, Chodavarapu H, Lazartigues E. Angiotensin converting enzyme 2: a new important player in the regulation of glycemia. IUBMB Life. 2013;65(9):731-8.

[36] Foureaux G, Nogueira BS, Coutinho DC, Raizada MK, Nogueira JC, Ferreira AJ. Activation of endogenous angiotensin converting enzyme 2 prevents early injuries induced by hyperglycemia in rat retina. Braz J Med Biol Res. 2015;48(12):1109-14.

[37] Ma D, Chen CB, Jhanji V, Xu C, Yuan XL, Liang JJ, et al. Expression of SARS-CoV-2 receptor ACE2 and TMPRSS2 in human primary conjunctival and pterygium cell lines and in mouse cornea. Eye (Lond). 2020;34(7):1212-9.

[38] Rahman N, Basharat Z, Yousuf M, Castaldo G, Rastrelli L, Khan H. Virtual Screening of Natural Products against Type II Transmembrane Serine Protease (TMPRSS2), the Priming Agent of Coronavirus 2 (SARS-CoV-2). Molecules. 2020;25(10).

[39] Szabo R, Bugge TH. Type II transmembrane serine proteases in development and disease. Int J Biochem Cell Biol. 2008;40(6-7):1297-316.

[40] Vaarala MH, Porvari KS, Kellokumpu S, Kyllönen AP, Vihko PT. Expression of transmembrane serine protease TMPRSS2 in mouse and human tissues. J Pathol. 2001;193(1):134-40.

[41] Antalis TM, Bugge TH, Wu Q. Membrane-anchored serine proteases in health and disease. Prog Mol Biol Transl Sci. 2011;99:1-50.

[42] Zhou L, Xu Z, Castiglione GM, Soiberman US, Eberhart CG, Duh EJ. ACE2 and TMPRSS2 are expressed on the human ocular surface, suggesting susceptibility to SARS-CoV-2 infection. Ocul Surf. 2020;18(4):537-44.

[43] Zhang BN, Wang Q, Liu T, Dou SQ, Qi X, Jiang H, et al. A special on epidemic prevention and control: analysis on expression of 2019-nCoV related ACE2 and TMPRSS2 in eye tissues. Zhonghua Yan Ke Za Zhi. 2020;56(6):438-46.

[44] Tikellis C, Johnston CI, Forbes JM, Burns WC, Thomas MC, Lew RA, et al. Identification of angiotensin converting enzyme 2 in the rodent retina. Current Eye Research. 2004;29(6):419-27.

[45] Schnichels S, Rohrbach JM, Bayyoud T, Thaler S, Ziemssen F, Hurst J. Can SARS-CoV-2 infect the eye? An overview of the receptor status in ocular tissue. Der Ophthalmologe. 2021;118(1):81-4.

[46] Sungnak W, Huang N, Bécavin C, Berg M, Queen R, Litvinukova M, et al. SARS-CoV-2 entry factors are highly expressed in nasal epithelial cells together with innate immune genes. Nature Medicine. 2020;26(5):681-7.

[47] Lange C, Wolf J, Auw-Haedrich C, Schlecht A, Boneva S, Lapp T, et al. Expression of the COVID-19 receptor ACE2 in the human conjunctiva. J Med Virol. 2020;92(10):2081-6.

[48] Roehrich H, Yuan C, Hou JH. Immunohistochemical Study of SARS-CoV-2 Viral Entry Factors in the Cornea and Ocular Surface. Cornea. 2020;39(12):1556-62.

[49] Ocansey S, Abu EK, Abraham CH, Owusu-Ansah A, Boadi-Kusi SB, Ilechie AA, et al. Ocular Symptoms of SARS-CoV-2: Indication of Possible Ocular Transmission or Viral Shedding. Ocul Immunol Inflamm. 2020;28(8):1269-79.

[50] Chen Y, Liu Q, Guo D. Emerging coronaviruses: Genome structure, replication, and pathogenesis. J Med Virol. 2020;92(4):418-23.

[51] Hui KPY, Cheung M-C, Perera RAPM, Ng K-C, Bui CHT, Ho JCW, et al. Tropism, replication competence, and innate immune responses of the coronavirus SARS-CoV-2 in human respiratory tract and conjunctiva: an analysis in ex-vivo and in-vitro cultures. The Lancet Respiratory Medicine. 2020;8(7):687-95.

[52] Sun C-B, Wang Y-Y, Liu G-H, Liu Z. Role of the Eye in Transmitting Human Coronavirus: What We Know and What We Do Not Know. Front Public Health. 2020;8:155-.

[53] Yang Y, Peng F, Wang R, Yange M, Guan K, Jiang T, et al. The deadly coronaviruses: The 2003 SARS pandemic and the 2020 novel coronavirus epidemic in China. J Autoimmun. 2020;109:102434.

[54] Coroneo MT. The eye as the discrete but defensible portal of coronavirus infection. The ocular surface. 2020:S1542-0124(20)30089-6.

[55] Huet E, Vallée B, Delbé J, Mourah S, Prulière-Escabasse V, Tremouilleres M, et al. EMMPRIN modulates epithelial barrier function through a MMP-mediated occludin cleavage: implications in dry eye disease. Am J Pathol. 2011;179(3):1278-86.

[56] Kitazawa K, Hikichi T, Nakamura T, Mitsunaga K, Tanaka A, Nakamura M, et al. OVOL2 Maintains the Transcriptional Program of Human Corneal Epithelium by Suppressing Epithelial-to-Mesenchymal Transition. Cell Rep. 2016;15(6):1359-68.

[57] Redzic JS, Armstrong GS, Isern NG, Jones DN, Kieft JS, Eisenmesser EZ. The retinal specific CD147 Ig0 domain: from molecular structure to biological activity. J Mol Biol. 2011;411(1):68-82.

[58] Karampelas M, Dalamaga M, Karampela I. Does COVID-19 Involve the Retina? Ophthalmology and Therapy. 2020;9(4):693-5.

[59] Landecho MF, Yuste JR, Gándara E, Sunsundegui P, Quiroga J, Alcaide AB, et al. COVID-19 retinal microangiopathy as an in vivo biomarker of systemic vascular disease? Journal of Internal Medicine. 2021;289(1):116-20.

[60] Virgo J, Mohamed M. Paracentral acute middle maculopathy and acute macular neuroretinopathy following SARS-CoV-2 infection. Eye (Lond). 2020;34(12):2352-3.

[61] Gascon P, Briantais A, Bertrand E, Ramtohul P, Comet A, Beylerian M, et al. Covid-19-Associated Retinopathy: A Case Report. Ocular Immunology and Inflammation. 2020;28(8):1293-7.

[62] Brandão-de-Resende C, Diniz-Filho A, de Almeida Brito F, Vasconcelos-Santos DV. SARS-CoV-2 and COVID-19 for the ophthalmologist. Clinical & Experimental Ophthalmology.n/a(n/a).

[63] Deng W, Bao L, Gao H, Xiang Z, Qu Y, Song Z, et al. Ocular conjunctival inoculation of SARS-CoV-2 can cause mild COVID-19 in rhesus macaques.

Nature Communications. 2020;11(1):4400.

[64] Zimmerman K, Kearns F, Tzekov R. Natural protection of ocular surface from viral infections - A hypothesis. Med Hypotheses. 2020;143:110082.

[65] Akpek EK, Gottsch JD. Immune defense at the ocular surface. Eye. 2003;17(8):949-56.

[66] Maurizio Rolando M, Manfred Zierhut, MD. The Ocular Surface and Tear Film and Their Dysfunction in Dry Eye Disease. 2001.

[67] Cholkar K, Dasari SR, Pal D, Mitra AK. Eye: anatomy, physiology and barriers to drug delivery. Ocular Transporters and Receptors2013. p. 1-36.

[68] Napoli PE, Nioi M, d'Aloja E, Fossarello M. The Ocular Surface and the Coronavirus Disease 2019: Does a Dual 'Ocular Route' Exist? Journal of clinical medicine. 2020;9(5):1269.

[69] Güemes-Villahoz N, Burgos-Blasco B, Arribi-Vilela A, Arriola-Villalobos P, Rico-Luna CM, Cuiña-Sardiña R, et al. Detecting SARS-CoV-2 RNA in conjunctival secretions: Is it a valuable diagnostic method of COVID-19? Journal of Medical Virology. 2021;93(1):383-8.

[70] Paulsen F, Garreis F, Schicht M, Bräuer L, Ali MJ, Sel S. [Anatomy and physiology of the nasolacrimal ducts]. Hno. 2016;64(6):354-66.

[71] Chen X, Yu H, Mei T, Chen B, Chen L, Li S, et al. SARS-CoV-2 on the ocular surface: is it truly a novel transmission route? Br J Ophthalmol. 2020.

[72] Belser JA, Rota PA, Tumpey TM. Ocular tropism of respiratory viruses. Microbiol Mol Biol Rev. 2013;77(1): 144-56.

[73] van Moorsel CH, van der Vis JJ, Benschop C, Ruven HJ, Quanjel M, Grutters JC. The MUC5B promotor polymorphism associates with severe Covid-19. medRxiv. 2020.

[74] Smith JCS, Erin L., Girish VY, Monet Lou, John KMS, Jason M. Cigarette smoke triggers the expansion of a subpopulation of respiratory epithelial cells that express the SARS-CoV-2 receptır ACE2. 2020.

[75] Lu W, Liu X, Wang T, Liu F, Zhu A, Lin Y, et al. Elevated MUC1 and MUC5AC mucin protein levels in airway mucus of critical ill COVID-19 patients. J Med Virol. 2021;93(2):582-4.

[76] Qing H, Li Z, Yang Z, Shi M, Huang Z, Song J, et al. The possibility of COVID-19 transmission from eye to nose. Acta Ophthalmol. 2020;98(3):e388.

[77] Siedlecki J, Brantl V, Schworm B, Mayer WJ, Gerhardt M, Michalakis S, et al. COVID-19: Ophthalmological Aspects of the SARS-CoV 2 Global Pandemic. Klin Monbl Augenheilkd. 2020;237(5):675-80.

[78] Abrishami M, Tohidinezhad F, Daneshvar R, Omidtabrizi A, Amini M, Sedaghat A, et al. Ocular Manifestations of Hospitalized Patients with COVID-19 in Northeast of Iran. Ocul Immunol Inflamm. 2020;28(5):739-44.

[79] Acharya S, Diamond M, Anwar S, Glaser A, Tyagi P. Unique case of central retinal artery occlusion secondary to COVID-19 disease. IDCases. 2020;21:e00867.

[80] Benito-Pascual B, Gegundez JA, Diaz-Valle D, Arriola-Villalobos P, Carreno E, Culebras E, et al. Panuveitis and Optic Neuritis as a Possible Initial Presentation of the Novel Coronavirus Disease 2019 (COVID-19). Ocul Immunol Inflamm. 2020;28(6):922-5.

[81] Cheema M, Aghazadeh H, Nazarali S, Ting A, Hodges J, McFarlane A, et al. Keratoconjunctivitis as the initial medical presentation of the novel coronavirus disease 2019 (COVID-19). Can J Ophthalmol. 2020;55(4):e125-e9.

[82] Chen L, Liu M, Zhang Z, Qiao K, Huang T, Chen M, et al. Ocular manifestations of a hospitalised patient with confirmed 2019 novel coronavirus disease. Br J Ophthalmol. 2020;104(6):748-51.

[83] Colavita F, Lapa D, Carletti F, Lalle E, Bordi L, Marsella P, et al. SARS-CoV-2 Isolation From Ocular Secretions of a Patient With COVID-19 in Italy With Prolonged Viral RNA Detection. Annals of internal medicine. 2020;173(3):242-3.

[84] Guan W-j, Ni Z-y, Hu Y, Liang W-h, Ou C-q, He J-x, et al. Clinical Characteristics of Coronavirus Disease 2019 in China. New England Journal of Medicine. 2020;382(18):1708-20.

[85] Guo D, Xia J, Wang Y, Zhang X, Shen Y, Tong JP. Relapsing viral keratoconjunctivitis in COVID-19: a case report. Virol J. 2020;17(1):97.

[86] Hong N, Yu W, Xia J, Shen Y, Yap M, Han W. Evaluation of ocular symptoms and tropism of SARS-CoV-2 in patients confirmed with COVID-19. Acta Ophthalmologica. 2020;98(5):e649-e55.

[87] Invernizzi A, Pellegrini M, Messenio D, Cereda M, Olivieri P, Brambilla AM, et al. Impending Central Retinal Vein Occlusion in a Patient with Coronavirus Disease 2019 (COVID-19). Ocular Immunology and Inflammation. 2020;28(8):1290-2.

[88] Khavandi S, Tabibzadeh E, Naderan M, Shoar S. *Corona* virus disease-19 (COVID-19) presenting as conjunctivitis: atypically high-risk during a pandemic. Cont Lens Anterior Eye. 2020;43(3):211-2.

[89] Lani-Louzada R, Ramos CdVF, Cordeiro RM, Sadun AA. Retinal changes in COVID-19 hospitalized cases. PLoS One. 2020;15(12):e0243346.

[90] Liang L, Wu P. There may be virus in conjunctival secretion of patients with COVID-19. Acta Ophthalmologica. 2020;98(3):223-.

[91] Lim LW, Tan GS, Yong V, Anderson DE, Lye DC, Young B, et al. Acute Onset of Bilateral Follicular Conjunctivitis in two Patients with Confirmed SARS-CoV-2 Infections. Ocul Immunol Inflamm. 2020;28(8):1280-4.

[92] Mahmut A, Boz AAE, Çınar BK, Çelik E, Yuvacı İs. Concomitant Ocular Diseases in Patients with SARS-CoV-2 Infection. Sakarya Tıp Dergisi.11(1): 137-41.

[93] Marquezan MC, Marquezam JP, Nascimento H, Chalita MR, de Freitas D, Belfort R. Conjunctivitis Related to not Severe COVID-19: A Case Report. Ocular Immunology and Inflammation. 2020:1-3.

[94] Meduri A, Oliverio GW, Mancuso G, Giuffrida A, Guarneri C, Venanzi Rullo E, et al. Ocular surface manifestation of COVID-19 and tear film analysis. Scientific Reports. 2020;10(1):20178.

[95] Navel V, Chiambaretta F, Dutheil F. Haemorrhagic conjunctivitis with pseudomembranous related to SARS-CoV-2. American Journal of Ophthalmology Case Reports. 2020;19:100735.

[96] Pereira LA, Soares LCM, Nascimento PA, Cirillo LRN, Sakuma HT, Veiga GLd, et al. Retinal

findings in hospitalised patients with severe COVID-19. British Journal of Ophthalmology. 2020:bjophthalmol-2020-317576.

[97] Pirraglia MP, Ceccarelli G, Cerini A, Visioli G, d'Ettorre G, Mastroianni CM, et al. Retinal involvement and ocular findings in COVID-19 pneumonia patients. Scientific Reports. 2020;10(1):17419.

[98] Savastano A, Crincoli E, Savastano MC, Younis S, Gambini G, Vico U, et al. Peripapillary Retinal Vascular Involvement in Early Post-COVID-19 Patients. Journal of clinical medicine. 2020;9.

[99] Scalinci SZ, Trovato Battagliola E. Conjunctivitis can be the only presenting sign and symptom of COVID-19. IDCases. 2020;20:e00774.

[100] Seah I, Agrawal R. Can the Coronavirus Disease 2019 (COVID-19) Affect the Eyes? A Review of Coronaviruses and Ocular Implications in Humans and Animals. Ocular immunology and inflammation. 2020;28(3):391-5.

[101] Sheth J, Narayanan R, Goyal J, Goyal V. Retinal vein occlusion in COVID-19: A novel entity. Indian Journal of Ophthalmology. 2020;68(10):2291-3.

[102] Valente P, Iarossi G, Federici M, Petroni S, Palma P, Cotugno N, et al. Ocular manifestations and viral shedding in tears of pediatric patients with coronavirus disease 2019: a preliminary report. Journal of American Association for Pediatric Ophthalmology and Strabismus. 2020;24(4):212-5.

[103] Wu P, Liang L, Chen C, Nie S. A child confirmed COVID-19 with only symptoms of conjunctivitis and eyelid dermatitis. Graefes Arch Clin Exp Ophthalmol. 2020;258(7):1565-6.

[104] Xia J, Tong J, Liu M, Shen Y, Guo D. Evaluation of coronavirus in tears and conjunctival secretions of patients with SARS-CoV-2 infection. Journal of Medical Virology. 2020;92(6):589-94.

[105] Ye Y, Song Y, Yan M, Hu C, Chen X, Yu J, et al. Novel coronavirus pneumonia combined with conjunctivitis: three cases report. Chin J Exp Ophthalmol. 2020;38(03):242-4.

[106] Zhang X, Chen X, Chen L, Deng C, Zou X, Liu W, et al. The evidence of SARS-CoV-2 infection on ocular surface. The Ocular Surface. 2020;18(3):360-2.

[107] Zhou Y, Duan C, Zeng Y, Tong Y, Nie Y, Yang Y, et al. Ocular Findings and Proportion with Conjunctival SARS-COV-2 in COVID-19 Patients. Ophthalmology. 2020;127(7):982-3.

[108] Zhou Y, Zeng Y, Tong Y, Chen C. Ophthalmologic evidence against the interpersonal transmission of 2019 novel coronavirus through conjunctiva. medRxiv; 2020.

[109] Danzi GB, Loffi M, Galeazzi G, Gherbesi E. Acute pulmonary embolism and COVID-19 pneumonia: a random association? Eur Heart J. 2020;41(19):1858.

[110] Iba T, Levy JH, Levi M, Connors JM, Thachil J. Coagulopathy of Coronavirus Disease 2019. Critical Care Medicine. 2020;48(9):1358-64.

[111] Chen Y-C, Chen S-N. Microvascular change in acute macular neuroretinopathy by using optical coherence tomography angiography. Taiwan journal of ophthalmology. 2019;9(2):118.

[112] Pryce-Roberts A, Talaei M, Robertson N. Neurological complications of COVID-19: a preliminary review. Journal of Neurology. 2020:1.

[113] Paniz-Mondolfi A, Bryce C, Grimes Z, Gordon RE, Reidy J, Lednicky J, et al. Central nervous system involvement by severe acute respiratory syndrome coronavirus-2 (SARS-CoV-2). Journal of medical virology. 2020;92(7):699-702.

[114] Casagrande M, Fitzek A, Püschel K, Aleshcheva G, Schultheiss H-P, Berneking L, et al. Detection of SARS-CoV-2 in Human Retinal Biopsies of Deceased COVID-19 Patients. Ocular Immunology and Inflammation. 2020:1-5.

[115] London A, Benhar I, Schwartz M. The retina as a window to the brain—from eye research to CNS disorders. Nature Reviews Neurology. 2013;9(1):44.

[116] Mammo Z, Heisler M, Balaratnasingam C, Lee S, Yu D-Y, Mackenzie P, et al. Quantitative Optical Coherence Tomography Angiography of Radial Peripapillary Capillaries in Glaucoma, Glaucoma Suspect, and Normal Eyes. American Journal of Ophthalmology. 2016;170:41-9.

[117] Mansoori T, Sivaswamy J, Gamalapati JS, Balakrishna N. Radial peripapillary capillary density measurement using optical coherence tomography angiography in early glaucoma. Journal of glaucoma. 2017;26(5):438-43.

[118] Jia Y, Simonett JM, Wang J, Hua X, Liu L, Hwang TS, et al. Wide-Field OCT Angiography Investigation of the Relationship Between Radial Peripapillary Capillary Plexus Density and Nerve Fiber Layer Thickness. Investigative Ophthalmology & Visual Science. 2017;58(12):5188-94.

[119] Sefic S, Kasumovic A, Matoc I, Halimic T, Voloder B, Muhamedagic L, et al. Assessment of Perfused Peripapillary Capillaries and Peripapillary Capillary Density Maps in Glaucoma Patients. Med Arch. 2020;74(4):275-8.

[120] Hooper LC, Chin MS, Detrick B, Hooks JJ. Retinal degeneration in experimental coronavirus retinopathy (ECOR) is associated with increased TNF-α, soluble TNFR2 and altered TNF-α signaling. Journal of Neuroimmunology. 2005;166(1):65-74.

Chapter 8

COVID-19 Conjunctivitis

Suzana Konjevoda, Samir Čanović and Ana Didović Pavičić

Abstract

The outbreak of new Cov-2 epidemic was detected in December 2019 in the city of Wuhan, China, caused by Severe Acute Respiratory Syndrome Coronavirus –2 and started its rapid spread througth the world. The World Health Organisation (WHO) declared a public health emergency of international concern (PHEIC) on the 30th of January 2020. -2 infection can present with spectrum of clinical manifestations, primary of upper respiratory tract and in some cases, especially in immunocompromised patients can cause changes in lower respiratory tract such as pneumonia and bronchitis. Conjunctivitis is not a common manifestation of SARS-Cov-2 infection. It should however be kept in mind that patients with ocular manifestations and symptoms can represent the COVID-19 cases. CoVs can produce several ocular manifestations from conjunctivitis, uveitis – anterior and posterior, retinitis and optic neuritis.

Keywords: SARS-CoV-2, eye infection

1. Introduction

The outbreak of new Cov-2 epidemic was detected in December 2019 in the city of Wuhan, China. It is caused by Severe Acute Respiratory Syndrome Coronavirus –2 (SARS-CoV-2) and started its rapid spread through the world [1]. The World Health Organization (WHO) declared a public health emergency of international concern (PHEIC) on the 30th of January 2020 [2].

CoV-2 infection, among other clinical presentations can also affect the eye and cause conjunctivitis, uveitis – anterior and posterior, retinitis and optic neuritis. In this chapter the CoV-2 ocular surface manifestation are divided in two different divisons- CoV-2 conjunctivits as an rare and uncommon manifestation of CoV-2 infection and ocular CoV-2 transmision since conjunctiva and conjunctival discharge are detected as a possible route of SARS-Cov-2 transmission.

The data about CoV-2 ocular manifestations are sparse. We analised the number of publications of conjunctivitis, SARS-CoV-2, COVID 19, ocular manifestations as key words was in PubMed, WoS, and Scopus. Published data are divided into two periods of time, year 2004 and 2005 in the outbreak of the first epidemic of CoVs and the period of recent ongoing epidemic since the outbreak in Dec 2019.

2. Conjunctivitis

CoV -2 infection can present with spectrum of clinical manifestations, primary of upper respiratory tract [3] and in some cases, especially in immunocompromised patients can cause changes in lower respiratory tract such as pneumonia

 IntechOpen

and bronchitis [4]. Conjunctivitis is not a common manifestation of SARS-Cov-2 infection. However it should be kept in mind that patients with ocular manifestations and symptoms can represent the COVID-19 cases [5]. Coronaviruses (CoVs) can produce several ocular manifestations from conjunctivitis, uveitis – anterior and posterior, retinitis and optic neuritis. The data on the topic are sparse and as the epidemic continues more data should be available and better understanding of the disease is to be achieved [6].

The first reports suggesting CoVs affecting the eye dates from year 2004 and 2005 in patients – primary children with respiratory illness and conjunctivitis. Retrospective studies showed that 17% of patients with CoV-NL63 infection with primary upper and lower respiratory tract illnes had developed conjunctivitis [7].

The route of how CoVs ends up in the eye is not yet clear. The possible ways are from infected droplets, migration from the upper respiratory tract through the nasolacrimal duct or hematogenous spread and infection of the lacrimal gland [8, 9]. Most of the data are from the epidemic in 2004 and since the epidemic died down the research did not continue and the questions remained unanswered. The question emerged again the light of the new ongoing epidemic.

In 2020 there has been a report of the first SARS-CoV-2 infected patient with also an ocular infection in Wuhan [10] and it emerged the need to research the topic again [11]. Majority of studies conducted come from China and the first study in Europe was performed by a group of authors from Spain [12]. The frequency of conjunctivitis in COVID-19 disease is not yet specified, with different data from 0.8% in some to 3% in other and up to 31.6% in different studies conducted in China [13–15].

The European, Spanish study showed that 11.6% of the patients diagnosed with COVID 19 presented with some symptoms of conjunctivitis [12].

3. Clinical presentation and differential diagnosis

Mucopurulent discharge, tearing and foreign body sensation, follicular reaction, conjunctival hyperemia and discharge are the most common symptoms of conjunctivitis. The median time of onset of ocular symptoms is 6 days and the duration of symptoms 3 days.

SARS-CoV2 conjunctivitis can be similar to other viral infections mostly adenoviral. SARS-CoV-2 is usually unilateral and unlike one of adenoviral aethyology, rarely bilateral [16]. The onset in both scenarios is abrupt, injection more severe in adenoviral, similar folicular reaction and chemosis. Petechial hemorrhage, corneal infiltrates and membrane and pseudomembrane formation is more often detected in adenoviral conjunctivitis and discharge is more prominent.

There is a low rate of positive PCR test for SARS-CoV-2 RNA in tears and conjunctival discharge in patients with conjunctivitis presuming the false negativity. Also since the symptoms could be mild and patients do not have visual impairment it can go unnoticed the prevalence can be underestimated.

4. Duration and therapy

The duration of SARS-CoV-2 conjunctivitis is usually 3–4 days and it is a rapid self-limited disease. It ceases with no specific treatment. There are no clinical evidence of efficacy of topical antibotic or corticosteroid therapy. It is sometimes used as a prevention of a bacterial superinfection but it is generaly not recomended. Lubricants, gels and ointments can be used as a symptomatic therapy. Potential sequelae are not yet enough investigated.

5. Ocular symptoms and other CoV-2 infection manifestations

The connection between ocular symptoms and severity of pulmonary disease is yet to be investigated. The data in some studies imply that patients with conjunctivitis are more often presented with more severe COVID-19 – higher white blood cells and neutrophile count, levels of procalcitonin, C-reactive protein and lactate dehydrogenase [17]. Some suggestions emphasize the importance of hosts characteristics and site of inoculation.

6. Transmission

Health care workers are at special risk for SARS-CoV-2 infection due to high incidence of long term end repeated exposure, protected as well as unprotected.

Conjunctiva and conjunctival discharge is a possible route of SARS-Cov-2 transmission.

Presence of virus particles in conjunctival swabs, tear swabs and conjunctival scrappings has been investigated in several studies with different outcomes. Case series from Singapore first detected SARS-CoV in tears of 3of 36 tested patients sampled within 9 days of onset of disease (in the early phase). This case series has important implications for the ophthalmology practice since reported with the detection of the SARS-CoV from tears [18].

Considering the new and ongoing epidemic several studies were conducted in China and analyzed tears and conjunctival secretions from SARS-Cov-2 infected patients. In study conducted in Wuhan 2.8% of tested patients (of 72 tested) were confirmed SARS-CoV-2 RNA in conjunctival discharge [19] while in the study conducted in Hangzhou (on 30 patients) only one sample tested positive on presence of visus in PCR results [20]. Study from Wuhan investigated 67 cases of probable or confirmed COVID-19 infection. They found positive PCR result in one sample of conjunctival swab and two possible positive samples. None of the tested patients had ocular symptoms. The sample was taken from one patient with symptoms of conjunctivitis and the PCR test was negative [21].

The study conducted in Italy (Lombardia) SARS-CoV-2 was found in 57.1% of patients on the ocular surface with a variability of viral load from both eyes [22]. The infectivity of the material was not determined but the results suggested that the test can be positive in conjunctival swab and negative in nasopharingeal swab.

Authors from Croatia emphasize the importance of early detection of possible ocular manifestations and the need for precaution in order to prevent transmission through ocular secretions [23].

Besides frequent hand washing they emphasize the need for immediate disinfection of ophthalmic instruments, especially those in direct contact with patient's mucosal membranes.

Considering the several study results we can presume that the conjunctiva and ocular surfaces are rearly detected in presence of SARS-Cov-2 but have to be considered and investigated in the future.

7. Conclusion

Ocular manifestations of SARS-CoV-2 infection including conjunctivitis are incommon. If present, conjunctivitis is usually selflimited disease with mild symptoms and of limited duration. Important but not yet investigated topic is a presence of CoV in conjunctival swabs in asymptomatic patients and in patients wit other manifestations of CoV-2 infection with no ocular symptoms. Potential viral transmision via conjunctival dicharge and secretions is yet to be investigated. The importance of precaution in contact with mucosal membranes including conjunctiva has to be emphasysed.

Author details

Suzana Konjevoda*, Samir Čanović and Ana Didović Pavičić
General Hospital Zadar, University of Zadar, Zadar, Croatia

*Address all correspondence to: suzana.konjevoda@gmail.com

References

[1] Organisation WH. Coronavirus disease 2019 (COVID19) situation report 32.https://who.int/docs/default-source/coronaviruse/situation-reports/20200221-sitrep-32-covid-19

[2] Organisation WH. Statement on the second meeting of the international health regulations (2005) emergency commettee regarding the outbreak of novel coronavirus (2019-n-Cov). https://www.who.int/news-room/detail/30-01-2020

[3] Corman VM, Muth D, niemeyer D, Drosten C. Hosts and sources of endemic human coronaviruse. Adv Virus Res. 2018;100:163-188

[4] Vassilara F, Spyridaki A, Pothitos G, Deliveliotou A, Papadopulos A. A rare case of human coronavirus 229E associated with acute respitarory distress syndrome in healthy adult. Case Rep Infect Dis. 2018;2018:6796839

[5] van Doremalen N, Bushmaker T, Morris DH, Holbrook MG, Gamble A, Williamson BN, et al. Aerosol and surface stability of SARS-CoV-2 as compared with SARS-CoV-1. N Engl J Med. 2020.

[6] Seah I, Agrawal R Can the Coronavirus Disease 2019 (COVID-19) Affect the Eyes? A Review of Coronaviruses and Ocular Implications in Humans and AnimalsOCULAR IMMUNOLOGY AND INFLAMMATION 2020, VOL. 28, NO. 3, 391-395 https://doi.org/10.1080/09273948.2020.1738501

[7] Vabret A, Mourez T, Dina J et al Human coronavirus NL63 France.Emerg Infect Dis.2005;11(8):1225-1229.

[8] Tong T, Lai TS. The severe acute respiratory syndrome coronavirus in tears. Br J Ophthalmol. 2005;89(3):392. doi:10.1136/bjo.2004.054130.

[9] ChanWM, Yuen KS, Fan DS, Lam DS, Chan PK, Sung JJ. Tears and conjunctival scrapings for coronavirus in patients with SARS. Br J Ophthalmol. 2004;88(7):968-969.

[10] Yan A Chinese expert who came down with Wuhan coronavirus after saying it was controllable thinks he was infected through his eyes China: South China morning post. https://www.scmp.com/news/china/article/3047394/chinese-expert-who-came-downwuhan-coronavirus-after-saying-it-was. 2020.

[11] Lu CW, Liu XF, Jia ZF. 2019-nCoV transmission through the ocular surface must not be ignored. Lancet. 2020;395(10224):e39.doi:10.1016/S0140-6736(20)30313-5.

[12] Güemes-Villahoz N, Burgos-Blasco B, García-Feijoó J, Sáenz-Francés F, Arriola-Villalobos P, Martinez-de-la-Casa JM2 Benítez-del-Castillo JM, Herrera de la Muela M Conjunctivitis in COVID-19 patients: frequency and clinical presentationGraefes Arch Clin Exp Ophthalmol. 2020 Aug 29 : 1-7.doi: 10.1007/s00417-020-04916-0

[13] Xia J, Tong J, Liu M, Shen Y, Guo D (2020) Evaluation of coronavirus in tears and conjunctival secretions of patients with SARS-CoV-2 infection. J Med Virol:1-6. 10.1002/jmv.25725

[14] Zhang X, Chen X, Chen L et al (2020) The evidence of SARS-CoV-2 infection on ocular surface. Ocul Surf. 10.1016/j.jtos.2020.03.01

[15] Wu P, Duan F, Luo C et al (2020) Characteristics of ocular findings of patients with coronavirus disease 2019 (COVID-19) in Hubei Province, China. JAMA Ophthalmol:1-8. 10.1001/jamaophthalmol.2020.1291

[16] Chen L, Liu M, Zhang Z et al (2020) Ocular manifestations of a hospitalised

patient with confirmed 2019 novel coronavirus disease. Br J Ophthalmol:1-4. 10.1136/bjophthalmol-2020-316304

[17] Wu P, Duan F, Luo C et al (2020) Characteristics of ocular findings of patients with coronavirus disease 2019 (COVID-19) in Hubei Province, China. JAMA Ophthalmol:1-8. 10.1001/jamaophthalmol.2020.1291

[18] Loon SC, Teoh SC, Oon LL, Se-Thoe SY, Ling AE, Leo YS, et al. The severe acute respiratory syndrome coronavirus in tears. Br J Ophthalmol. 2004;88:861-3. Medline:15205225 doi:10.1136/bjo.2003.035931

[19] Zhang X, Chen X, Chen L, Deng C, Zou X, Liu W, et al. The infection evidence of SARS-COV-2 in ocular surface: a singlecenter cross-sectional study.

[20] Xia J, Tong J, Liu M, Shen Y, Guo D. Evaluation of coronavirus in tears and conjunctival secretions of patients with SARSCoV-2 infection. J Med Virol. 2020.

[21] Zhou Y, Zeng Y, Tong Y, Chen C. Ophthalmologic evidence against the interpersonal transmission of 2019 novel coronavirus through conjunctiva. medRxiv preprint doihttps://doi.org/10.1101/2020.02.11.20021956

[22] Azzolini C, Donati S, Premin E, Baj A, Siracusa C, Genoni A, Grossi PA, Azzi L, Sessa F, Dentali F, Severgnini P, Minoja G, cabrini L, Charavalli M, Veronesi G, Catcano G, Maffioli LS, Tagliabue A, SARS-CoV-2 on Ocular Surfaces in Cohort od Patients With COVID-19 From the Lombardy Region, *JAMA Ophthalmol.* Published online March 4, 2021. doi:10.1001/jamaophthalmol.2020.5464

[23] Konjevoda S, Canovic S, Pastar Z, Tabain I, Savic V, Barbic Lj, Dzelalija B, Vukojevic K, Stevanovic V, Mardesic S, Kosovic I, Vilibic-Cavlek T Ophthalmic manifestations of novel coronaviruses: precautionary measures and diagnostic possibilities; JoGH, 2020 ISGH